Neurology for the Speech-Language Pathologist

Neurology for the Speech-Language Pathologist

Third Edition

Russell J. Love, Ph.D.
Professor of Hearing and Speech Sciences,
Vanderbilt University School of Medicine,
Nashville, Tennesse

Wanda G. Webb, Ph.D.
Assistant Professor of Hearing and Speech Sciences,
Vanderbilt University School of Medicine,
Nashville, Tennesse

Foreword by
Howard S. Kirshner, M.D.
Professor and Vice Chair,
Department of Neurology,
Vanderbilt University School of Medicine,
Nashville, Tenessee

Illustrations by
Donna B. Halliburton
Additional illustrations by
Paul Gross

Butterworth–Heinemann
Boston   Oxford   Johannesburg   Melbourne   New Delhi   Singapore

Library of Congress Cataloging-in-Publication Data

Love, Russell J.
  Neurology for the speech-language pathologist / Russell J. Love, Wanda G. Webb ; foreword by Howard S. Kirshner ; illustrations by Donna B. Halliburton ; additional illustrations by Paul Gross.— 3rd ed.
    p.   cm.
  Includes bibliographical references and index.
  ISBN 0-7506-9686-9 (alk. paper)
  1. Language disorders—Pathophysiology. 2. Neurology. I. Webb, Wanda G. II. Title.
  [DNLM: 1. Brain—physiology. 2. Brain—physiopathology.
3. Communicative Disorders—physiopathology. WL 300 L897n 1996]
  RC423.L68   1996
  616.85′5—dc20
  DNLM/DLC
  for Library of Congress   96-20156
                                                                 CIP

British Library Cataloguing-in-Publication Data

A catalogue record for this book is available from the British Library.

The publisher offers discounts on bulk orders of this book.

For information, please write:
Manager of Special Sales
Butterworth–Heinemann
313 Washington Street
Newton, MA 02158-1626

Tel: 617-928-2500
Fax: 617-928-2620

For information on all medical publications, contact our World Wide Web home page at: http:/www.bh.com/med

10 9 8 7 6 5 4

Printed in the United States of America

To Barbara and Joe

Contents

FOREWORD   Speech Pathology and Neurology:
Intersecting Specialties   ix
Howard S. Kirshner, M.D.

Preface to Third Edition   xi
Preface to Second Edition   xii
Preface to First Edition   xiii

1 Introduction to Speech-Language Neurology   1

2 The Organization of the Nervous System I   17

3 The Organization of the Nervous System II   47

4 Neuronal Function in the Nervous System   67

5 Neurosensory Organization of Speech and Hearing   83

6 The Neuromotor Control of Speech   106

7 The Cranial Nerves   139

8 Clinical Speech Syndromes of the Motor System   167

9 The Central Language Mechanism and Its Disorders   195

10 Language Mechanisms in the Developing Brain   256

11 Clinical Speech Syndromes and the Developing Brain   272

APPENDIX A   Prevalence of Neurological Disorders   300

APPENDIX B   Medical Conditions Related to Communication Disorders   303

APPENDIX C   Bedside Neurological Examination   308

APPENDIX D   Screening Neurologic Examination for Speech-Language Pathology   310

Glossary   314

Index   322

Speech Pathology and Neurology: Intersecting Specialties

Howard S. Kirshner, M.D.

Neurology is the study of the effects of disease in the nervous system—brain, spinal cord, cerebellum, nerves, and muscles—on human behavior. The neurologist examines specific functions—including higher cortical functions; cranial nerve functions; motor, sensory, and cerebellar functions—all to localize disorders to specific areas of the nervous system. These lesion localizations, along with the clinical history of how the deficit developed and the results of laboratory tests, allow a precise diagnosis of the disease process.

Speech and communication are among the most complicated functions of the human brain, involving a myriad of interactions between personality, cognitive processes, imagination, language, emotion, and lower sensory and motor systems necessary for articulation and comprehension. These functions involve brain pathways and mechanisms, some well understood and others only beginning to be conceptualized. The brain mechanisms underlying higher functions such as language are known largely through neurological studies of human patients with acquired brain lesions. Animal models have shed only limited light on these complex disorders.

Stroke has historically been a great source of information since this "experiment of nature" damages one brain area while leaving the rest of the nervous system intact. For over a century, patients with strokes and other brain diseases have been studied in life, and the clinical syndromes have then been correlated with brain lesions found at autopsy. Recently, new methods of brain imaging have made possible the simultaneous study of a lesion in the brain and a deficit of communication in the same patient. These advances in brain imaging, including computerized tomography, magnetic resonance imaging, and positron emission tomography, have brought about a burgeoning of knowledge in this area.

In this book, Drs. Love and Webb have laid the factual groundwork for the understanding of the nervous system in terms of the organization of the brain, descending motor and ascending sensory pathways, and cranial nerves and muscles. Understanding these anatomic systems makes possible the understanding and classification of the syndromes of aphasia, alexia, dysarthria, and dysphonia, as well as the effects of specific, localized disease processes on human speech and communication. All of these subjects are clearly and accurately reviewed. The speech pathologist who studies this book should have a much improved comprehension of the brain mechanisms disrupted in speech- and language-impaired patients, and, thereby, a greater understanding of the disorders of speech and language themselves.

Perhaps the most important byproduct of this book should be a closer interaction between neurologists and speech pathologists. Neurologists understand the anatomic relationships of the brain and its connections, but they often fail to use speech and language to their full limits in assessing the function of specific parts of the nervous system. A careful analysis of speech and language functions can supplement the more cursory portions of the standard neurological examination devoted to these functions. Thus, detailed aphasia testing supplements the neurologist's bedside mental-status examination, and close observation of palatal, lingual, and facial motion during articulation supplements the neurologist's cranial nerve examination. The neurologist's diagnosis of the patient's disorder, on the other hand, should aid the speech pathologist in understanding the nature and prognosis of the speech and language disorder. The neurologist and speech pathologist should ideally function as a team, each complementing the other. In order for this teamwork to occur, however, each specialist must comprehend the other's language. To this end, Drs. Love and Webb have made the language of the neurologist understandable to speech pathologists. As a neurologist who has worked closely with both of them, I applaud them for this important accomplishment.

Preface to the Third Edition

We have made several changes in this edition to clarify, condense, and expand material. We have traced the enormous growth and development of interest and appreciation of neurology in speech-language pathology, plus we have added flowcharts of the corticobulbar pathways and the sensory pathways. We have also clarified aspects of the visual and auditory systems and included new material on evoked electrical potentials research in speech, specific language impairment, dementia, and right hemisphere deficits. Last, we have combined the material in Chapters 2 and 9 into a single chapter on the basic neuroanatomy of the nervous system. We hope these changes make for a more readable and timely book.

We are indebted to those anonymous reviewers of the second edition who suggested some of these changes. We hope we have met their expectations. We also appreciate the encouragement and guidance given to us by the medical editors at Butterworth-Heinemann. Finally, we express our gratitude to Kathy Hollis for her excellent typing and assistance with composition as we struggled to get the new edition on computer. Were it not for her, we would both probably still be sitting at our desks staring helplessly at the computer screen.

R.J.L.
W.G.W.

Preface to the Second Edition

Our goals in this second edition have been to update various sections of the book to make the material more current and accessible to the student. Approximately 30 percent of the illustrations have been redrawn to increase their clarity. The reader will find expanded coverage of neuroimaging techniques, dysphagia, and neurologic models and new discussions of subcortical aphasia, progressive aphasia, subcortical dementia, traumatic brain injury, attention deficit–hyperactivity disorder, and autism. Numerous minor corrections have been made, and references have been updated where necessary.

R.J.L.
W.G.W.

□ □ □
□ □ □
□ □ □

Preface to the First Edition

The spur for this book was a time-honored one. We found the current crop of textbooks inappropriate to the needs of our students. The senior author in particular has spent considerable effort in recent years attempting to adapt neurology textbooks designed for medical students to the needs of students in speech-language pathology. The results of these efforts often have been frustrating and less than ideal. Therefore, this book is designed as an introduction to neuroanatomy, neurology, and neuropsychology for the student and practicing clinician interested in neurogenic communication disorders. We hope it will be helpful to students without medical training. It is not designed to replace the excellent textbooks now available that have been prepared for courses in adult aphasia, motor speech disorders, and developmental neurologic speech and language problems in children. Rather, it is hoped that this book will serve as a primary textbook for an introductory course in the neurology of speech and language, or as a supplementary source in those usually standard courses in the curriculum that deal with neurogenic communication disorders. This book is aimed at advanced undergraduates and beginning graduate students as well as the working speech-language pathologist.

For authors primarily trained in the field of speech-language pathology rather than neurology, a project like this demands reliance on colleagues in neurology to assist in the development of the work. Howard S. Kirshner, M.D., Department of Neurology, Vanderbilt University School of Medicine, went above and beyond the call of duty in bringing his expertise to bear on this project. He not only read the text for accuracy, but also made important suggestions concerning the organization and clarity of the book. He was extremely patient with our attempts to oversimplify a complex area of knowledge that is rarely grasped completely by the individual who has not had some training in the biological sciences. We are indebted to him for his careful attention to the manuscript, but we wish to indicate that we alone are responsible for errors of fact and flaws in organization and clarity in the text. We are indebted as well to several members of the editorial staff, past and present, of Butterworth-Heinemann. These include David Coen, Arthur Evans, Julie Stillman, and Margaret Quinlin. Finally, no book can be successfully completed without competent secretarial support. We wish to thank Tammy Richardson, Betty Longwith, Dot Blue, Sherri Culp, Solveig Hultgren, Julie Michie, and Gloria Proctor.

Textbooks grow from seeds of inspiration usually planted by outstanding teachers. We would particularly like to acknowledge Harold Westlake, Ph.D., Professor Emeritus, School of Speech, Northwestern University, and the late Joseph Wepman, Ph.D., University of Chicago. Both of these scholar-clinicians provided a vision of the role of the speech-language pathologist in the study, diagnosis, and management of neurologic communication disorders. Without their inspiration and contribution as role models, this book probably would not have been written.

R.J.L.
W.G.W.

1

□ □ □
□ □ □
□ □ □

Introduction to Speech-Language Neurology

"We must admit that the divine banquet of the brain was, and still is, a feast with dishes that remain elusive in their blending, and with sauces whose ingredients are even now a secret."

—MacDonald Critchley, *The Divine Banquet of the Brain*, 1979

Why Neurology?

Language and speech are universally acquired by every child who is free of disease or disorder, and every student of communication disorders realizes that the source of all speech and language behavior is the brain. The 1990s have been labeled by the United States Congress as the "Decade of the Brain." Significant research from language and the neurology of speech promises a new era of understanding of the age-old problems of speech and language disorders (Kirshner, 1995). The work of the linguist, the cognitive psychologist, and the neuroscientist as well as the speech-language pathologist has brought to the field of communication sciences and disorders an accelerated knowledge of the specialized brain mechanisms that underlie speech and language and their disorders.

Widespread interest in the study of neurogenic issues has increased among speech and language students as opportunities for clinical experiences and employment in hospitals, rehabilitation centers, and other health care agencies have increased in recent years. As people live longer and longer, there is a greater incidence of hearing, speech, and language disorders such as aphasia, dysarthria, and apraxia. With improving medical technology, traumatically brain-injured infants, children, and adults are now saved from death much more frequently than in the past. The speech and language disorders of these survivors present new and greater challenges to the speech pathologist.

1

In 1986, when the first edition of this textbook appeared, only some 50 percent of undergraduate and graduate training programs in communication disorders offered specific course work in neurology with an emphasis on speech and language mechanisms. As of this writing, only a decade later, the majority of the 296 programs in the field provide such course work.

Accompanying the exploding interest among neurologists in communication sciences and disorders has been a parallel increase in the number of practicing speech-language pathologists. In the past four decades, membership in the American Speech-Language and Hearing Association has risen from 2,203 in 1952 to over 65,000 in 1995. Although not all of these individuals are interested in neurologic disorders, many are, and for those who wish to study and specialize in neurologic speech and language disorders, there is a certification body, the Academy of Neurologic Communication Disorders and Sciences, that accepts qualified members. It is possible to specialize in adult neurologic impairment, child neurologic impairment, or both. (For further information, contact the Academy of Neurologic Communication Disorders and Sciences, Suite 300, 1250 24th Street, NW, Washington, DC 20037.)

Recent Contributors to the Study of Neurologic Communication Disorders

During the past four decades, two towering figures have dominated the field of language and speech. One, a neurologist, was Norman Geschwind (1926–1984). He almost single-handedly resurrected the early neurologic literature of Europe focusing on language disorders and related deficits. Geschwind brought this body of knowledge to the attention of the American medical audience when interest in aphasia and related disorders was waning in medicine. He particularly highlighted the value of identifying lesions in the connective pathways of the brain as well as diagnosing lesions in the traditional localized cortical areas of the brain that had been associated with language disorders for over a century. His masterwork, "Disconnection Syndromes in Animals and Man" was published in *Brain* over 30 years ago (Geschwind, 1965).

Geschwind taught brilliantly at Harvard University Medical School for many years and inspired generations of students to pursue neurology as a specialty and to concentrate on disorders of higher cerebral function. This area is now known as "behavioral neurology." Aphasic disorders and other related defects, such as agnosia and apraxia, were considered minor aspects of a general neurologic practice until Geschwind highlighted them in neurology and related fields.

Thanks to Geschwind's original and incisive thinking, the study of language and its disorders was returned to its rightful place of importance among the vast range of neurological diseases. His thinking was so innovative that it influenced many other scientific disciplines, particularly linguistics, psychology, and philosophy. Geschwind was one of the few physicians who have been honored by having their scientific papers collected and published before their death (Geschwind, 1974).

The second towering figure in the latter half of the 20th century in the field of neurology of speech and language has been Noam Chomsky (1928–), a linguist of international renown. Chomsky is credited with creating a scientific revolution in the understanding of syntax and other components of language (Harris, 1993), and he has been called a major intellectual force, a "modern master" of creative and scientific thought (Pinker, 1994).

Beginning in 1957 with his monograph, *Syntactic Structures*, Chomsky has developed a theory of grammar, stressing mental processes, that replaced the structural analysis of language based on the mechanistic and behavioral viewpoint exemplified by the writings of Bloomfield (1933). Chomsky disputes the traditional idea that language is essentially a system of habits established by training and forcefully argues that every human being has the innate capacity to use language. Innate grammatical processes, he believes, are triggered by external stimuli but function autonomously. The concept of innateness implies a biologic, neurologic, and genetic basis for language.

Chomsky's definition of grammar differs from that of the structuralist linguists in that it is concerned not only with a specific and formal description of language, but also with neurologic language processes as they work in the human brain. The details of these aspects of language, however, are not clearly explained in Chomsky's writings, and it can be difficult, even with knowledge of transformational-generative grammar, to reconcile the details of the newer linguistic theory of Chomsky with the older neurologic theory of Geschwind and his followers.

The very recent literature, however, is beginning to synthesize the linguistic and neurologic positions in explaining disordered communication. Steven Pinker (1994), a cognitive psychologist and linguist, writes that language may be considered an "instinct" in the same sense that Charles Darwin conceived of "animal instincts." Pinker asserts that grammar is a perfect example of a biological trait determined by the Darwinian principle of natural selection and that it is genetically based. In addition, Pinker states that the intricately structured neural circuits that support language and speech are "laid down by a cascade of precisely timed genetic events" (1994, p. 362). A genetic nature of language is supported by cases of inherited disturbance that appear to be accompanied by specific defects of grammar (Gopnik & Crago, 1991).

Even earlier than Pinker's work, a biological defense of Chomsky's concept of innateness appeared in a well-known but somewhat controversial book by Eric Lenneberg (1921–1975), *The Biological Foundations of Language* (1967). Lenneberg placed language development clearly in a developmental neurology context. One of the highlights of this book was Lenneberg's attempt to define a critical period for the acquisition of early language. Lenneberg maintained that the acquisition of syntax was paced by the rate of cerebral maturation and the lateralization of language mechanisms. He asserted that the rapid acquisition of language starts at approximately 2 years of age as the brain begins to grow rapidly and slows at puberty (at about 12 years of age), when cerebral growth reaches a plateau. Although often criticized, the concept of critical periods is consistent with the importance of biological and neurological mechanisms for language development. Hurford (1991) has supported Lenneberg's claims.

Although the concepts of Lenneberg, Geschwind, and particularly Chomsky concerning neurologic aspects of language have been widely criticized, they have focused interest on the need to understand brain function in detail when studying speech and language disorders. The work of these three neurological theorists is discussed further in later chapters.

Before moving on, we wish to mention a speech-language pathologist who has provided insights into the field of neurologic communication disorders from the vantage point of the therapy room. Although many speech-language pathologists have collaborated with neurologists to make extremely important contributions, we have chosen Nancy Helm-Estabrooks as a major model for clinicians. Helm-Estabrooks (1940–   ) was employed at the Boston Veterans Administration Hospital for most of her career as a speech-language pathologist. There she was strongly affected by the excitement generated by Norman Geschwind and his students as they developed the field of behavioral neurology.

Helms-Estabrooks has worked closely with various neurologists and neuropsychologists and is recognized worldwide for her innovative contributions, particularly in testing and therapy techniques for patients with neurogenic disorders. An example of her work is the *Manual of Aphasia Therapy*, written with the internationally known neurologist, Martin L. Albert (Helm-Estabrooks & Albert, 1991).

The clinical neurologist must work closely with the speech-language pathologist in evaluating the communication disorders of the neurologic client (see Foreword, pp. ix–x). It is clearly not the responsibility of the speech-language pathologist to make the final diagnosis of a neurologic disorder. Nevertheless, it is the undeniable responsibility of the speech-language pathologist to assess all relevant aspects of speech, language, and related disorders in those clients with a known or suspected neurologic disorder.

The speech-language pathologist must understand the results of speech and language assessment in terms of the underlying neurologic mechanisms. Further, the speech-language pathologist must be conversant with current methods of neurologic diagnosis and treatment as they apply to persons with communication disorders. The neurologist's point of view toward speech and language disorders should be familiar to every clinician. In turn, neurologists must be knowledgeable about the assessment methods and therapy procedures of the communication disorders specialist. The understanding of each other's work is particularly crucial since neurology and the study of speech and language disorders have developed independently for many years and are only now beginning to interact more closely. This increased interaction will certainly result in additional benefits for members of both professions and the people they serve.

Historical Roots: Development of a Brain Science of Speech-Language

Speech-language pathology has many of its roots in neurology. In 1861, the French physician Pierre Paul Broca (1824–1880) studied the brains of two patients who had sustained language loss and motor speech disorders. This study allowed him to localize human language to a definite circumscribed area of the left hemisphere, thereby laying the foundation for a brain science of speech and language. Broca's discovery went far beyond the now classic description of an interesting brain disorder called *aphasia*. Possibly foremost among his conclusions were the assertions that the two hemispheres of the brain are asymmetrical in function and that the left cerebral hemisphere contains the language center in most humans. Important implications of brain asymmetry are even now coming to light, some 13 decades later. Asymmetry of function is more pervasive than originally thought. It extends well beyond language to other brain areas and their functions.

Another conclusion that has had everlasting importance for neurology since Broca's death is that specific behavioral functions appear to be associated with clearly localized sites in the brain. The corollary of this observation is that behavioral dysfunction can point to lesions at specific sites in the nervous system. The concept of localization of function in the nervous system has been demonstrated repeatedly by clinical and research methods since Broca first articulated it over a century ago. This observation was so profound that it became a significant historical force in the establishment of the medical discipline of clinical neurology. Much of clinical neurology is dependent on the physician's ability to lateralize and localize a lesion in the nervous system.

Very important for speech-language pathology was the fact that Broca's discovery stimulated a period of intensive search for a workable explanation of the brain mechanisms of speech and language. Probably no period in the history of neurologic science has so advanced the understanding of communication and its disorders as those years between the date of Broca's discovery and World War I.

One of the first and foremost outcomes of this intensive study of speech-language brain mechanisms was the establishment of neurologic substrata for modalities of language deficit other than the expressive oral language described by Broca. In 1867 William Ogle published a case that demonstrated that a cerebral writing center was independent of Broca's center for oral language.

Carl Wernicke (1848–1905) in 1874 identified an auditory speech center in the temporal lobe; it was associated with comprehension of speech as opposed to Broca's area in the frontal lobe, which was an expressive speech center. Lesions in Broca's area produced a motor aphasia, in Wernicke's area a sensory aphasia. In 1892 Joseph Dejerine identified mechanisms underlying reading disorders. Disorders of cortical sensory recognition, or the *agnosias*, were named by Sigmund Freud in 1891, and in 1900 Hugo Liepmann comprehensively analyzed the *apraxias*, disorders of executing motor acts resulting from brain lesion.

Early Language Models

Of the many neurological models of the cerebral language mechanisms that were generated soon after Broca's great discovery, Wernicke's 1874 model has best withstood the test of time. Wernicke stressed the importance of cortical language centers associated with the various language modalities, but he also emphasized the importance of association fiber tracts connecting areas or centers. Like his teacher Theodore Meynert (1833–1892), he understood that the connections in the brain were just as important as the centers for a complete picture of language performance (Meynert, 1885). In addition, Wernicke organized the symptoms of language disturbance in such a way that they could be used diagnostically to predict the lesion site in either connective pathways or centers in the language system. Ironically, the Wernicke model was eclipsed until the last half of the 20th century, when it was revitalized and expanded by Norman Geschwind and his followers (Geschwind, 1974).

Wernicke's model came under criticism by the English neurologist Henry Head in 1926. He lumped Wernicke with a cadre of early neurologists he considered the more flagrant of the "diagram makers," implying that they constructed language models that were highly speculative and not supported by empirical evidence. Current methods of neurologic investigation, including electrical cortical stimulation, isotope localization of lesions, computerized tomography, and regional blood flow studies in the brain, have generally vindicated Wernicke's model of language.

Neurologic speech mechanisms, as opposed to language mechanisms, also received attention in the late 19th century. In 1871 the famous French neurologist Jean Charcot (1825–1893) described the "scanning speech" that he associated with "disseminated sclerosis," now known as multiple sclerosis (Charcot, 1890). The term *scanning*, probably inappropriate, has also been widely used to describe speech with cerebellar or cerebellar pathway lesions (see Chapter 8). In 1888 an English neurologist, William Gowers (1846–1915), surveyed the neurologic speech disorders, known as *dysarthrias*, in a well-known textbook titled *A Manual of Diseases of the Nervous System*.

World War I

World War I had a profound influence on the study of speech and language mechanisms resulting from neurologic insult. With a large population of head-injured young men with penetrating skull wounds, some neurologists felt an urgency for treatment. A handful of dedicated neurologists provided therapy for these traumatic language disorders because the profession of speech pathology was not yet born. Not until the next decade did the profession really begin. Lee Edward Travis has the distinction of being the first individual in the United States to specialize in the field of speech and language disorders at the doctoral level. In 1927 he became the first director of the speech clinic at the University of Iowa. His special interest was in stuttering, which he began to study in a neurologic context. Influenced by the neuropsychiatrist Samuel Terry Orton (1879–1948), Travis researched the hypothesis that stuttering was the result of brain dysfunction, specifically an imbalance or competition between the two cerebral hemispheres to control the normal bilateral functioning of the speech musculature. Orton's hypothesis of dysfunctioning neural control of the speech musculature has generally been discredited, but his hemisphere competition theory of stuttering still surfaces from time to time in different guises to explain certain communication disorders.

Although several of the founders of speech pathology in the United States believed that psychological explanations were more rewarding for understanding speech and language problems, there were notable exceptions.

In particular, Harold Westlake of Northwestern University; Robert West of the University of Wisconsin; Jon Eisenson, formerly of California State University; and Joseph Wepman of the University of Chicago were all advocates of neurologic principles in communication disorders.

Modern Times

World War II, bringing in its wake thousands of servicemen with traumatic aphasia, utilized neurologists, psychologists, and speech pathologists in treatment programs for the first time. This effort produced a series of books and articles on aphasia rehabilitation; perhaps the most notable for the neurologically oriented speech-language pathologist was Wepman's *Recovery From Aphasia* (1951). It served as a textbook of language disorders for the growing number of students in the field and often served as their first introduction to study of a major neurologic communication disorder.

The study of neurologic speech mechanisms was greatly advanced after World War II by the work of Wilder G. Penfield (1891–1976) and his colleagues in Canada. Penfield, a neurosurgeon, used the technique of electrical cortical stimulation to map cortical areas directly, particularly speech and language centers. In 1950 in *The Cerebral Cortex of Man* (written with Theodore Rasmussen) and in 1959 in *Speech and Brain Mechanisms* (written with Lamar Roberts), he documented his observations on cerebral control of speech and language function and wrote on the concepts of subcortical speech mechanisms and infantile cerebral plasticity.

The decades of the 1960s and 1970s were marked by several advances of neurologic concepts in communication and its disorders. As already mentioned, newer linguistic theory, particularly that proposed by Noam Chomsky (1972, 1975), emphasized the universal features and innate mechanisms reflected in language, and the biological aspects of language and speech were highlighted by the linguist and psychologist Eric Lenneberg (1967), who specifically placed language acquisition in the context of developmental neurology. The split-brain studies reported by Roger Sperry and his colleagues (1969), in which the commissural tracts between the hemispheres were severed, indicated specific functions of the right hemisphere as different from the left.

Major anatomical differences in the right and left language centers were also demonstrated in the human brain. Most significant are larger areas in the left temporal lobe in the fetus, infant, and adult (Geschwind & Levitsky, 1968; Wada, Clark, & Hamm, 1975; Witelson & Pallie, 1973). These differences suggest an anatomical basis for cerebral dominance for language and contradict a theory of progressive lateralization of speech centers.

Throughout the 1960s and 1970s considerable attention was paid to neurologic speech disorders. Neurologists and speech pathologists in the Mayo Clinic Neurology Department (Darley, Aronson, & Brown, 1969a, 1969b, 1975) documented the acoustic-perceptual characteristics of the major dysarthrias in a viable classification scheme. This work has stimulated widespread study of the various adult dysarthrias in the speech science laboratories of the country.

The 1960s and 1970s were also marked by the development of three psychometrically sound and widely used aphasia tests: the *Minnesota Test of Differential Diagnosis of Aphasia* (Schuell, 1965); the *Porch Index of Communicative Ability* (Porch, 1967, 1971); and the *Boston Diagnostic Aphasia Examination* (Goodglass & Kaplan, 1972).

Brain Imaging

The cortical areas believed to be critical for language function have been established by what is called the *clinicopathologic method* in neurology. Developed into a powerful technique by the great French neurologist Jean Charcot, it is the method of establishing a relationship between the site of a lesion and the behavioral functions that are lost or modified. The underlying assumption is that the lesioned area is related to the lost or disordered function. This simple logic is very important in clinical neurology: it forms the basis of neurologic diagnosis and is the foundation of the historically traditional neurological examination.

In the mid-1970s, the clinicopathologic technique of diagnosis of the site of neurologic lesions was revolutionized by modern technology that, through relatively noninvasive means, vastly clarified the actual sites of lesions and made diagnoses more valid and reliable. Objective neurodiagnostic tests, such as computerized tomography (CT scans), positron emission tomography (PET scans), single photon emission tomography (SPECT scans), and magnetic resonance imaging (MRI scans), and other clinical neurodiagnostic tests have established the value of the clinicopathologic method in medicine. The four scanning techniques are the most widely used in clinical neurodiagnosis.

Computerized tomography and MRI scans permit study of the structure of the human brain with a degree of detail that is occasionally comparable with the detail revealed by postmortem examination. In fact, MRI, which generates fine cross-sections of brain structure without penetrating radiation, may even go beyond postmortem examination because it allows views of multiple slicings of the brain.

The CT scan, probably the most widely used diagnostic imaging technique in neurology, yields a three-dimensional representation of the brain—unlike the conventional X-ray, which provides a two-dimensional projection of a three-dimensional object. The body appears on X-ray films as overlapping structures that are sometimes difficult to distinguish. The CT scanner uses an X-ray beam that is passed through the brain from one side of the head, and the radiation not absorbed by the intervening tissue is absorbed by a series of detectors revolving around the subject's head. The data from the radiation detectors allow a calculation of the density of tissue in a particular slice of brain. A computer then reconstructs a two-dimensional cross-sectional picture of the brain observed by the camera. Several cross-sections may be printed out corresponding to different planes through the head. Contrast substances are sometimes injected into the patient to increase the density of damaged tissue. This enhancement technique allows clearer visualization and more accurate diagnosis.

Magnetic resonance imaging generates cross-sectional images using radio waves and a strong magnetic field to detect the distribution of water molecules in living tissue. The technique allows very accurate assessment of brain tissue densities, and an excellent pictorial image can be generated by the computer. Generally, MRI is more sensitive to abnormalities than the CT scan. It is more expensive, however.

Damasio and Damasio (1989) point out that the analysis of CT and MRI images is sometimes difficult in that the number of brain slices provided for viewing may vary from institution to institution and from patient to patient. The number of slices may even vary in the same patient as scanning devices are improved over time.

These factors sometimes lead to difficulty in accurate localization of lesions. Although precise accuracy in localization may not be critical to the clinician who needs only to know the nature of a lesion and its rough extent, it may be vital to the neuroscientist who wants to correlate lesion with dysfunction. To improve such correlations, brain templates have been developed to increase the accuracy of reading and comparing various types of brain scans.

Computerized tomography and MRI are unable directly to detect certain forms of cellular and subcellular brain pathology. Dynamic neuroimaging procedures employing emission tomography (PET and SPECT) are helpful in cases where imaging of brain structures alone is not decisive. For instance, in some cases of early dementia, CT and MRI scans appear normal, but language and neuropsychological testing reveal serious cerebral dysfunction.

Positron emission tomography is a visual technique in which the subject is given a radioactively labeled form of glucose, which is metabolized by the brain. The radioactivity is later recorded by a special detector. Unlike CT and MRI scans, a PET scan measures metabolic activity in different brain areas. More active areas will metabolize more glucose, and more radioactivity will be focused in these areas. Thus, regional three-dimensional quantification of glucose and oxygen metabolism or blood flow in the human brain is achieved. This technique is advantageous in that glucose metabolism is a more direct measure of the function of neural tissue than is cerebral blood flow, particularly in patients whose regulatory vascular mechanisms are affected by cerebral injury or disease. PET scan studies have been used to research higher mental functions during different cognitive and language tasks and appear to offer an excellent tool for the study of language in the human brain. This technology is expensive because it requires a cyclotron or atomic accelerator. To date, only major medical centers employ this technology.

Single photon emission tomography uses the mechanism of CT scan reconstruction, but instead of detecting X-rays, the instrument detects single photons emitted from an external tracer. Radioactive compounds that emit gamma rays are injected into the subject. As these biochemicals reach the brain, emissions are picked up that are converted into patterns of metabolism or blood flow in three-dimensional cross-sections of the brain. The picture resolution of SPECT is less than that of PET, but the equipment is less expensive because a cyclotron is not required. This technology is employed at small medical centers.

Thus, in only a century and a quarter there have been dramatic gains in knowledge about brain function as it relates to speech and language. Also in this time, a new discipline, *speech-language pathology*, has been born, experienced tremendous growth, and earned respect as a profession. Today's speech-language pathologist is obligated to continue to advance the profession by being knowledgeable in neuroanatomy and neurologic disease as they affect human communication.

How to Study

Most students in speech-language pathology receive a limited introduction in their undergraduate careers to the neurosciences. Often they have not been exposed to course work in the biological sciences. The majority of students are, of course, enrolled in courses designed to acquaint them with the anatomy and physiology of speech, but usually these courses focus on speech musculature. Students often do not receive an adequate introduction to neuroanatomy and neurophysiology of speech and language. It is assumed that students will learn these details in courses in aphasia, adult dysarthria, and rehabilitation of speech in cerebral palsy. Students find a neuroscience course taken as advanced undergraduates or beginning graduate students difficult.

Students often say that neurology courses are difficult because they believe they must learn the technical term for each hill and valley in the complex anatomy of the brain. In addition, the technical terms are unfamiliar ones, usually derived from Greek and Roman roots. We will concentrate on crucial terminology for an understanding of speech and language, but we will not burden the student with neuroanatomical terminology that does not affect speech and language directly. A glossary is provided at the end of the book.

Part of the strategy in mastering any textbook in the biological sciences is to give the study of drawings, diagrams, and tables in the text as much time as the narrative sections of the textbook. If the reader can come away from a study of this textbook with a set of working mental images of the structures and pathways of the nervous system that are important to communication, and can recall them at critical times, then one of the purposes of this textbook will be realized.

The reader, of course, must also master the verbal material in the text. An integration of verbal material with eidetic imagery means that students must call on all of their brain power, bringing into play the special capacities of both the right and left hemispheres of the brain. We now know that the left hemisphere is specialized for its capacities of verbal analysis and reasoning, whereas the right hemisphere is specialized for its imagery functions. Utilization of functions of both hemispheres will facilitate learning in neurology.

With our emphasis on imagery as one of the better ways to learn neurology, it should be no surprise that we urge readers to use as a teaching aid their own drawings of structures and pathways. Even crude sketches, carefully labeled, will teach the necessary anatomic relationships and will fix pathways, structures, and names in the mind.

Directions

Several terms are used to designate direction in neuroanatomy. Some of these terms are used synonymously. *Anterior* means toward the front, and *posterior* indicates toward the back. *Superior* refers to upper; *inferior* means lower. The term *cranial* or *cephalic* can be used in place of superior. The word *rostral*, meaning near the mouth or front end, may sometimes be substituted for *cranial* or *cephalic*.

Medial means toward the medial plane, and *lateral* means further from the median plane. *Ventral* means toward the belly or front; *dorsal* is toward the back. *Ventral* is sometimes used to indicate structures lying at the base of the brain (Figure 1–1). Table 1–1 describes terms used for the connective pathways in the nervous system.

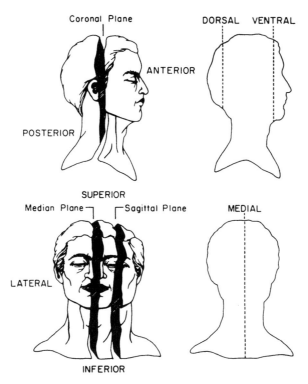

Figure 1–1 Diagram of the major terms of position and the basic planes of reference in the body.

Table 1–1 Terms for Connective Pathways in the Nervous System

Bundle: A group of fibers; a fasciculus

Column: A pillar of fibers

Fasciculus: A small bundle

Funiculus: A cord; a cord of nerve fibers in a nerve trunk

Lemniscus: A ribbon; a ribbon of fibers

Tract: A large group of nerve fibers; a pathway

Anatomical Orientation

In order to aid this visualization process of learning, we have used many drawings throughout the text. When viewing drawings in textbooks or creating your own set of anatomic sketches, you must constantly orient yourself in terms of the standard anatomical positions and planes. The human body itself may be defined in terms of an anatomical position—one in which the body is erect, the head, eyes, and toes pointed forward. The limbs are at the side of the body and the palms face forward. From this fundamental position, other positions, planes, and directions may be defined. These positions, planes, and directions apply to the brain as well as other sections of the body. The following planes and sections are traditionally defined:

- The *median* plane, or section, passes longitudinally through the brain and divides the right from the left.
- A *sagittal* plane divides the brain vertically at any point and parallels the medial plane.
- A *coronal*, or frontal, section is any vertical cut that separates the brain into front and back halves.
- A *horizontal* plane divides the brain into upper and lower halves and is at right angles to the median and coronal planes.
- A *transverse* cut is any section that is at right angles to the longitudinal axis of the structure.

Summary

The brain is the source of all speech and language behavior. Hence, current knowledge concerning its anatomy and functioning must be studied and absorbed by the speech-language pathologist. The study of the relationship between the brain and speech and language function has a rich history in the past century and a quarter, and the disciplines of speech-language pathology and neurology have often cooperated in the study of neurologically based communication disorders. In the study of neuroanatomy and neurology, clinicians must take advantage of diagrams and drawings and must initially orient themselves to the anatomical directions and terminology used in neuroanatomy texts. Employing both verbal reasoning (left-hemisphere function) and visual imagery (right-hemisphere function) will contribute to a successful experience.

References and Further Readings

Bloomfield, L. (1933). *Language.* New York: Holt, Rinehart and Winston.

Broca, P. (1861). Remarques sur le siège de la faculté du langage articulé, suivies d'une observation d'aphémie (perte de la parole). *Bulletin, Société D'Anatomie, (2nd series) 330–337.* Translated in D. A. Rottenberg & F. H. Hockberg (1977), *Neurologic classics in modern translation.* New York: Hafner Press.

Charcot, J. M. (1890). *Oeuvres complète de J. M. Charcot.* Paris: Lecrosnier et Babe.

Chomsky, N. (1957). *Syntactic structures.* The Hague, Netherlands: Mouton.

Chomsky, N. (1972). *Language and mind.* New York: Harcourt and Brace.

Chomsky, N. (1975). *Reflections on language.* New York: Pantheon Books.

Damasio, H., & Damasio, A. R. (1989). *Lesion analysis in neuropsychology.* New York: Oxford University Press.

Darley, F. L., Aronson, A. E., & Brown, J. R. (1969a). Differential diagnostic patterns of dysarthria. *Journal of Speech and Hearing Research,* 12, 246–249.

Darley, F. L., Aronson, A. E., & Brown, J. R. (1969b). Clusters of deviant speech dimensions in the dysarthrias. *Journal of Speech and Hearing Research,* 12, 462–469.

Darley, F. L., Aronson, A. E., & Brown, J. R. (1975). *Motor speech disorders.* Philadelphia: W. B. Saunders.

Dejerine, J. (1892). Contribution a étude anatomopathologique et clinique des différentes variétés de cectie verbal. *Mémoires de la Société de Biologie,* 27, 1–330.

Freud, S. (1953). *On aphasia: A critical study.* Translated by E. Stengel. New York: International Universities Press.

Geschwind, N. (1965). Disconnection syndromes in animals and man. *Brain,* 88, 237–294; 585–644.

Geschwind, N. (1974). *Selected papers on language and the brain.* Boston: D. Reidel.

Geschwind, N., & Levitsky, W. (1968). Human brain: Right-left asymmetries in temporal speech region. *Science,* 168, 186–187.

Goodglass, H., & Kaplan, E. (1972). *Assessment of aphasia and related disorders.* Philadelphia: Lea & Febiger.

Gopnik, M., & Crago, M. (1991). Family aggregation of developmental language disorder. *Cognition,* 39, 1–50.

Gowers, W. R. (1888). *A manual of diseases of the nervous system.* Philadelphia: Blakiston.

Harris, R. A. (1993). *The linguistics wars.* New York: Oxford University Press.

Head, H. (1926). *Aphasia and kindred disorders* (2 vols.). London: Cambridge University Press.

Helm-Estabrooks, N., & Albert, M. L. (1991). *Manual of aphasia therapy.* Austin, TX: Pro-ed.

Hurford, J. R. (1991). The evolution of the critical period of language acquisition. *Cognition,* 40, 159–201.

Kirshner, H.S. (Ed.) (1995). *Handbook of neurological speech and language disorders.* New York: Marcel Dekker.

Lenneberg, E. (1967). *Biological foundations of language.* New York: Wiley.

Liepmann, H. (1900). Das Krankheitbild der apraxie ("motorischen asymbolie") *Monatsschrift für Pyschiatrie und Neurologie,* 8, 15–40.

Meynert, T. (1885). *Psychiatry*. Translated by B. Sachs. New York: Putnam.

Ogle, W. (1867). Aphasia and agraphia. *St. George's Hospital Reports, 2*, 83–122.

Orton, S. T. (1937). *Reading, writing and speech problems in children*. New York: W. W. Norton.

Penfield, W., & Rasmussen, T. (1950). *The cerebral cortex of man*. New York: Macmillan.

Penfield, W., & Roberts, L. (1959). *Speech and brain mechanisms*. Princeton, NJ: Princeton University Press.

Pinker, S. (1994). *The language instinct*. New York: William Morrow.

Porch, B. (1967, 1971). *The Porch index of communicative ability*. Palo Alto, CA: Consulting Psychologists Press.

Schuell, H. (1965). *The Minnesota test for differential diagnosis of aphasia*. Minneapolis: University of Minnesota Press.

Sperry, R. W., Gazzaniga, M. S., & Bogen, J. E. (1969). Interhemispheric relationships: The neocortical commissures; syndromes of hemispheric disconnection. In P. J. Vinken & G. W. Bruyn (Eds.), *Handbook of clinical neurology* (vol. 4). Amsterdam: North Holland.

Travis, L. E. (1931). *Speech pathology*. New York: Appleton-Century-Crofts.

Wada, J. A., Clark, R., & Hamm, A. (1975). Cerebral asymmetry in humans. *Archives of Neurology, 2*, 239–246.

Wepman, J. (1951). *Recovery from aphasia*. New York: Ronald Press.

Wernicke, C. (1874). Der aphasische Symptomenkomplex. Breslau: Cohn and Weigert. Translated in G. H. Eggert (1977), *Wernicke's works on aphasia: A sourcebook and review*. The Hague, Netherlands: Mouton.

Whitaker, H. A. (1976). Neurobiology of language. In E. C. Carterette & M. P. Friedman (Eds.), *Handbook of perception* (vol. 7), *Language and speech*. New York: Academic Press.

Witelson, S. F., & Pallie, W. (1973). Left hemisphere specialization for language in the newborn: Neuroanatomical evidence of asymmetry. *Brain, 96*, 641–647.

2 ⬜⬜⬜ ⬜⬜⬜ ⬜⬜⬜

The Organization of the Nervous System I

> *"The brain is the organ of destiny. It holds within its humming mechanism secrets that will determine the future of the human race. Speech might be called the human brain's first miracle.... Speech it was that served to make man what he is, instead of one of the animals."*
>
> —Wilder Graves Penfield, *The Second Career*, 1963

The Human Communicative Nervous System

The nervous system is the source of all communication in humankind. Only humans can talk. Their special talent for speaking identifies them as unique in the animal kingdom. The special human capacity for speech, or oral language, is the result of an aggregate of intricate nervous mechanisms that have developed in the human brain through a series of dramatic evolutionary changes. Over a period of thousands of years, there has been created in the human brain a novel representation and organization of neural structures and processes that result in what may be called the human communication nervous system. How does this nervous system differ from the communicative nervous system of other animals? A clear answer to this old question is beginning to emerge from attempts to teach the great apes, particularly chimpanzees, different types of communication systems. Attempts to teach oral speech to chimpanzees have been notably unsuccessful; on the other hand, attempts to teach chimpanzees using visual and gestural representations of human language have been undeniably successful. Chimpanzees have been taught to use colored plastic chips to represent morphemes and in other cases have mastered American Sign Language to the extent that they can communicate adequately and even creatively in rudimentary sign language. Whether these nonverbal languages are characteristically human is open to question, but it is clear that humans and chimpanzees share some characteristics of communication. It is highly likely that the chimpanzee uses cortical structures of the brain to master visual and gestural components of human language.

What are the differences between the human brain and that of the chimpanzee? It has been suggested that overall brain size, which reflects the total volume of the cerebral cortex, the total number of nerve cells in the brain, and the degree of dendrite growth or proliferation of the processes of the nerve cell, is crucial to both information-processing and communication-processing in the brain.

The chimpanzee's ability is reflected by its average brain weight of 450 grams, as compared with an average weight of 1,350 grams for the human brain. Generally, a lack of uniqueness has been found in the parietal, occipital, and temporal lobes of both chimpanzees and humans. In the frontal lobe of the brain, however, humans are distinguished by Broca's area, which has been associated with the control of expressive oral speech. With the exception of Broca's area, the primary difference between the human and chimpanzee cortex is quantitative, with the temporal lobe, the inferior parietal lobe, and the frontal lobe anterior to Broca's area being larger in humans. The temporal lobe, the inferior parietal lobe, and the unique Broca's lobe area, as we will learn in later chapters, are those portions of the cerebral cortex that make speech possible. These particular species-specific brain structures, plus the human's special vocal tract and the significant increase in the size of the information- and communication-processing cortex, make the oral speech of humans unique in the animal world (Wallman, 1992).

Divisions of the Nervous System

In order to understand the human communicative nervous system thoroughly, one must first have a basic understanding of the organization of the nervous system as a whole. First, think of the nervous system as separate from the other tissues and structures of the body. Imagine the major parts of the nervous system as if they were displayed on a dissection table spread out for your study. You should see in your mind's eye an oval-shaped brain with a tail-like appendage, called the *spinal cord*, hanging from its base. A series of nerves attached to the base of the brain are called the *cranial nerves*. Another set of nerves, called the *spinal nerves*, project from both sides of the spinal cord (Figure 2–1). Of all these parts—the brain, cord, and nerves—the brain is by far the most important for communication. It is within the brain that the evolutionary neural mechanisms of the communicative nervous system are developed.

The nerves that exit from the brain merely transmit sensory or motor information to and from the brain to control the speech, language, and

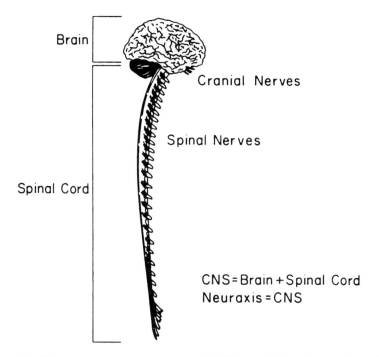

Figure 2–1 The central nervous system (CNS), including the brain and spinal cord. The CNS is synonymous with the term *neuraxis*.

hearing mechanisms. The nerves that are attached to the spinal cord innervate muscles of the neck, trunk, and limbs and bring sensation from these parts to the brain.

From this oversimplified first mental image of the structure and function of the communicative nervous system, we hope to develop a more precise and complex picture of the several aspects of the anatomy, physiology, and diagnosis of neurogenic speech, language, and hearing disorders.

Anatomically the human nervous system has two major divisions: the central nervous system (CNS) and the peripheral nervous system. Chapter 3 deals with the anatomy of the peripheral nervous system.

The Central Nervous System

As you inspect the dissected nervous system displayed in Figure 2–1, you will see that it can be divided naturally into two gross divisions: *brain* and *spinal cord*. The brain and spinal cord taken together are called the *central nervous system* or *neuraxis*.

The brain is gray, shaped like an oval melon, and slightly soft to the touch. The average brain weighs about 1,350 grams or approximately

3 pounds. The brain normally is housed in the part of the bony skull called the *cranium*. A synonym for *brain* is *encephalon*. The largest mass of brain tissue is identified as the *cerebrum*. The human cerebrum, through its evolutionary development from the brains of lower animals, includes three parts: the *cerebral hemispheres*, the *basal ganglia*, and the *rhinencephalon*.

The cerebral hemispheres are the two large halves of the brain; they are readily discernible, even if you merely glance quickly at a brain on display. The cerebral hemispheres are connected by a mass of white matter called the *corpus callosum*. During development the cerebral hemispheres become enormously enlarged and overhang the structures deep in the brain called the *brainstem*. The cerebral hemispheres are extremely crucial for speech, particularly the left hemisphere, in which we find the major neurologic mechanisms of speech and language.

Cerebral Lobes

The cerebral hemispheres are identical twins in looks, although the functions of the various parts may differ dramatically on the left and right sides of the brain. Each cortical mantle of a hemisphere has been divided anatomically into four different primary lobes—the *frontal*, *temporal*, *parietal*, and *occipital* lobes. These lobes can be located on the brain surface by using certain landmarks, the gyri and sulci. A *gyrus* is an elevation on the surface of the brain caused by the folding-in of the cortex. A *sulcus* is a groove-like depression on the brain surface that separates the gyri. Another name for a sulcus is *fissure*. You should seek to become very adept at locating the gyri, sulci, and lobes shown in Figures 2–2 through 2–4.

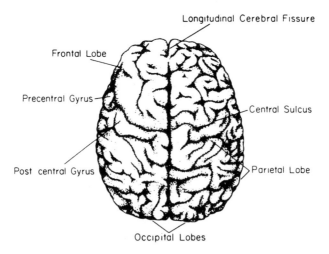

Figure 2–2 Superior view of the cerebral hemispheres.

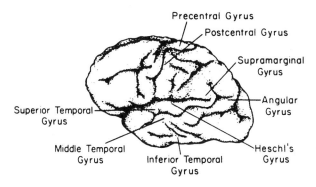

Figure 2–3 Lateral view of the left cerebral hemisphere.

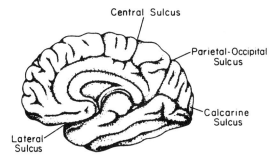

Figure 2–4 Medial view of the right cerebral hemisphere.

The frontal lobe is bounded anteriorly by the *lateral sulcus* or *Sylvian fissure* and posteriorly by the *central sulcus* or *Rolandic fissure*. The frontal lobe accounts for about one third of the surface of the hemisphere. In the frontal lobe there is a long gyrus immediately anterior to the central sulcus. This very prominent gyrus is called the *precentral gyrus*, and it makes up the majority of what is known as the *primary motor cortex*. You will also read and use the term *motor strip* for this area. The cells in this area are responsible for voluntary control of skeletal muscles on the opposite, or contralateral, side of the body. This fact has important clinical significance, which we will discuss later.

Motor pathways making up the *pyramidal tract* descend into the brain and spinal cord from starting points in the primary motor area. Immediately anterior to the primary motor area is the *premotor* or *supplementary motor area*. Stimulation studies of this area show that sequential muscular movement is also produced here, but that a stronger stimulus must be used than in the primary motor area.

The connections between the controlling area on the motor strip and the voluntary muscles served are arranged so that it is possible to draw a map of motor control on the cerebral cortex and show how the muscles are innervated from the cortex. This map is referred to as a *homunculus*, or "little man" (Figure 2–5). As you can see, the areas are represented in an almost upside-down or inverted fashion. You can also see that the area of cortical representation given to a particular part does not appear to be strongly related to the size of that part of the body, as the leg and arm are given smaller areas than the hand or mouth. Rather, it is those body parts that require the most precision in motor control that are apportioned the larger cortical areas.

Another important area of the frontal left lobe, known as *Broca's area*, is located in the inferior (third) frontal gyrus of the lobe (Figure 2–6). In most people, Broca's area is vital for the production of fluent, well-articulated speech. Ablation of the corresponding area in the nondominant hemisphere, on the other hand, usually has no effect on speech.

The parietal lobe is bounded anteriorly by the central sulcus, inferiorly by the posterior end of the lateral sulcus, and posteriorly by an imaginary border line. The primary sensory, or somesthetic, area is found in the parietal lobe, the major portion of which is the *postcentral gyrus* (Figure 2–2). This gyrus lies directly posterior to the central sulcus, or Rolandic fissure. On this sensory cortex can be mapped the sensory control of various parts of the body. Somesthetic sensations (pain, temperature, touch, and the like) are sent to the sensory cortex from the opposite side of the body. This arrangement is a mirror image of the motor strip and is sometimes called the *sensory strip*.

Located in the parietal lobe are also two other gyri with which speech-language pathologists should become familiar. The first is the *supramarginal gyrus*, which curves around the posterior end of the lateral Sylvian fissure. The second gyrus lies directly posterior to the supramarginal gyrus and curves around the end of the prominent sulcus in the temporal lobe, the superior temporal sulcus. This gyrus is called the *angular gyrus* (Figure 2–3). Damage in the area of the angular gyrus in the dominant hemisphere may cause word-finding problems (anomia), reading and writing deficits (alexia with agraphia), as well as left-right disorientation, finger agnosia (inability to identify the fingers), and difficulty with arithmetic (acalculia).

The temporal lobe is the seat of auditory processing in the brain. It is bounded superiorly by the lateral fissure and posteriorly by an imaginary line that forms the anterior border of the occipital lobe. There are three prominent gyri on the temporal lobe: the superior, middle, and inferior *temporal gyri* (Figure 2–3). If one pulls apart the two borders of the lateral

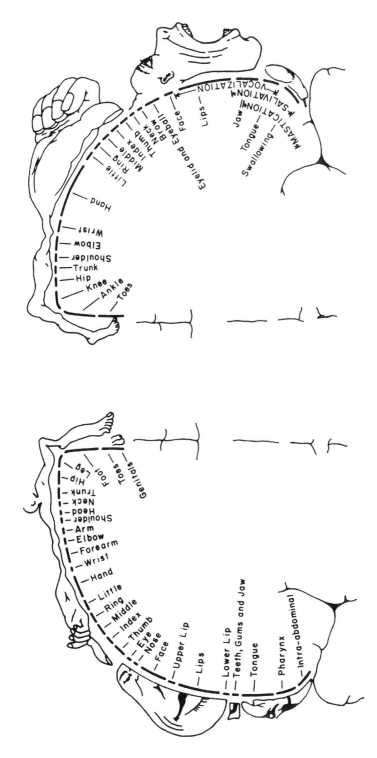

Figure 2-5 Homunculi or "maps" of the cortical sensory and motor control of the parts of the body. Source: Adapted from W. Penfield and T. Rasmussen, *The Cerebral Cortex of Man: A Clinical Study of Localization of Function* (New York: Macmillan, 1950). Reprinted with permission of the literary executors of the Penfield Papers and Princeton University.

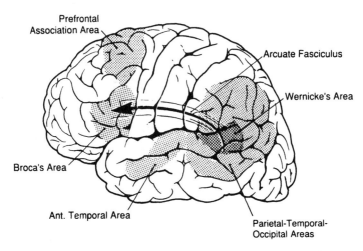

Figure 2–6 Primary language and association areas of the cortex (Ant., anterior).

fissure, a structure called the *insula* or the *Island of Reil* may be seen. Fiber connections to the insula are not well-defined, but the insula is thought to have major connections to the *viscera* (internal organs). Lesions in this area may contribute to language disorder. The primary auditory cortex is situated in the superior temporal gyrus in the inferior wall of the lateral fissure. *Heschl's gyrus*, or the anterior transverse temporal gyrus, represents the cortical center for hearing (Figure 2–3). The posterior part of the superior temporal gyrus is the auditory association area, best known as *Wernicke's area*, which is very important to the development and use of language.

The *occipital lobe*, which occupies the small area behind the parietal lobe and is marked by imaginary lines rather than prominent sulci, is concerned with vision. Two sulci that can be found on the medial surface of the brain and that help locate the occipital lobe are the *parietal-occipital sulcus* and the *calcarine sulcus* (Figure 2–4).

The portions of the cortex on the various lobes that are not assigned as primary motor or sensory areas—such as the primary motor or sensory strip, the primary auditory area, and the primary visual area—are categorized as *association cortex*. This type of cortical area makes up most of the hemisphere. Association cortex has a different cellular makeup than the primary sensory and motor areas. There appear to be multiple inputs and outputs in the association areas, and many of them are apparently independent of the primary motor and sensory areas. Three main association areas that are widely recognized are the *prefrontal, anterior temporal,* and *parietal-temporal-occipital areas* (Figure 2–6).

Cerebral Connections

Your knowledge of the cerebral hemispheres should also include the types of fibers found in these areas. *Association fibers* connect areas within the hemisphere. *Commissural fibers* connect an area in one hemisphere with an area in the opposite hemisphere. The *corpus callosum* is the largest set of commissural fibers in the brain. Association fibers form *association tracts* between areas. Short association tracts are within lobes and long ones are between lobes. One association tract with which you should be familiar is the *arcuate fasciculus*. *Fasciculus* means "little bundle," and the arcuate fasciculus is a bundle of nerve fibers within the CNS. It travels from the posterior temporal lobe forward via another set of fibers, the *superior longitudinal fasciculus*, to the motor association cortex on the frontal lobe (Figure 2–7). Lesions in the area of the arcuate fasciculus are thought to cause a certain major syndrome of aphasia called *conduction aphasia*.

Corpus Callosum

A commissural pathway called the *corpus callosum* is of crucial importance to speech-language functions (Figure 2–8). This pathway serves as the major connection between the hemispheres and conveys neural information from one hemisphere to the other. The corpus callosum is the largest of the side-to-side interconnections between the two hemispheres. In general, the corpus callosum connects analogous areas in the two hemispheres. The anterior and posterior commissures are small bundles of interhemispheric fibers located anteriorly and posteriorly to the

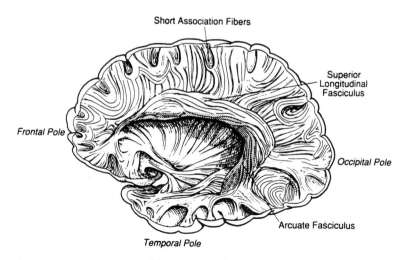

Figure 2–7 Association fiber tracts of the left cerebral hemisphere.

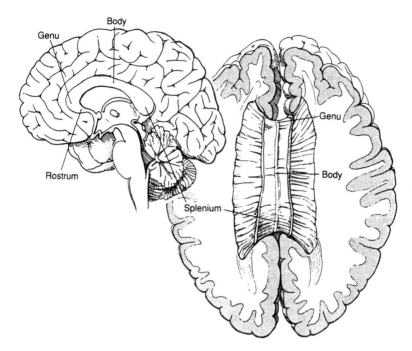

Figure 2–8 The corpus callosum, in a medial view and transverse section. It is the largest of the commissures connecting the two hemispheres.

corpus callosum. The anterior commissure connects the temporal lobe with the *amygdaloid nucleus,* a small subcortical structure. The anterior commissure also connects the occipital lobe in one cerebral hemisphere to the temporal lobe in the other hemisphere. This connection has significance in visual-auditory associations.

Split-Brain Research

The corpus callosum and its role in the transfer of information from one hemisphere to another has attracted wide attention in recent years. The large bundle of tissue may be cleanly and completely severed surgically without damage to other tissue. This operation, called a *commissurotomy,* has been performed on patients who were plagued by chronic and severe epileptic seizures that could not be controlled by massive doses of anticonvulsive medication. A seizure that begins in one cerebral hemisphere may easily travel across the corpus callosum to the other hemisphere, producing a bilateral generalized seizure. Neurosurgeons reasoned that sectioning the corpus callosum would contain the seizure to one hemisphere.

Results of the early commissurotomies were even more beneficial than had been anticipated. Not only did the surgery contain seizures to a single hemisphere, but they also reduced seizures overall because of the severing of apparent reciprocal actions between the hemispheres.

The surgery was not only helpful in seizure control, but it also provided information on the differing psychological functions of each hemisphere and on the role of the corpus callosum in the brain mechanisms for speech and language. The split-brain patients clearly showed asymmetry for speech and language functions, indicating that the corpus callosum plays a decisive role in transmitting language heard in the right ear (and received at the right Heschl's gyrus) to the left hemisphere, where it is processed by the major mechanisms for speech and language.

Experiments on split-brain patients suggested that the right hemisphere was responsible for spatial, tactile, and constructional tasks. These experiments led to speculations that the two hemispheres function in very different ways, each having its own cognitive style. The left hemisphere is characterized as logical, analytical, and verbal, the right as intuitive, holistic, and perceptual-spatial, but there is no doubt that they are integrated in intact brain function.

Cortical Localization Maps

For over a century, neuroanatomists have divided and classified the human cortex into different areas. These tireless attempts to fractionate the cortex followed the unparalleled achievement of Paul Broca in 1861; Broca demonstrated that different cortical regions were associated with different mental functions, one of which was expression of speech. The localization systems that followed have most frequently been based on cell study of the cortex. These are called *histological* methods. They allow the development of cytoarchitectural diagrams or maps based on the varied cell structures of the cortex. The most popular map, developed by a German neurologist, Korbinian Brodmann (1868–1918), is represented in Figure 2–9. Note that each area of the cortex is numbered, providing a much more convenient way to specify a cortical site than by a complex description of gyri and sulci. Brodmann's map is open to criticism on the grounds that it chops the cortex into innumerable specific centers, implying that cortical areas have sharply defined limits, but it has provided a convenient tool in clinical practice with which to indicate cortical localization.

Specific Cortical Areas

The cortical areas have been divided into three major divisions: (1) primary motor projection areas, (2) primary sensory reception areas, and (3) association areas, which cover 86 percent of the cortex.

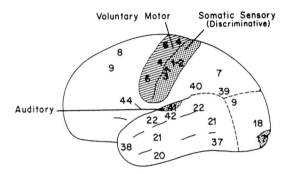

Figure 2-9 Left hemisphere with major architectonic cortical subdivisions of K. Brodmann as indicated by numbers. This numbering system is still in use. Source: Redrawn and reproduced with permission from W. Penfield and L. Roberts, *Speech and Brain Mechanisms.* Copyright (c) 1959 by Princeton University Press.

The primary motor projection areas are the bilateral cortical strips in the frontal lobes in which voluntary movement patterns are initiated. The motor strip also serves as a source of descending motor pathways, projecting to lower levels of the nervous system.

The primary sensory reception area registers sensory impulses relayed from the periphery to the thalamus and upward to the cortex. The pathways from thalamus to cortex are called *thalamic radiations.* An example of a primary reception area is Heschl's gyrus in the superior temporal lobe.

Association Area Functions

The association areas are generally adjacent to primary motor and sensory areas. The association areas elaborate information received at the primary motor and sensory areas. Motor association areas are sites where motor plans, programs, and commands are formulated. The association area adds meaning and significance to the sensory or motor information received in the primary motor or sensory areas. The matching of present sensory information with past sensory information drawn from memory probably takes place in the association areas. In addition, certain sensory association areas blend and mingle sensory information from several association areas to establish a higher level of cortical sensory information. This results in a complex level of awareness that is above and beyond mere recognition of sensory data. This level of sensory awareness is known as *perception.* For example, if someone places a door key in your hand in the dark of the night, you must recognize its shape and judge its size, weight, texture, and metallic surface in order to match this information with your memories and concepts of keys. Only when you can identify your perception of the key can you name the key and relate its function if asked. The everyday sensory recognition of objects relies on complex sensory integration of multiple sensations enhanced by memory and conceptual knowledge of objects with similar qualities. This complex activity of knowing is known as *gnosis*.

Cortical Motor Functions

The primary projection cortex is known as the *motor area* or motor strip. In Brodmann's system, it is area 4. The motor area is located on the anterior wall of the central sulcus and the adjacent precentral gyrus. Figure 2–5 shows the areas devoted to the motor control of the different parts of the body. Recall that this area allows contralateral motor control of the limbs. The inverted arrangement of motor control areas on the bilateral motor cortices reveals that cortical control for the muscles and functions of the speech mechanism is represented at the lower end of the motor area on the lateral wall of the cerebrum. The large areas given over to motor control of the oral mechanism contribute to the coordination of its rapid and precise movements during talking, singing, and changes in facial expression.

Anterior to the motor area is the *premotor area* (area 6). The area is considered a supplement to the primary motor projection cortex and is related to the extrapyramidal system. If areas 4 and 6 are ablated, spasticity in the limbs results. There is a third motor area, discovered by Wilder G. Penfield, on the ventral surface of the precentral and postcentral gyri. It is called the *supplementary*, or *secondary*, *motor area* (SMA).

In recent years the SMA has received considerable attention. Its primary function appears to be control of sequential movements, and speech production is a prime example of sequential movement. The supplementary area now appears to be the principle cortical structure in a neural network that initiates speech. Electrical stimulation produces vocalization in both humans and monkeys. Regional blood flow studies reveal highly dramatic activation in silent counting and spoken recitation. In addition, the SMA, along with the anterior cingulate area, forms a link with midbrain dopamine centers. Dopamine is the facilitative neurotransmitter for this network (Kirshner, 1995, pp. 468–469).

Cortical Motor Speech Association Areas

Surrounding the foot of the motor and premotor cortices are areas considered motor association areas. These areas are numbered 44, 45, 46, and 47 in the Brodmann system. They have been called the *opercular gyri*. Areas 44 and 45 include (1) the pars opercularis, (2) the pars triangularis, and (3) the pars orbitalis. Areas 44 and 45 in the left hemisphere are sometimes called the *frontal operculum*. Area 44 is known best as

Broca's area. Although its function is controversial, Broca's area is usually associated with the formation of motor speech plans for oral expression. The cytoarchitecture of the area is similar in both right and left hemispheres, but traditional theory maintains that only the left is involved with speech formulation. Regional cerebral blood flow and metabolic rate studies have suggested that right cortical areas may also be activated during some speech and language activities.

Primary Somatosensory Cortex

This cortical area (areas 3, 2, and 1) is on the postcentral gyrus and is a primary receptor of general bodily sensation. Thalamic radiations carry sensory data from skin, muscles, tendons, and joints of the body to the primary somatosensory cortex. Lesions of this cortex produce partial sensory loss (paresthesia); rarely is there complete sensory loss (anesthesia). Symptoms of a lesion cause numbness and tingling in the opposite side of the body. Widespread destructive lesions produce gross sensory loss with inability to localize sensation.

Primary Auditory Receptor Cortex

Heschl's gyrus (areas 41 and 42), described earlier, is the primary auditory cortical reception area. The area is found in each temporal lobe, but the left Heschl's area appears to be somewhat larger in most humans. The significance of this neuroanatomic difference is not completely clear, but it may be related to language dominance.

Primary Visual Receptor Cortex

The primary visual receptor cortex is in the occipital lobe along the calcarine fissure, which can be seen from the medial surface of the hemisphere and is not obvious on the outside of the brain. The area, 17 in the Brodmann scheme, is also known as the *striate area*. It receives fibers from the optic tract. Areas 18 and 19, which adjoin area 17, are sensory association areas and are important regions for visual perception and for some visual reflexes, such as visual fixation. Lesions in the area cause visual hallucinatory symptoms. Lesions of the optic pathways cause various degrees of blindness. This partial blindness is considered a visual-field defect.

Primary Olfactory Receptor Cortex

The cortical area that allows you to appreciate the fragrance of a rose is deep in the temporal lobe and is called the olfactory area (area 28, medial surface). It includes an area called the *uncus* and the nearby parts of the *parahippocampal gyri* of the temporal lobe. The olfactory nerves, the end organs for smell, lie in a bony structure in the nose. The nerves end in the olfactory bulb, which is an extension of brain tissue in the nasal area. The bulbs are supported by an olfactory stalk. Destruction of the olfactory system causes *anosmia,* or lack of smell. Irritative lesions produce olfactory hallucinations or *uncinate fits.*

Sensory Association Areas

The sensory association areas, where elaboration of sensation occurs, can best be considered as extensions of the primary sensory receptor areas. They are also known as secondary association areas or unimodal association areas because only one type of sensory input is processed there. Their margins are necessarily vague and it is sometimes controversial as to what the exact functions of certain areas are. The sensory association areas are richly connected to the receptor areas by a host of association fibers, but these association fibers are often difficult to follow because of the vast number of relays in the cortical association system. Areas 5 and 7 in the parietal lobe are related to general somesthetic sensation. Areas 42 (part of Heschl's gyrus) and 22 (Wernicke's area) are related to language comprehension. Areas 18 and 19 are visual association areas.

Recall that we said that the function of the sensory association areas was that of gnosis or knowing. A deficit in the sensory association function is known as *agnosia,* a perceptual-cognitive deficit presumed to follow a destructive cerebral lesion; *agnosia* means "lack of recognition." Lesions in auditory association areas affecting the appreciation of incoming sound will produce language disorders. Areas surrounding Heschl's gyrus are involved in adding meaning to sound and providing comprehension of language. Lesions in area 42 destroy the ability to appreciate the meaning of sound, and lesions in area 22 compromise the ability to understand spoken language.

The inability to comprehend spoken language can be identified as an *auditory verbal agnosia* if we employ a diagnostic nomenclature that assumes that there are lesions in sensory association areas that produce an agnosia. This defect is sometimes distinguished from an *auditory agnosia,* which refers to the inability to recognize a nonverbal sound like the blare of an automobile horn or the roar of a lawn mower's motor. More commonly, lesions in the left temporal association areas have been identified with classic syndromes of language disorder. Temporal lobe lesions affecting comprehension of language are often labeled *sensory aphasia* because the foremost sign in this well-known aphasic syndrome is the inability to recognize oral language. Bilateral lesions of areas 18 and 19 produce *visual agnosia* or the inability to recognize objects visually. *Tactile agnosia* is associated with lesions of the parietal lobe areas 5 and 7.

Another highly significant association area related to language disorder is the *angular gyrus*. This gyrus extends around the posterior end of the superior temporal gyrus, which is usually designated area 39. Lesions in this area have been associated with defects in recognition of the printed word, and reading, writing, and word-recall deficits are often present.

Area 40 is the *supramarginal gyrus*, found in the inferior portion of the parietal lobe, which is known as the *inferior parietal lobule*. This gyrus circles the posterior end of the Sylvian fissure. When the supramarginal gyrus and its underlying association pathway in the left hemisphere are damaged, the patient finds it difficult to formulate written language. The disorder is *agraphia*. Other specific cortical areas have been identified as possible contributors to language mechanisms, but those listed here have received wide acceptance.

Other Cortical Association Areas

Mesulam (1985) and Benson (1994) have provided support for the associative function of other areas of the brain that are architecturally considered to be cortical areas. Their discussions of these areas focus on patterns formed by regions of cortex sharing common functions. Beyond the primary association areas and the secondary motor and sensory association areas that we just discussed, neuroanatomists of this school believe that there are three other functionally associative areas.

The limbic system or limbic lobe was named by Pierre Paul Broca who thought of it as the fifth lobe of the brain. This "lobe" is on the medial surfaces of the two hemispheres. If you look at the medial surfaces of the hemispheres with the brainstem removed, you will observe an arch-like pattern of cortex surrounding the nonconvoluted central portions of the brain. This internal circular arch is called the *limbic lobe* (or *limbic system*), and it is formed by several smaller structures (Figure 2–10), including the (1) subcallosal gyrus; (2) gyrus cingula; (3) isthmus; (4) hippocampal gyrus; and (5) uncus. Mesulam includes in the limbic system structures that are cortical-like in archetype. *Cortical-like* refers to the fact that their formations are part cortical and part subcortical nuclear in architecture. These structures are the *amygdala*, the *substantia innominata*, and the *septal area*. They are part of the basal forebrain and are formed by the simplest and most undifferentiated type of cortex in the forebrain.

A second associative area of cortex is composed of the paralimbic areas. Mesulam points out that gradual increases in complexity of the cortex can be found in these areas when compared with the limbic system formations. The paralimbic areas include (1) the caudal orbitofrontal cortex; (2) the insula; (3) the temporal pole; (4) the parahippocampal gyrus; and (5) the cingulate complex. These structures form an uninterrupted girdle around the medial and basal aspects of the cerebral hemispheres.

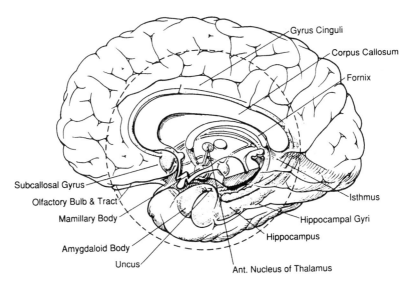

Figure 2–10 The limbic lobe: medial view of the left cerebral hemisphere. The circled area is the limbic lobe or Broca's lobe (Ant., anterior).

One structure of particular interest in the paralimbic area is the *insula*. It is located deep to the temporal lobe and may be seen by pulling apart the two borders of the lateral fissure. The insula is also known as the *Island of Reil*. Mesulam and Mufson (1982) found the insula to be the major relay of somatosensory information into the limbic system in the monkey brain. Ongoing research by Dronkers (1993) has implicated the insula in disorders of motor programming for speech.

The third association area proposed by Mesulam is the portion of isocortex called *heteromodal cortex*. Neuronal responses in this area of cortex are not confined to any single sensory modality and damage to this type of cortex leads to non–modality-specific behavioral deficits. The inputs to these areas originate from secondary (or unimodal) sensory areas or other heteromodal areas. Regions of the brain that are referred to as higher order associative areas, multimodal cortex, or polysensory areas are regions of heteromodal cortex. As Mesulam points out, the primary research identifying specific brain areas as to type of cortex has been done on monkey brains. The major heteromodal areas identified in the monkey brain are (1) the prefrontal region, including the anterior portion of Brodmann area 8, posterior area 9, and areas 45, 46, and possibly 47; and (2) the inferior parietal lobule, extending into the banks of the superior temporal lobule. The inferior parietal lobule includes the angular gyrus, supramarginal gyrus, superior portion of the second temporal gyrus, part of Wernicke's area, and the anterior portion of the superior parietal lobe. Other regions of the temporal lobe may have mixed modality functions (Benson, 1994).

If one accepts the premise of Mesulam, Benson, and others that cortical functioning is hierarchical and that there is a vast network of interrelated functional systems with different, but similar, neuroanatomical substrates, then the study of the functional systems (such as language, memory, vision, etc.) and their disorders must be tempered with the knowledge that brain function is highly complex, with interdependent systems throughout, and only partially understood. While we study the functional subunits of brain operations, attempts to analyze and synthesize the integration of the neural systems that control human behavior continues at a rapid pace.

Association Pathways

It is obvious that each of the cortical centers involved in speech and language must be interconnected to function fully. Association pathways connect the cerebral lobes and the centers within a given lobe. Two distinct patterns of association fibers are found: short fibers and long fibers. Short fibers pass from gyrus to gyrus and are found close to the cortical mantle. Long fibers connect remote regions and make up distinct bundles of fibers.

The uncinate fasciculus is a hook-like configuration of fibers that passes from the frontal lobe to the temporal pole. The occipital-frontal fasciculus is in the white matter and passes from the occipital lobe to the frontal lobe. It travels through the insula and has at times been considered a primary connection in the central mechanism for language. Another long association pathway, the inferior longitudinal fasciculus, passes from temporal to occipital cortex.

The superior longitudinal fasciculus makes connections from frontal lobe to parietal, occipital, and temporal lobes in a fan-like fashion. This fasciculus connects the anterior speech mechanism of Broca's area with the posterior regions such as Wernicke's area and the angular and supramarginal gyri. A part of the superior longitudinal bundle contains fibers that interconnect the major cortical language regions. These significant fibers make up the arcuate fasciculus, which gets its name from its arched appearance (see Figure 2–7).

The cerebral interconnections, like the commissures and fasciculi, are crucial in the theory of human language function and dysfunction. Many of the classic aphasic syndromes appear to be the result of lesions that disconnect one language area from another or disconnect the hemispheres or the cerebral lobes.

Subcortical Structures

The basal ganglia are masses of gray matter deep within the cerebrum, below its outer surface or *cerebral cortex*. The division of the structures known as basal ganglia has been very confusing in the literature. Various anatomists categorize the structures differently. For our purposes we will think of the basal ganglia as consisting of three main parts: the *caudate nucleus,* the *globus pallidus,* and the *putamen* (Figure 2–11). Some neuroanatomists also include a structure called the *claustrum.* The *substantia nigra* and *subthalamic nuclei* are functionally related but not a part of the basal ganglia. The three main parts are often grouped together and referred to as the *corpus striatum.* The putamen and globus pallidus are sometimes grouped and called the *lentiform nucleus.*

The *rhinencephalon* is part of what is called the "old brain." The prefix *rhino* means "nose," so it is easy to see that the functions of the old animal brain dealt primarily with the sense of *olfaction* or smell. Since smell is a much more crucial sense for animals in their adaptation to the environment than it is to humans, the old brain is relatively large in animals and the cerebral hemispheres are less well-developed. Right now, however, concentrating too much on the structures of the cerebrum will distract you from your main task at the moment—conceptualizing the major subdivisions of the CNS or neuraxis.

Cerebellum and Brainstem

The brain contains two other major parts in addition to the large cerebrum: the *cerebellum* and the *brainstem.* Both structures are extremely important to an understanding of the neurology of speech.

The word *cerebellum* means "little brain," and the cerebellum is indeed a much smaller structure than the cerebrum, weighing only about one eighth as much. The cerebellum is located at the rear of the brain,

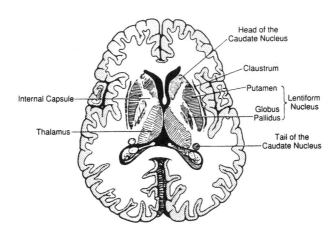

Figure 2–11 Horizontal section of the cerebrum showing the basal ganglia.

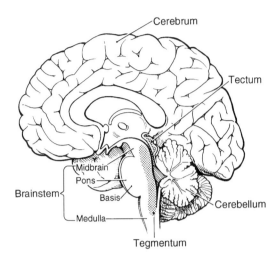

Figure 2–12 Medial view of the right cerebrum, brainstem, and cerebellum. Also seen are the tectum, tegmentum, and basis, which are the internal longitudinal division of the brainstem.

below and at the base of the cerebrum (Figure 2–12). It resembles a small orange wedged into the juncture of the attachment of the spinal cord to the melon-shaped cerebrum. The cerebellum, a recent evolutionary addition to the nervous system, provides fine coordination to the movements of the body. It appears to play a particularly important role in coordinating the extremely rapid and precise movements needed for the normal articulation of speech.

The Brainstem

The third major part of the brain is the *brainstem* (Figure 2–13). The brainstem and its subdivisions cannot be viewed directly unless the cerebral hemispheres are cut away and we are allowed to see the internal structures of the brain. The brainstem appears as a series of structures that seem to be an upward extension of the spinal cord, thrust upward into the brain between the cerebral hemispheres. Often the parts of the brainstem are depicted as extending as vertical segments one above the other, but in fact the parts of the brainstem do not sit in a vertical plane. The upper structures are crowded together to fit within the cranium.

A confusing point for the speech student is that the structures that define the brainstem are not universally agreed on. We have chosen a definition of the brainstem that is reasonably popular and that fits logically into the neuroanatomy and physiology of communication. We include four

Diencephalon

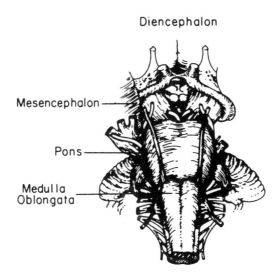

Figure 2–13 Ventral view of the brainstem.

structures in our definition of the brainstem. From the caudal (tail) end of the neuraxis to the rostral (head) end of the nervous system, the brainstem structures are as follows:

- Medulla oblongata
- Pons
- Mesencephalon (midbrain)
- Diencephalon (thalamus)

The following variations in the definitions of the brainstem are found in many neurology textbooks. The basal ganglia, described earlier as part of the cerebrum, are classified by some experts as part of the brainstem. Other authorities only include the medulla oblongata and the pons as brainstem structures; they consider the mesencephalon and diencephalon to be cerebrum. As a compromise, some neurologists have designated the diencephalon and mesencephalon as *upper brainstem* and the pons and medulla oblongata as *lower brainstem*. The brainstem also has three longitudinal internal divisions: the tectum, the tegmentum, and the basis (see Figure 2–12).

Before describing the brainstem structures, we will review what we have discussed so far so that you may check your mental picture of the nervous system. The nervous system is made up of the brain and the spinal cord. The major anatomical units of the CNS are the cerebrum, the cerebellum, the brainstem, and the spinal cord. The brainstem has four major subdivisions, which we now describe.

Medulla Oblongata

This is the most caudal brainstem structure. Older terminology identified it as the *bulb*. The medulla oblongata is a rounded bulge that is an enlargement of the upper spinal cord (Figures 2–12 and 2–13). It contains ascending and descending tracts plus the nuclei of several of the nerves that control phonation, velopharyngeal closure, swallowing, and articulation. It is extremely important for the control of speech production. There is a *median fissure* (furrow) on the anterior surface. On either side of this fissure are landmark swellings called *pyramids*. Other landmarks are oval elevations called *olives*, produced by the *olivary nuclei*, which are important way stations on the pathways of the auditory nervous system. The olives are posterior to the pyramids. The *inferior cerebellar peduncles* (feet) are also found on the medulla. The peduncles connect the cerebellum to the brainstem at the level of the medulla.

Pons

Just above the medulla in the neuraxis is the pons, a massive rounded structure that serves in part as a connection to the hemispheres of the cerebellum. The connections to the cerebellum are made by a number of transverse fibers on the anterior surface of the pons. The pons is aptly named, since the Latin term for bridge is *pons*, and the pons is a bridge to the cerebellum (Figures 2–12 and 2–13).

Mesencephalon

This area, immediately above the pons, is also called the *midbrain* (Figures 2–12 and 2–13). The midbrain is the narrowest part of the brainstem. The midbrain contains the *tectum* or roof, one of the three longitudinal divisions of the brainstem. On the tectum are four swellings, or little hills, called *colliculi*: two *inferior colliculi* and two *superior colliculi* (Figures 3–10 and 5–5). The tectum and the four colliculi are known collectively as the *corpus quadrigemia*. The inferior colliculi serve as way stations in the central auditory nervous system, and the superior colliculi are way stations in the visual nervous system.

The *crus cerebri* is a massive fiber bundle found at the base of the midbrain (Figure 3–10). It includes corticospinal, corticobulbar, and corticopontine pathways. The base of the midbrain also contains the *substantia nigra*, which plays a key role in motor control as it sends dopaminergic efferent fibers to the striatum. The external aspect of the basis of the midbrain is called the cerebral peduncle (Figure 3–10). The tegmentum of the midbrain contains all the ascending and many of the descending systems of the spinal cord or lower brainstem.

Diencephalon

Above the midbrain is a double oval structure, the dien-cephalon (Figure 2–13). It is almost completely hidden from the surface of the brain and is made up of two structures, the *thalamus* and the *hypothalamus*. The thalamus is placed ventrally (toward the belly), and the hypothalamus is placed dorsally (toward the back) (Figure 3–10). The thalamus is a large, rounded structure consisting of gray matter. It is made up of two egg-like masses that lie on either side of the third *ventricle*, one of the large openings in the brain through which the cerebrospinal fluid (CSF) flows. The posterior end of the thalamus expands in a large swelling, the *pulvinar*. Wilder G. Penfield, a famous 20th century neurosurgeon was the first to ascribe special subcortical speech and language functions to this thalamic structure.

The thalamus integrates sensation in the nervous system. It brings together and organizes sensation from the classic sensory pathways. Its nuclei act as thalamic relays, sending sensory information upward to sensory areas on the cerebral cortex. The to-and-fro sensory pathways between the thalamus and cerebral cortex are so numerous, and the two structures so interdependent, that it is sometimes difficult to assign a sensory deficit to the thalamus or the sensory cortical areas of the cerebrum.

The hypothalamus forms part of the *third ventricle*. The lower part of its lateral wall and the floor of the third ventricle make up the hypothal-amus. Two other important landmarks on the base of the brain are found on the floor of the third ventricle: the *optic chiasm* and the *mammillary bodies*. The optic chiasm is the point at which optic nerves cross over. The mammillary bodies are two nipple-shaped protuberances that contain nuclei important to hypothalamic function.

The hypothalamus controls several aspects of emotional behavior, such as rage and aggression, as well as escape behavior. In addition, it aids in regulation of body temperature, food and water intake, and sexual and sleep behavior. The hypothalamus exerts neural control over the pituitary gland, which releases *hormones* involved in many bodily functions.

The Spinal Cord

We said earlier that the two natural anatomic divisions of the nervous system are the brain and the spinal cord. Up to now we have been describing some of the important structures of the brain. Now, moving to the more caudal, or lower, end of the nervous system, we will describe the spinal cord.

Recall our mental image of the dissection of the nervous system. Looking at the brain, one sees a long pigtail of flesh hanging from its base. This is the spinal cord. It is normally found in an opening in the center of the bony vertebral column. The spinal cord is strictly defined. It is what is caudal to the large opening at the base of the skull called the *magnum foramen*; the nervous tissue encased in the skull proper is brain.

A cross-section of the spinal cord reveals an *H*-shaped mass of gray matter in the center of the spinal segment. As in other parts of the CNS, the gray matter contains neuronal and glial cell bodies, axons, dendrites, and synapses. The ventral or anterior portion of the cord mediates motor output. The anterior horn cell of the ventral gray matter is the point of synapse of the descending motor tracts with the ventral roots of the spinal cord. The dorsal or posterior portion of the cord mediates sensory input from the spinal cord. The dorsal root relays sensory information to the cord. Each lateral half of the spinal cord also has white matter columns: a dorsal or posterior column, a ventral or anterior column, and a lateral column. This white matter is composed of myelinated and unmyelinated nerve fibers as well as glial cells. The myelinated fibers form bundles or fasciculi that rapidly conduct nerve impulses that ascend or descend for varying distances. Bundles of white matter with a common function are called *tracts*. Major anatomic landmarks of a cross-section of the spinal cord are shown in Figure 2–14. You will be referring often to this drawing when studying sensory and motor pathways later.

Inspecting the cord closely on the dissection table, you can see a series of thin, regularly placed filaments extending from each side of the cord. These are the *spinal nerves*. Branching off the spinal nerves are the *peripheral nerves*, which go to muscles, glands, and skin. The spinal nerves and the extensions (the peripheral nerves), along with their branches, are one

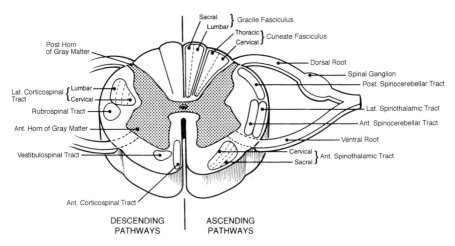

Figure 2–14 Cross section of the spinal cord (Post., posterior; Lat., lateral; Ant., anterior).

part of the *peripheral nervous system* (PNS). If we add the cranial nerves, we have a complete definition of the PNS.

The spinal cord is divided into five regions (Figure 2–15). Each of these regions is named for a section of the 31 spinal vertebrae that surround the spinal cord itself. The regions of the cord are (1) cervical, (2) thoracic, (3) lumbar, (4) sacral, and (5) coccygeal. There are eight cervical nerves, 12 thoracic nerves, five lumbar nerves, five sacral nerves, and one coccygeal nerve. There are, however, only seven cervical vertebrae, yet there are four coccygeal vertebrae.

The spinal cord does not extend the complete length of the vertebral column. In the adult it terminates at the level of the lower border of the first lumbar vertebra. In the child, it is longer, ending at the upper border of the third lumbar vertebra.

Close inspection of the form and quantity of gray versus white matter reveals variations at the different levels of the spinal cord. The proportion of gray to white is greatest in the lumbar and cervical regions where the major motor and sensory neurons for the arms and legs are found. In the cervical regions the dorsal column (mediating sensory input) is somewhat narrow and the ventral column (mediating motor output) is broad and expansive. Both columns are broad and expansive in the lumbar region, and in the thoracic region both are narrow. There is laminar

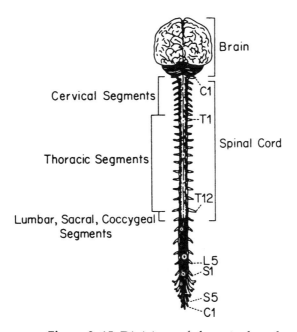

Figure 2–15 Divisions of the spinal cord.

organization in the gray matter with 10 layers identified. Each layer is made up of neurons that respond to different sensory stimuli or innervate different muscle fibers.

Combined with a careful sensory examination, testing of muscle functions can be most valuable to the physician in assessing the extent of a lesion. Most muscles are innervated by axons from several adjacent spinal roots. This peripheral nerve innervation pattern is discussed in Chapter 3.

Reflexes

Reflexes are subconscious automatic stimulus response mechanisms. The behavior of lower animals is primarily governed by reflexes. In humans, reflexes are basic defense mechanisms to sensory stimulation that is painful or potentially damaging. If, for instance, you accidentally touch a hot stove, it is not necessary to send the sensation of pain up the sensory tracts to the cortex. You simply suddenly withdraw your finger. Motor commands from the cortex need not be sent down motor tracts to allow you to move. The rapid response to noxious stimuli is processed quickly at the spinal level by a mechanism called the *simple reflex arc*. The reflex arc contains a *receptor* and an *afferent neuron*, which transmits an impulse along the peripheral nerve to the CNS where the nerve synapses through an intercalated neuron with a lower motor or *efferent neuron*. From this point, an impulse is sent to an efferent nerve, then an efferent impulse passes outward in the nerve, which moves the *effector;* that is, the muscle or gland. A response is then elicited (Figure 2–16).

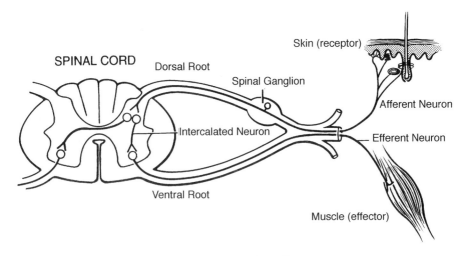

Figure 2–16 A simple reflex arc.

There are several types of reflexes: superficial or skin reflexes; deep tendon or myotactic reflexes; visceral reflexes; and pathologic reflexes. Reflexes occur at different levels in the nervous system: spinal level; bulbar level; midbrain level and righting reflexes; and cerebellar level. Reflex assessment is a vital tool for assessing the intactness of various sensory motor systems, and reflexes will be discussed in more detail in Chapters 6 and 11.

Development of the Nervous System

Now that you are somewhat familiar with the terminology utilized in discussing the central and peripheral nervous systems and are becoming acquainted with structures, we would like to discuss the way in which these structures are formed. The embryological development of the nervous system is a fascinating sequence of events occurring over a very brief period of time.

The spinal cord and brain (with the exception of the cerebellum) reach development of their full number of neurons by the 25th week of gestation. This includes the almost 10 billion cells of the cerebral cortex. The complete mature cortex contains 50 to 100 billion cells, which are primarily glial cells that continue to develop after birth. Dendrites of the neuronal cells begin to develop a few months before birth but are quite primitive in the newborn.

In the first year of life dendritic processes develop on each cortical neuron to establish an individual cell's amazing number of connections with other neurons. The average number of connections that a single cell will make with other cells is about 10,000, with a range of 1,000 to 10,000 (Netter, 1983). This pattern of increasing interconnection among neurons continues until young adulthood, at which time the pattern is reversed as neurons begin to die.

Early Development

On the 18th day of embryonic development, the neural plate, neural tube, and neural crest develop from the ectodermal layer of the embryonic disk. The neural plate begins to enfold in the third week and somites are formed along the groove. These somites will differentiate into muscle, bone and connective tissues—that is, *nonneural tissue*. The groove formed on the neural plate continues to open, and the neural tube is formed and separates from the ectoderm. Certain cells that are not included in the wall or in the superficial ectoderm migrate to become the neural crest. These cells will differentiate into *neural tissue*, sensory nerves, dorsal root ganglia, Schwann cells, and visceral motor cells.

A longitudinal groove known as the *sulcus limitans* forms on either side of the lumen of the neural tube and divides it into a dorsal half, the *alar plate*, and a ventral half, the *basal plate*. The alar plate is the site of sensory and coordinating neuronal cell bodies. These are located in a gray matter layer called the *mantle plate* (see below). Similarly, the cell bodies of motor control neurons are located in the basal plate and are also found in a mantle layer. This basal plate mantle layer is located in parts of the developing brain that become the spinal cord, medulla oblongata, and the midbrain. The basal plate does not participate in formation of areas anterior to the midbrain. Therefore, the diencephalon and telencephalon arise from the alar plate, breaking the sensory-motor division between the alar and basal plate that is carried out in the rest of nervous system development.

Cellular differentiation begins very early in development. There are initially three cell layers: the ependymal, mantle, and marginal layers. The marginal layer lacks cell bodies. As development of the nervous system continues, the layers form distinct zones, maintaining the same name as the layers.

Spinal Cord

By the end of the fourth week of development, the neural tube is closed. After closure there is an enlarged rostral region containing three subdivisions of the brain and a narrow caudal region, the primitive spinal cord. The marginal zone of this caudal region becomes the white matter of the spinal cord. The mantle zone of the alar plate forms the sensory region of the spinal cord and brainstem, and the gray matter differentiates into the nuclei associated with sensory input from spinal, peripheral, and cranial nerves. The mantle zone of the basal plate in spinal cord development differentiates into the motor nuclei of the spinal nerves with the gray matter being made up of cell bodies of efferent neurons that innervate muscles and glands.

Until the third month of development, the spinal cord extends the entire length of the developing vertebral column. At this time the dorsal (sensory) and ventral (motor) roots of the spinal cord extend out laterally from the spinal cord and unite in the intervertebral foramina to form the spinal nerves. The vertebral column elongates at a more rapid rate than the spinal cord, thus making the spinal cord shorter than the vertebral column. At birth the end of the cord, called the *conus medullaris*, is located at the level of the third lumbar vertebra. In the adult it is located approximately between the first and second lumbar vertebrae. As the differential growth of the two structures takes place, the nerve roots located between the conus medularis and the intervertebral foramina elongate. The lumbar, sacral, and coccygeal nerve roots become directed downward at an angle. This elongated bundle of nerve fibers is known as the *cauda equinas* (horse's tail).

The Brain

The three subdivisions of the brain developed by the fourth week are the hindbrain or rhombencephalon; midbrain or mesencephalon; and forebrain or prosencephalon. The central canal dilates into a rudimentary ventricular system, and in the thin roof of the ventricles the choroid plexus develops to produce CSF. By about the sixth week of development these divisions have further divided and significant brain development can be noted. The rhombencephalon divides into the myelencephalon, which later becomes the medulla oblongata, and the metencephalon, which is the future pons and cerebellum. The midbrain or mesencephalon does not divide. The prosencephalon divides into the diencephalon, which later becomes the thalamic complex and the third ventricle. The other division of the prosencephalon is the telencephalon.

It is at about the third month that the telencephalon divides into three parts. The rhinencephalon will contain the olfactory lobes. The second division, the striatal area, is the site of the basal ganglia, which are groups of neuronal cell bodies.

It is only in higher vertebrate and human development that the third division of the telencephalon develops. This division is the suprastriatal structure called the neopallium. This is what we see as the cerebral hemispheres and what we call the *cortex*. The smooth surface of the hemispheres begin to convolute at about 20 weeks of gestation and by week 24 gyri and sulci gradually appear. The first sulcus to appear is the lateral sulcus with its floor, the insula, gradually covered up by further development and enfolding. This folding-in of the tissue allows the outer layer of neurons (the cortex) to increase greatly, eventually reaching an approximate dimension of 2,300 cm^2 without the brain becoming too large for the skull.

The cortex begins to stratify into layers, and at about 6 months of gestation the demarcation of the cortex into layers or lamina is present. The allocortex or archicortex, which is found primarily in the limbic system cortex, is composed for the most part of three layers. The mesocortex is found as transition cortex between the archicortex and the neocortex. It contains three to six layers and is found in regions such as the insula and the cingulate gyrus. The neocortex or isocortex of the cerebral hemispheres is composed of six layers. All six layers can be microscopically differentiated early in development, but the final differentiation of the outer three layers is not complete until middle childhood. The organization of these six layers, or the *cytoarchitecture,* is as follows from the inner to the outermost layer: multiform (VI); internal pyramidal (V); external granular (IV); external pyramidal (III); external granular (II); and molecular (I). There are five different kinds of cells that make up the layers. The cells are different depending on which layer is being examined. The two pyramidal layers contain the pyramidal cells with layer V containing the large pyramidal cells.

The cortex is also organized into vertical columns of interconnected neurons. Each column seems to be a functional unit of cells that share a common function.

Summary

The human communicative nervous system is a novel representation and organization of neural processes and structures; it allows humans to communicate at a complex level unique in the animal world. The speech-language pathologist must be knowledgeable in the area of neurology and neurological disease to participate in the treatment of communication disorders. The nervous system is organized into brain, spinal cord, and nerves. This chapter presented an overview of the central nervous system, which includes the brain and spinal cord. At the end of Chapter 3, the structures reviewed herein are outlined for your continued study.

References and Further Readings

Benson, D. F. (1994). *The neurology of thinking.* New York: Oxford University Press.

Broca, P. (1861) Remarques sur le siège de la faculté du langage articulé suivis d'une observation d'aphémie. *Bulletin de la Société d'Anatomie,* 6, 330–364.

Geschwind, N., & Galaburd, A. M. (1986). *Cerebral localization.* Boston: Harvard University Press.

Kirshner, H. S. (Ed.) (1995). *Handbook of neurological speech and language disorders.* New York: Marcel Dekker.

Mesulam, M. M. (1985). *Principles of behavioral neurology.* Boston: F.A. Davis.

Netter, F. H. (1983). *Nervous system (atlas and annotations): Vol. 1. The Ciba collection of medical illustrations.* Summit, NJ, Ciba Pharmaceutical Company.

Wallman, J. (1992). *Aping language.* New York: Cambridge University Press.

Waxman, S. G., & deGroot, J. (1995). *Correlative neuroanatomy.* (22nd ed.). Norwalk, CT: Appleton and Lange.

3

□ □ □
□ □ □
□ □ □

The Organization of the Nervous System II

"The charm of neurology...lies in the way it forces us into daily contact with principles. A knowledge of the structure and function of the nervous system is necessary to explain the simplest phenomena of disease and it can only be attained by thinking scientifically."

—Henry Head

The central nervous system is the controlling influence in the human communicative nervous system. However, the central nervous system would not be functional, nor necessary, without the lower level structures reviewed in this chapter.

The Peripheral Nervous System

The peripheral nervous system includes (1) the cranial nerves with their roots and rami (branches); (2) the peripheral nerves; and (3) the peripheral parts of the autonomic nervous system. The cranial nerves exit from the neuraxis at various levels of the brainstem and the uppermost part of the spinal cord. Ordinarily the peripheral nerves include the spinal nerves plus their branches.

Spinal peripheral nerves are described as mixed nerves, meaning that they carry both sensory and motor fibers. Each spinal nerve is connected to the spinal cord by two roots: the anterior root and the posterior root. The anterior root of the spinal nerve consists of bundles of nerve fibers that transmit nerve impulses away from the central nervous system. These nerve fibers are called *efferent fibers*. Those efferent fibers that go to the muscles and make them contract are called motor fibers. The motor fibers of the spinal nerves originate from a group of cells or motor nuclei in the spinal cord called the *anterior* (or *ventral*) *horn cells*. The anterior horn cells are the point of synapse, or connection, with the spinal nerves as they leave the neuraxis. When nerve impulses have left the neuraxis, they have reached what the great British neurophysiologist Charles Sherrington (1857–1952) called the "final common pathway"—the terminal route of all neural impulses acting on the muscles.

The posterior root of the spinal nerve consists of *afferent fibers* that carry information to the central nervous system about the sensations of touch, pain, temperature, and vibration. They are called sensory fibers. The cell bodies of the sensory fibers are a swelling on the posterior root of the spinal nerve called the *posterior root ganglion*.

The motor and sensory roots leave the spinal cord at the intervertebral foramina, where the roots unite to form a spinal nerve. At this point the motor and sensory fibers mix together.

The organization of the spinal roots allows us to understand some clinical principles when there is damage to the spinal cord or spinal nerves. First, recall that we can make the generalization that the anterior or ventral half of the spinal cord is devoted to motor or efferent activity, and the posterior or dorsal half is devoted to sensory or afferent activity. A lesion, or damaged area, will impair motor or sensory activities at the cord level depending on the specific site of the lesion. Naturally, large lesions in the spinal cord will impair both sensory and motor functions.

You will recall that, in early embryologic development, somites are formed and differentiated into nonneural tissue. This somitic differentiation results in segmentally distributed "zones" for the skin called *dermatomes* and, for the skeletal muscles, *myotomes*. The sensory component of each spinal nerve is distributed to a dermatome. Similarly, myotomes are innervated by motor axons forming a specific spinal nerve. Figure 3–1 shows the segmental distribution of underlying muscle innervation. The pattern of cutaneous innervation generally follows the same distribution.

If there is a high spinal cord injury or lesion at the level of the cervical cord, speech production may be affected because the respiratory muscles are controlled by spinal nerves exiting from the intervertebral foramina of the cervical and thoracic region. If respiration is stopped, death may follow with a lesion above the third, fourth, and fifth cervical nerves. These nerves, called the *phrenic nerves*, innervate some of the breathing muscles, particularly the diaphragm. Spinal cord injuries involving the caudal portion of the cord do not affect speech production but are of interest to the speech-language pathologist, who may work with spinal cord–injured patients on language or other related problems. These injuries are instructive in understanding the effect of lesions at various levels of the nervous system. Injuries in the spinal cord may produce partial or complete loss of function at the level of the lesion. Function is also completely or partially impaired below the level of the lesion. Spinal cord injuries must be considered serious because they impair functions beyond those controlled directly at the lesion point.

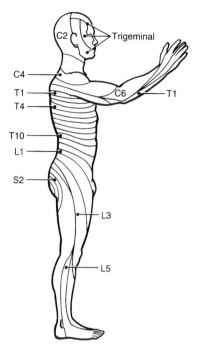

Figure 3–1 Segmental myotome distribution of underlying muscle innervation. Not evident in this figure is the fact that *dermatomes* for C5, C6, C7, C8, and T1 are confined to the arm and that the thumb, middle finger, and fifth digit are within the C6, C7, and C8 dermatomes, respectively.

The Cranial Nerves

The cranial nerves, in contrast to the spinal nerves, are of more significance to the speech pathologist since all of the cranial nerves have some relation to the speech, language, and hearing process, and seven of the 12 nerves are directly related to speech production and hearing. On dissection, the 12 pairs of cranial nerves look like thin cords, gray-white in color. They consist of nerve fiber bundles surrounded by connective tissue. Like the spinal nerves, they are relatively unprotected and may be damaged by trauma. The cranial nerves leave the brain and pass through the foramina of the skull to reach the sense organs or muscles of the head and neck with which they are associated. Some are associated with special senses such as vision, olfaction, and hearing. Cranial nerves innervate the muscles of the jaw, face, pharynx, larynx, tongue, and neck. Unlike the spinal nerves, which attach to the cord at regular intervals, the cranial nerves are attached to the brain at irregular intervals. They do not all have dorsal (sensory) and ventral (motor) roots. Some have motor function, some have sensory functions, and some have mixed functions. Their origin, distribution, brain and brainstem connections, functions, and evolution are complicated. (The cranial nerves are discussed in detail in Chapter 7.) It is traditional to designate them with Roman numerals, as follows: cranial nerve I, olfactory; cranial nerve II, optic; cranial nerve III, oculomotor; cranial nerve IV, trochlear; cranial nerve V, trigeminal; cranial nerve VI, abducens; cranial nerve VII, facial: cranial nerve VIII, acoustic-vestibular; cranial nerve IX, glossopharyngeal; cranial nerve X, vagus; cranial nerve XI, spinal accessory; and cranial nerve XII, hypoglossal (Figure 3–2).

Autonomic Nervous System

The innervation of involuntary structures such as the heart, the smooth muscles, and the glands is accomplished through the *autonomic nervous system*. Although this system has primarily indirect effects on speech, language, and hearing, you must be familiar with its contribution to total body function in order to understand how involuntary but vital functions such as hormonal secretions, visual reflexes, and blood pressure are controlled within the nervous system.

The autonomic nervous system is distributed throughout both the central nervous system and the peripheral nervous system. The enteric nervous system, which is formed by neuronal plexuses in the gastrointestinal tract, is considered to be a division of the autonomic nervous system. The major divisions of the autonomic nervous system, however, are the *sympathetic* and *parasympathetic divisions*, which have almost antagonistic functions. The sympathetic system is the body's alerting system, sometimes referred to as the *fight-or-flight system*. This part of the autonomic nervous system is responsible for such preparatory measures as accelerating the heart rate, causing constriction of the peripheral blood vessels, raising the blood pressure, and redistributing the blood so that it

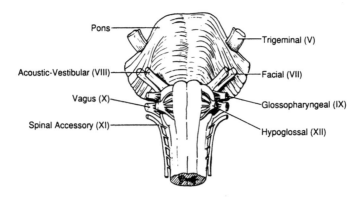

Figure 3–2 Cranial nerves exiting from the brainstem.

leaves the skin and intestines to be used in the brain, heart, and skeletal muscles if needed. It serves to raise the eyelids and to dilate the pupils. The sympathetic part will also decrease peristalsis (the propelling contractions of the intestine) and will close the sphincter.

The parasympathetic part of the autonomic nervous system has an almost opposite calming effect on bodily function. It serves to conserve and restore energy by slowing the heart rate, increasing intestinal peristalsis, and opening the sphincters. As a result of parasympathetic action, other functions, such as increased salivation and increased secretion of the glands of the gastrointestinal tract, may take place.

Rarely is autonomic activity solely sympathetic or parasympathetic. Both parts work together in the autonomic nervous system along with the endocrine system to maintain the stability of the body's internal environment or *homeostasis*. The endocrine system is a group of glands and other structures that release internal secretions called *hormones* into the circulatory system. These hormones influence metabolism and other body processes. The endocrine system includes such organs as the pancreas, the pineal gland, the pituitary gland, the gonads, the thyroid, and the adrenal glands. These work more slowly than the autonomic nervous system.

The autonomic nervous system is composed of both efferent (conducting away from the central nervous system) and afferent (conducting toward the central nervous system) nerve fibers. Both kinds of fibers travel routes that include either synapsing on or passing through a ganglion—a group of nerve cell bodies, usually outside the central nervous system. Before reaching the ganglion, the fiber is referred to as *preganglionic*. After synapsing on or passing through the ganglion, it becomes *postganglionic* fiber. All fibers of the sympathetic part course through or synapse on a chain of ganglia running adjacent to the cerebral bodies called the *sympathetic trunk*. Therefore, the sympathetic postganglionic neurons are located at some distance from the organs affected. The parasympathetic postganglionic fibers are scattered throughout the body and are located either in the wall of the organs or in close proximity to them. Its activity is therefore more localized than that of the sympathetic system.

The integration of the autonomic activity with endocrine and somatic responses, allowing homeostasis to be maintained, is regulated by the hypothalamus. There is evidence for a network of central neuronal circuits that includes not only the hypothalamus but also the insula, the amygdala, and an area in the midbrain called the *periaqueductal gray*. These structures receive input from the *nucleus solaritarius*, a prominent nucleus of the medulla that receives input from all of the visceral organs. Input is also received from other nuclei in the brainstem and spinal cord. This network is referred to as the *central autonomic network* (Heimer, 1994) and probably is responsible for adjustments to basic cardiovascular and respiratory functions as they relate to a range of body activities such as food intake, emotional behavior, and mental activity.

As stated earlier, the autonomic nervous system is of importance to the speech-language pathologist because of its indirect effect on communication functioning. If you have ever experienced the sweaty palms, dry mouth, blushing, and upset stomach associated with anxiety before delivering a speech, you have some idea of the power of the autonomic nervous system. Those indirect effects may make a great deal of difference in how well one communicates!

The Protection and Nourishment of the Brain

Up to this point we have been concerned with the three major controlling mechanisms of the human body: the central nervous system, the peripheral nervous system, and the autonomic nervous system. The brain and the spinal cord, which make up part of these systems and house most of their mechanisms, must be protected in some way and must be nourished to continue to function. The following is a discussion of the protection and nourishment of these structures.

The Meninges

Since the spinal cord and the brain are the major coordinating and integrating structures for all physical and mental activities of the body, it is fortunate that they are very well-protected. The brain and the spinal cord are covered by layers of tissue called the *meninges*. Within certain layers of these meninges there is a cushioning layer of fluid called *cerebrospinal fluid*.

The meninges are three membranes that cover both the brain and the spinal cord. Moving from the outermost to the innermost covering, they are known as the *dura mater* ("tough mother"), the *arachnoid mater*, and the *pia mater* (Figure 3–3).

The dura mater actually consists of two layers that are closely united except where, in certain spots, they separate to form the venous sinuses. The dura mater of the spinal cord is continuous with that of the brain through the opening in the skull called the *foramen magnum*. In the brain, the dura mater is marked by complex folds that divide the contents of the cranial cavity into different cerebral subdivisions. These folds are the *falx cerebri* (between the cerebral hemispheres), the *tentorium cerebelli* (projecting between the cerebellar hemispheres), and the *diaphragma sella* (forming the roof of the sella turcica) (Figure 3–4). These folds serve to brace the brain

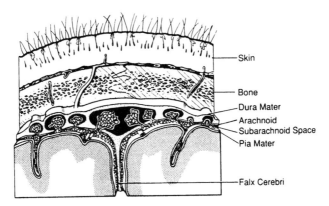

Figure 3–3 Cerebral meninges. Source: Redrawn and reproduced with permission from R. Snell, *Clinical Neuroanatomy for Medical Students* (Boston: Little, Brown and Company, 1980).

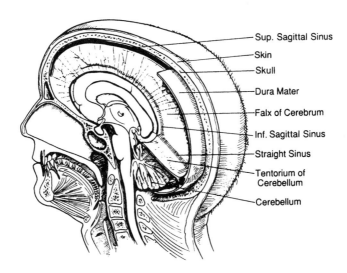

Figure 3–4 Folds of the dura mater (Sup., superior; Inf., inferior).

against rotary displacement. They receive blood from the brain through the cerebral veins and receive cerebrospinal fluid from the subarachnoid space. The blood ultimately drains into the internal jugular veins in the neck.

Beneath the dura mater is a space called the *subdural space*, which is filled with fluid. Immediately below this fluid is the second membrane covering, the arachnoid mater. This membrane bridges over the sulci or folds of the brain. In some areas it projects into the venous sinuses to form arachnoid villi, which aggregate to form the arachnoid granulations where cerebrospinal fluid diffuses into the bloodstream.

Separating the arachnoid and the third membrane, the pia mater, is the *subarachnoid space*, filled with cerebrospinal fluid. All cerebral arteries and veins as well as the cranial nerves pass through this space. The pia mater adheres closely to the surface of the brain, covering the gyri (ridges) and going down into the sulci. The pia mater also fuses with the ependyma (a cellular membrane lining the ventricles) to form the choroid plexuses of the ventricles.

The Ventricular System

The ventricular system of the brain has three parts: the lateral ventricles, the third ventricle, and the fourth ventricle. These are actually small cavities within the brain that are joined to each other by small ducts and canals (Figure 3–5). Each ventricle contains a tuft–like structure called the *choroid plexus*, which is concerned mainly with the production of cerebrospinal fluid.

The lateral ventricles are paired, one in each hemisphere. Each is a C-shaped cavity and can be divided into a body, located in the parietal lobe, and anterior, posterior, and inferior horns, extending into the frontal, occipital, and temporal lobes, respectively. The lateral ventricle is connected to the third ventricle by an opening called the intraventricular foramen or the foramen of Munro. The choroid plexus of the lateral ventricle projects into the cavity on its medial aspect.

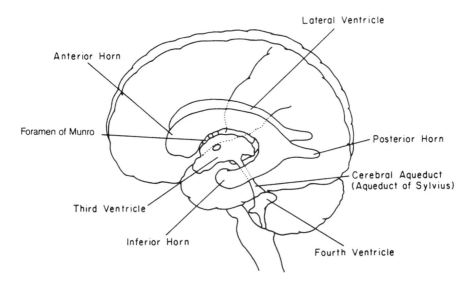

Figure 3–5 The ventricular system.

The third ventricle is a small slit between the thalami. It is connected also to the fourth ventricle, through the cerebral aqueduct or the aqueduct of Sylvius. The choroid plexuses are situated above the roof of the ventricle.

The fourth ventricle sits anterior to the cerebellum and posterior to the pons and the superior half of the medulla. It is continuous superiorly with the cerebral aqueduct and the central canal below. The fourth ventricle has a tent-shaped roof, two lateral walls, and a floor. There are three small openings in the fourth ventricle, the two lateral foramina of Luschkea and the median foramen of Magendie. Through these openings the cerebrospinal fluid enters the subarachnoid space. The choroid plexus of the fourth ventricle has a *T*-shape. The ventricular system serves as a pathway for the circulation of the cerebrospinal fluid (Figure 3–6). The

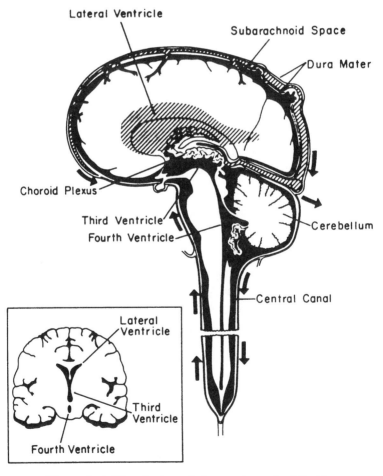

Figure 3–6 Circulation of the cerebrospinal fluid.

choroid plexuses of the ventricles appear to secrete the cerebrospinal fluid actively, although some of the fluid may originate as tissue fluid formed in the brain substance.

Cerebrospinal Fluid

The brain and the spinal cord are suspended in a clear, colorless fluid called *cerebrospinal fluid*, which serves as a cushion between the central nervous system and the surrounding bones, thereby protecting the brain against direct trauma. This fluid aids in regulation of intracranial pressure, nourishment of the nervous tissue, and removal of waste products.

The path of circulation of the cerebrospinal fluid is illustrated in Figure 3–6. It flows from the lateral ventricles into the third ventricle, to the fourth ventricle, and into the subarachnoid space. It then travels to reach the inferior surface of the cerebrum and move superiorly over the lateral aspect of each hemisphere. Some of it moves into the subarachnoid space around the spinal cord.

The cerebrospinal fluid is important in medical diagnostic procedures. The pressure of the fluid can be measured; if it is abnormally high, intracranial tumor or hemorrhage, hydrocephalus, meningitis, or encephalitis may be suspected. Chemical and cell studies may be made on cerebrospinal fluid that is drawn out of the nervous system through a procedure called a *lumbar puncture* or *spinal tap*. This route also may be used to inject drugs to combat infection or to induce anesthesia.

The Blood Supply of the Brain

The blood serves the brain much as food serves the body: to nourish it by supplying its most important element, oxygen. The brain uses about 20 percent of the blood of the body at any one time and requires approximately 25 percent of the oxygen of the body to function maximally. Initially, blood is delivered to the brain through four main arteries. There are two large *internal carotid arteries*, one on either side of the neck. These are a result of bifurcation, or splitting, of the common carotid artery from the heart. The other two main arteries supplying the brain are the *vertebral arteries* (Figure 3–7).

The Internal Carotid Arteries and Their Branches

The internal carotid arteries ascend in the neck and pass through the base of the skull at the carotid canal of the temporal bone. Each artery then runs horizontally forward and perforates the dura mater.

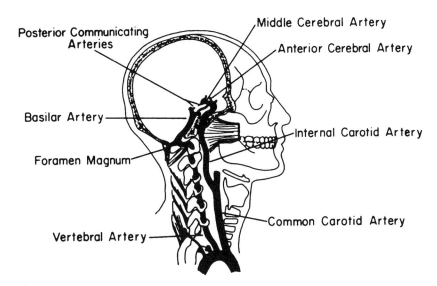

Figure 3–7 Cerebral arteries. Source: Redrawn and reproduced with permission from R. Snell, *Clinical Neuroanatomy for Medical Students* (Boston: Little, Brown and Company, 1980).

After entering the subarachnoid space, the artery turns posteriorly and, at the medial end of the lateral sulcus, divides into the *anterior* and *middle cerebral arteries*. Other cerebral arteries are also given off by the internal carotid artery. The *ophthalmic artery* supplies the eye, the frontal area of the scalp, the dorsum of the nose, and the ethmoid and frontal sinuses. The *posterior communicating artery* runs posteriorly above the oculomotor nerve and joins the posterior cerebral artery, forming part of the *circle of Willis*. The *anterior communicating artery* joins the two anterior cerebral arteries together in the circle of Willis.

Through these cortical branches, the internal carotid artery provides the blood supply to a very large portion of the cerebral hemisphere. The anterior cerebral artery supplies the medial surface of the cortex as far back as the parietal-temporal-occipital sulcus. It also supplies the so-called leg areas of the motor strip. Branches of this artery supply a small portion of the caudate nucleus, lentiform nucleus, and internal capsule.

The middle cerebral artery is the largest branch of the internal carotid. Its branches supply the entire lateral surface of the hemisphere except for the small area of the motor strip supplied by the anterior cerebral artery, the occipital pole, and the inferolateral surface of the hemisphere, which is supplied by the posterior cerebral artery. The middle cerebral artery's central branches also provide the primary blood supply to the lentiform and caudate nuclei and the internal capsule.

The Vertebral Artery and Its Branches

The vertebral artery passes through the foramina in the upper six cervical vertebrae and enters the skull through the foramen magnum. It passes upward and forward along the medulla and at the lower border of the pons and joins the vertebral artery from the opposite side to form the *basilar artery*. Prior to the formulation of the basilar artery, several branches are given off, including the following:

- The meningeal branches, which supply the bone and dura of the posterior cranial fossa
- The posterior spinal artery, which supplies the posterior third of the spinal cord
- The anterior spinal artery, which supplies the anterior two thirds of the spinal cord
- The posterior inferior cerebellar artery, which supplies part of the cerebellum, the medulla, and the choroid plexus of the fourth ventricle
- The medullary arteries, which are distributed to the medulla

After the basilar artery is formed by the union of the opposite vertebral arteries, it ascends and then divides at the upper border of the pons into the two *posterior cerebral arteries*. These arteries supply the inferolateral surface of the temporal lobe and the lateral and medial surfaces of the occipital lobe (that is, the visual cortex). They also supply parts of the thalamus and other internal structures (Figure 3–8).

Other branches of the basilar artery include the following:

- The pontine arteries, which enter the pons
- The labyrinthine artery, which supplies the internal ear

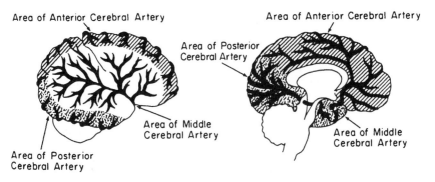

Figure 3–8 Distribution of the cerebral arteries of the lateral and mesial surfaces of the left cerebral hemisphere.

- The anterior inferior cerebellar artery, which supplies the anterior and inferior parts of the cerebellum
- The superior cerebellar artery, which supplies the superior portion of the cerebellum

The Circle of Willis

The circle of Willis, or the circulus arteriosus, is formed by the anastomosis of the two internal carotid arteries with the two vertebral arteries. The anterior communicating, anterior cerebral, internal carotid, posterior communicating, posterior cerebral, and basilar arteries are all part of the circle of Willis (Figure 3–9). This formation of arteries allows distribution of the blood entering from the internal carotid artery or vertebral artery to any part of both hemispheres. Cortical and central branches arise from the circle and further supply the brain.

The bloodstreams from the internal carotid artery and vertebral artery on both sides come together at a certain point in the posterior communicating artery. At that point the pressure is equal and they do not mix. Should, however, the internal carotid artery or the vertebral artery be occluded or blocked, the blood will pass forward or backward across that point to compensate for the reduced flow. The circle of Willis also allows blood to flow across the midline of the brain if an artery on one side is occluded. The circle of Willis thereby serves a safety valve function for the brain, allowing collateral circulation (or flow of blood through an

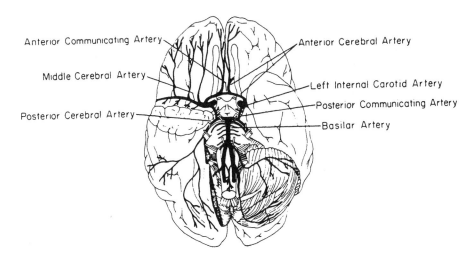

Figure 3–9 Circle of Willis. Source: Redrawn and reproduced with permission from R. Snell, *Clinical Neuroanatomy for Medical Students* (Boston: Little, Brown and Company, 1980).

alternate route) to take place if the flow is reduced to one area. The state of one's collateral circulation will help determine the outcome after a vascular lesion occurs and affects blood flow to the brain.

General Principles of Neurologic Organization

Now that we have surveyed the general anatomic organization of the nervous system for communication, it is appropriate to extract some fundamental principles of neurologic organization that are particularly crucial to the understanding and diagnosis of communication disorders. We will build on these principles in later chapters.

Contralateral Motor Control

The first principle to remember is that major movement patterns in humans have contralateral neurologic control in the brain. The arms and legs are represented in the motor strip of the cerebral cortex in a contralateral fashion. In other words, the cerebral hemisphere on one side of the body controls movements of the arm and leg on the other side of the body. This contralateral motor control is brought about by the crossing of the major voluntary motor pathway at the level of the lower brainstem. Auditory and visual sensory systems also have some contralateral organization, and this fact will become clinically important as you read Chapters 5 and 6.

If a patient sent to the speech-language pathologist has a severe language disorder and some paralysis of the right arm and leg, it suggests that the brain lesion causing this motor deficit is probably in the left cerebral hemisphere. The severe language disturbance accompanying the right limb paralysis serves as a confirming sign of left-sided brain lesion (discussed later). Why the nervous system is organized in such a manner as to provide contralateral motor control of the limbs is not completely known, but the fact illustrates that knowledge of principles of neurological organization can be used to locate and lateralize causative lesions seen in neurology and speech pathology.

Ipsilateral Motor Control

If a lesion occurs in the nervous system below the crossing of the major descending motor pathways, the effect is observed below the level of the lesion on the same side of the body where the lesion occurs. In many spinal cord injuries, paralysis and sensory loss occur below the point of injury. Thus, a second important principle is to determine whether effects of lesions are ipsilateral or contralateral.

Bilateral Speech Motor Control

For the most part, the midline muscles of the body in the head, neck, and trunk tend to be represented bilaterally and the nerve fibers supplying these regions, with certain exceptions, descend from both cerebral hemispheres. This bilateral neural control provides smooth, symmetrical movement for those muscles used in speaking—the lips, tongue, soft palate, jaw, abdominal muscles, and diaphragm. The principle of bilateral control of speech muscles suggests that serious involvement of the speech muscles usually results from diseases that affect bilateral neurologic mechanisms. With unilateral damage to the nervous system, effects on speech are generally less serious, and compensatory mechanisms are made available from the other side of the midline speech system.

Representation of the body is found in an inverted fashion on the motor areas of the cerebral cortex. Pathways that are concerned with movements of the lower limbs originate in the upper parts of the motor strip, whereas movements of the head and neck originate at the lower end of the motor strip, just above the Sylvian fissure. The area surrounding the left Sylvian fissure contains major areas for language processing. The anatomic relationship of motor speech areas and language suggests that it is not uncommon for speech and language disturbances to coexist because of the close proximity of their control areas on the cortex.

Unilateral Language Mechanisms

An impressive facet of cerebral asymmetry is that language mechanisms, for the most part, are unilaterally controlled in the brain, as compared with the bilateral speech muscle mechanism. Among the adult population, over 95 percent of right-handed people have their language mechanisms in the left cerebral hemisphere. Language dominance the world over is primarily in the left brain. Left-handers are more variable. Some are right-brained for language, others have bilateral representation of language. The obvious clinical principle suggested by these facts is that major language disturbance is a neurologic sign of left cerebral injury and that the left hemisphere has special anatomical properties for language.

Scheme of Cortical Organization

Although later chapters will detail the specifics of cortical localization, it is helpful for the student and clinician to have in mind a general scheme of organization of the cortex, since it is the site of most language functions. Although any such scheme is oversimplified and exaggerated, it nevertheless provides a crude but workable framework for conceptualizing functional localization.

The right and left hemispheres may be designated as nonverbal and verbal, and the anterior and posterior portions may be characterized as motor and sensory areas. The central sulcus divides the cerebral hemispheres into anterior and posterior regions. In humans, approximately half of the volume of the cerebral cortex is taken up by the frontal cortex. The frontal lobe contains the primary motor cortex, the premotor cortex, and Broca's area, the primary motor speech association area. In the anterior portion of the frontal lobes are the prefrontal areas, which are generally concerned with behavioral control of both cognitive and emotional functions. Lesions here produce slowed behavior, lacking in spontaneity. Difficulties in making mental shifts occur, and perseveration and rigidity are observed, as are a lack of self-awareness and a tendency toward concreteness. In brief, the frontal lobe appears to excel in the control, integration, and regulation of emotional and cognitive behavior.

In contrast, the posterior cortex appears dominated by the control, integration, and regulation of sensory behavior. The defects arising from the posterior cortex are related to the specific sensory association areas that are implicated by a lesion.

The occipital lobe, as noted earlier, contains the primary visual cortex and visual association areas. Deficits in the primary cortex result in blind spots in the visual field, and total destruction of the cortex produces complete blindness. Visual imperception and agnosias (see Chapter 9) are associated with the visual association areas.

The left parietal lobe is associated with constructional disturbances and visuospatial defects. Disorders of recognition, called *agnosias*, are common. The inferior parietal lobe concerns itself with language association tasks, and lesions there cause defects in reading and writing.

The temporal lobe on the left is concerned with hearing and related functions. It contains the primary auditory and auditory association areas. Auditory memory storage and complex auditory perception are among the functions of the temporal lobe. An area known as the *speech zone* surrounds the Sylvian fissure and appears to contain the major components of the language mechanism. Damage in the speech zone produces the aphasias.

With a clinical knowledge of primary sensory and related association areas and behavioral correlates to these areas, the speech-language pathologist is able to infer the approximate location of a lesion from the patient's behavioral symptoms and to recognize the well-known speech-language syndromes associated with cortical dysfunction. The general clinical principle is that specific cortical deficits can be associated with specific behavioral syndromes.

Summary

A vast amount of information is provided in Chapters 2 and 3. Figure 3–10 is a summary drawing of the levels of the central nervous system to help you organize the information you learned in Chapter 2. You will also refer to this drawing while reading subsequent chapters. In an additional effort to help you review and organize what you have learned, we have prepared an outline of the most important structures discussed in both chapters. For each item, ask yourself the following questions:

- What is it?
- Where is it?
- What does it do?

When appropriate, go back and see if you can label drawings of some of the various structures for which illustrations were used. The effort you put into doing this will be rewarded as you grow knowledgeable about and comfortable with the information in these chapters—information that is basic to your understanding of subsequent chapters.

  I. The human nervous system
    A. Central nervous system
      1. Brain
        a. Cerebral hemispheres
          (1) Four lobes
          (2) Fissures
          (3) Sulci
          (4) Gyri
          (5) Association cortex
          (6) Connecting fibers
        b. Basal ganglia
          (1) Corpus striatum
            (a) Caudate nucleus
            (b) Lentiform nucleus: putamen, globus pallidus
          (2) Claustrum
        c. Cerebellum
        d. Brainstem
          (1) Medulla oblongata
            (a) Pyramids
            (b) Olives
            (c) Peduncles

           (2) Pons
           (3) Mesencephalon
               (a) Tectum
               (b) Colliculi

2. Spinal cord
   a. Spinal nerves
   b. Peripheral nerves
   c. Five regions
3. Meninges
   a. Dura mater
   b. Arachnoid mater
   c. Pia mater
4. Ventricles
   a. Choroid plexuses
   b. Cerebrospinal fluid
5. Blood supply
   a. Internal carotid artery and its branches
   b. Vertebral artery and its branches
   c. Circle of Willis

B. Peripheral nervous system
  1. Spinal peripheral nerves
     a. Anterior horn cell
     b. Efferent fibers
     c. Afferent fibers
  2. Cranial nerves
     a. Twelve pairs

C. Autonomic nervous system
  1. Parasympathetic division
  2. Sympathetic division

II. Clinical principles of neurologic organization
   A. Contralateral motor control
   B. Ipsilateral motor control
   C. Bilateral speech motor control
   D. Unilateral language mechanisms
   E. Scheme of cortical organization

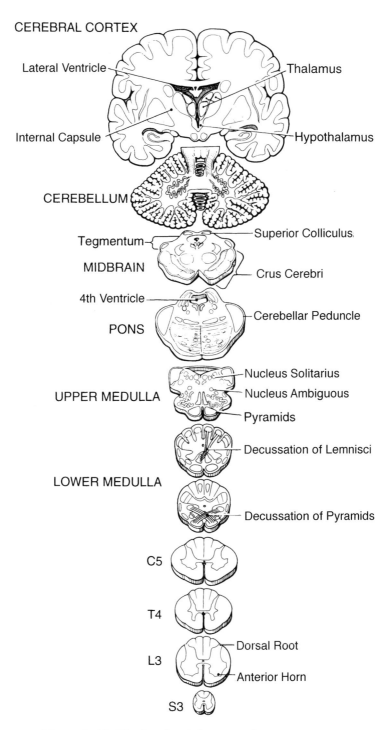

CEREBRAL CORTEX

Lateral Ventricle

Thalamus

Internal Capsule

Hypothalamus

CEREBELLUM

Tegmentum

Superior Colliculus

MIDBRAIN

Crus Cerebri

4th Ventricle

Cerebellar Peduncle

PONS

Nucleus Solitarius

UPPER MEDULLA

Nucleus Ambiguous

Pyramids

Decussation of Lemnisci

LOWER MEDULLA

Decussation of Pyramids

C5

T4

Dorsal Root

L3

Anterior Horn

S3

Figure 3–10 The levels of the central nervous system.

References and Further Readings

Angevine, J. B., & Cotman, C. W. (1981). *Principles of neuroanatomy.* New York: Oxford University Press.

Heimer, L. (1994). *The human brain and spinal cord. Functional neuroanatomy and dissection* (2nd ed.). New York: Springer-Verlag.

Liebman, M. (1983). *Neuroanatomy made easy and understandable.* Baltimore: University Park Press.

Snell, R. S. (1980). *Clinical neuroanatomy for medical students.* Boston: Little, Brown and Company.

4 □ □ □
□ □ □
□ □ □

Neuronal Function in the Nervous System

"But strange that I was not told
That the brain can hold
In a tiny ivory cage
God's heaven and hell."

—Oscar Wilde, *Poems and Fairy Tales of Oscar Wilde*, 1932

Neuronal Physiology

The Neuron

The *neuron*, or nerve cell, is the basic anatomic and functional unit of the nervous system, underlying all neural behavior including speech, language, and hearing. Each neuron consists of a cell body known as a *soma* or *perikaryon*. Neurons vary greatly in size, but most of the billions of neurons of the central nervous system are small (Figure 4–1). Each neuron contains a cell nucleus and one to a dozen projections of varying length. These projections receive stimuli and conduct neural impulses. Those receiving neural stimuli, called *dendrites*, are the shorter and more numerous projections of the nerve cell. Generally, the dendrites of a neuron are no more than a few millimeters in length.

The other process of a neuron is the *axon*, a longer single fiber that conducts nerve impulses away from the neuron to other parts of the nervous system, glands, or muscle. Axons range in length from several micrometers to more than 2 meters. The diameter of individual axons varies greatly, and their conduction velocity ranges from 2 to 100 meters per second, depending on the fiber size. The larger the diameter, the greater the conduction velocity. In a physiologic sense, the term axon refers to a nerve fiber that conducts impulses away from a nerve cell body. Any long nerve fiber, however, may be referred to as an axon, regardless of the direction of the flow of nervous impulses.

Neurons do the "work" of the nervous system by transmitting electrical signals or *neural impulses* to glands, muscles or to other neurons. In the peripheral nervous system many neuromuscular (i.e., neuron to muscle

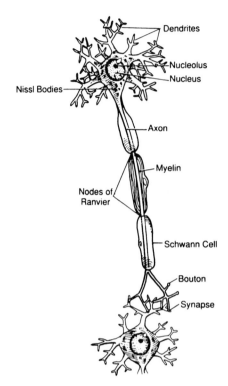

Figure 4–1 Schematic drawing of a neuron, myelinated axon, and synapse.
Source: Redrawn and reproduced with permission from M. Liebman, *Neuroanatomy Made Easy and Understandable* (2nd ed.). (Baltimore: University Park Press, 1983).

fiber) transmissions take place. In the brain itself, most of the neurons conduct neural impulses to other neurons, which are clustered very close together, providing a high neuronal density in the cerebrum. This high density creates an almost unlimited capacity for complex neuronal activity. This neuronal activity, or brain activation, produces our perceptions and thoughts, as well as nerve signals for voluntary muscle movement. Activation is the result of rapid biochemical and biophysical changes at the cellular level, in the neurons and glial cells of the brain (Roland, 1993).

The transmission of neural impulses is a complex process and its components are discussed below. A simplified summary of the process may be helpful prior to the discussion. For a neural impulse to be generated, the membrane of a neuron must open for a brief time to allow positively charged sodium ions to flow into the cell, which is normally negatively charged. This flow of ions will effect a change in polarization (or a depolarization) if continued and the cell will become positively charged. The positive charge causes an action potential or electrical charge to be emitted.

This action potential essentially is the neural impulse. The action potential travels down the axon until it reaches the area of synapse (literally, "union") with another neuron, a muscle or a gland. The area on this axon is called the presynaptic terminal of the membrane. The action potential causes a release of a substance called a neurotransmitter into the postsynaptic terminal of the membrane of the other neuron. At this point another action potential may be effected or other types of potentials may occur. These processes are given expanded explanation below.

Cellular Electrical Potentials

Like other cells of the body, the neuron is enclosed by membranes made up of protein and lipid layers. The intracellular portion of the neuron contains a high concentration of potassium and a low concentration of sodium and chloride in relation to the extracellular fluids. In the extracellular fluids, the concentrations are reversed. Sodium and chloride are found in high concentrations, about 10 times the intracellular concentrations. Potassium is found in low concentrations. The difference in chemical concentrations produces ionic differences across the membrane of the cell. These ionic differences create small electrical potentials across the surface membrane of the neuron and produce a flow of electric current. The electrical charge within the nerve cell is strongly negative compared with the outside of the cell. The term *resting potential* is employed to describe the differences in potential across the cell membranes.

Changes in electrical potential are conducted along the membranes of both the cell body and the nerve fibers. During the transmission of neural impulses, the primary mechanism is a change in the resting potential and a propagation of electrical current across the membrane. The conduction of the nerve impulse is actually brought about by an abrupt change in electrical potential, known as the *action potential*. The flow of current that occurs during the action potential is called the *action current* (Figure 4–2)

Action Potential

The action potential develops as the result of a rapid depolarization of the cell membrane, and there is a decrease in negativity inside the nerve cell relative to the outside of the cell. During the action potential, there is a transient reversal of the polarity of the electrical potential. At the peak of the action potential, the inside of the cell becomes positive with respect to the outside. The action potential is thus brought about by an initial inward current developed by a flow of sodium from the exterior to the interior of the cell.

The action current is propagated along the nerve fiber for long distances without change in the wave form and at a constant velocity. This means that all the neuronal signals of coded information that are transmitted in

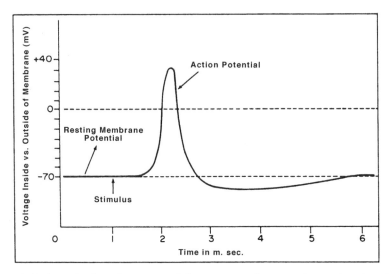

Figure 4-2 A typical action potential. Source: Redrawn and reproduced with permission from S. Rose, *The Conscious Brain* (New York: Knopf, 1973).

the nervous system are conveyed by a series of uniformly sized impulses. The information transmitted in the nervous system is therefore signaled by the frequency of the action potentials rather than by their amplitude. The action potential functions in an all-or-nothing manner. A stimulus sets up either a full-sized impulse or nothing.

During the passage of an action potential across a nerve cell membrane, the membrane becomes incapable of responding to another stimulus. This period of unresponsiveness is called an *absolute refractory period*. The absolute refractory period is relatively short, lasting approximately 0.8 milliseconds. Following the absolute refractory period, an action potential may be produced by a very intense stimulus initially and then by stimuli of less intensity. The period after the absolute refractory period is called the *relative refractory period*.

The Synapse

The Neuromuscular Synapse

As the electrical nerve impulse, in the form of an action potential, moves along an axon, it comes to a point where it must be transmitted to another neuron, a gland, or a muscle. This point is known as a *synapse*. Until it was realized that small junctures occur at the synapse, it was assumed that neurons were connected in one continuous network.

The transmission of a neural impulse across the synaptic juncture or gap is primarily a chemical process, sometimes an electrical process, and very occasionally a combination of both. The transmission of nerve impulses to muscle impulses in the peripheral nervous system was the first well-established example of chemical synaptic transmission. About 50 years ago, many neurophysiologists believed that the impulse transmission of one thousandth of a second was too fast for any type of chemical mediation. It was held that an electrical nerve impulse directly excited the muscle fiber. The large electrical mismatch, however, between the tiny nerve fiber and the large muscle fiber indicated that an electrical explanation would be faulty by at least two orders of magnitude. In the 1930s, it was established that synaptic transmission in nerve-to-muscle synapses was due entirely to chemical mediation by a substance called *acetylcholine* (ACh).

Chemical Transmission

In peripheral nerve-to-muscle transmission, or neuromuscular transmission, the nerve is known to be a structure on the muscle surface, making contact with the muscle fiber but not fusing with it. There is a special structural enlargement of the muscle fiber at the synaptic junction called the *motor endplate*. Near the motor endplate is the nerve terminal, or *synaptic knob* (Figure 4–3). With the advent of electron microscopy, a series of vesicles on the nerve terminal were identified. These became known as *synaptic vesicles*, and they release chemical transmitters at the synapse. In addition to the synaptic vesicles, a space known as the *synaptic cleft* has been observed. The synaptic cleft is the junction in the synapse across which transmission occurs. In the peripheral nervous system, electrical currents generated by the action of the transmitter substance, acetylcholine, flow across the synapse to the membrane known as the postsynaptic membrane. In nerve-to-muscle impulses, this is the membrane of the motor endplate. From the endplate, the impulse triggers muscle contraction.

In brief, the primary mechanism of the synapse occurs when a nerve impulse causes some of the synaptic vesicles to liberate their neurotransmitter substance into the synaptic cleft. In the nerve-to-muscle transmission, the vesicles contain acetylcholine, which is prepackaged with about 10,000 molecules in each vesicle. Neurotransmitters are released in what are called quanta, or small packets. The acetylcholine transmitters act to change the direction of depolarization. This, in turn, sets up an impulse on the motor endplate. An impulse is then generated along the muscle fiber, which sets off a complex series of events for muscle contraction.

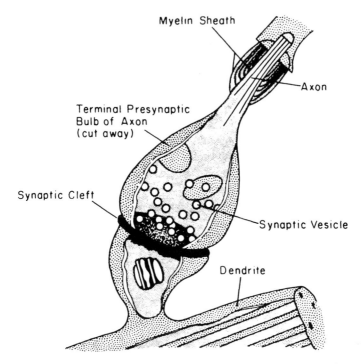

Figure 4–3 Reconstruction of what a synapse may look like in three dimensions. Source: Redrawn and reproduced with permission from *Biological Bases of Behavior, Unit 1,* London: Open University.

The chemical transmitters in either the peripheral nervous system or the central nervous system are removed by either reuptake or destruction by enzymes. Specific enzymes have been found to be involved for different types of transmitters.

Transmission Disorders

Disorders of chemical transmission can cause neurologic disorders. In the neuromuscular disease known as *myasthenia gravis*, the patient shows muscle weakness on sustained effort. Neuromuscular transmission appears to fail after continuous muscle contraction as a result of reduced availability of acetylcholine at the myoneural junction. Antibodies interfere with the transmission of the acetylcholine. These antibodies are an autoimmune disease reaction to postsynaptic receptor protein, with an involvement of the postsynaptic membranes.

The prime symptom of weakness often affects the speech muscles. The nerve innervating the larynx and palate is sometimes the first to be affected by the disease. The weakened vocal folds do not close appropriately, and the voice becomes breathy and weak in intensity. A hypernasal voice quality may develop after sustained speaking because of weakness of the soft palate. As the speech deteriorates, the tongue, lips, and respiratory muscles may be involved. Speech symptoms will be discussed further in Chapter 8.

Certain drugs—prostigmine and Tensilon—will temporarily relieve the symptoms promptly and aid the neurologist in diagnosing the disease. Treatment to reduce the antibodies blocking the acetylcholine transmission is effective in reversing the neuromuscular problem in the muscles of the body as well as the speech muscles.

Synaptic Excitation and Inhibition

Synaptic transmission in the brain, as opposed to neuromuscular transmission, is the result of synaptic action between neuron and neuron rather than nerve fiber and muscle fiber. Neurons connected to each other are called *interneurons*. The basic synaptic mechanism, however, is much the same. Synaptic vesicles release transmitter substances, and action potentials are triggered. The main neurotransmitter types are amino acid transmitters (e.g., GABA, glutamate, and glycine); amine transmitters (e.g., acetylcholine, dopamine, adrenaline, histamine, and serotonin); and peptide transmitters (e.g., neuropeptide, vasopressin, and cholecystokinin). Neurotransmitters may have excitatory or inhibitory effects on the postsynaptic membrane, but most serve to modulate the excitability of the neuron.

Excitatory and inhibitory potentials are established before and after the action potential. Before an action potential in the postsynaptic nerve fiber is triggered, there is an intervening potential developed called the *postsynaptic potential*. This potential may be either excitatory (E) or inhibitory (I). The excitatory postsynaptic potential (EPSP) persists for several milliseconds and may be strong enough to trigger an action potential, or it may summate in space and time to achieve the necessary voltage to trigger an action potential. Several individual nerve endings converging on one postsynaptic membrane may summate, or several subthreshold events may summate over time to evoke an action potential in an all-or-none manner.

The inhibitory postsynaptic potential (IPSP) is almost a mirror image of EPSP. The peak voltage is in the opposite direction, and the duration is almost the same except for minor alterations. The EPSP acts to depolarize the membrane, and the membrane potential may be driven beyond a threshold to trigger the action potential. The IPSP stabilizes the membrane potential so that the action potential is not triggered.

An action potential may be triggered when a series of impulses of the EPSP type arrive at a neuron. If the impulses occur in rapid succession, the action potential is more likely than when a single impulse or a few impulses arrive at the neuron. Excitatory states that assist the conduction of action potentials along a chain of neurons are called *facilitation*.

Both the EPSP and the IPSP are graded responses that will summate, resulting in plasticity and variability of function at the synapse. The individual synapse is subject to an almost infinite number of influences that affect the rate of firing in individual neurons. This fact allows for the notion of a probabilistic aspect in neuronal functioning in the brain.

Synaptic plasticity has been discussed by scientists studying learning. By this is meant short- or long-term changes in synaptic effectiveness that may, in part, account for an increase in skill or knowledge over time. There are two different theories regarding synaptic changes during learning. Hebb (1949) proposed that the postsynaptic neuron receives excitation simultaneously from two different axon terminals, increasing the effectiveness of one or both of the synapses. Kandel and Tauc (1965) hypothesized that the second axon joins with the first axon at the presynaptic terminal and causes increased neurotransmitter release to occur, thereby increasing synapse effectiveness.

Scientists studying learning have looked at long-term potentiation (LTP) which is a long-lasting increase in synaptic efficacy following afferent stimulation (Roland, 1993). These studies have been done primarily in the hippocampus and have shown that metabolic changes within the hippocampal cells do occur with stimulation, thus enabling the cells to become more receptive to synaptic input, though there is no data to show that the change is permanent. These studies do support the notion, however, that there may be a neuronal basis for producing a change in brain-behavior relationships through increased stimulation and experiential learning.

Principles of Neuronal Operation

The central nervous system is constantly bombarded by volleys of sensory nerve impulses. The excitatory and inhibitory influences of the nervous system provide for a process of selectivity of impulses for transmission at the level of the synapse. This selectivity of transmission of nerve impulse may be the basic function of the synapse. The synapse allows transmission in an all-or-none manner also. In other words, all that can be transmitted is either a full-sized response for the condition of the axon, or nothing.

Further, the central nervous system is characterized by the principle of divergence. Charles Sherrington observed that within the human nervous system there are numerous branchings of all axons with a great opportunity for wide dispersal of impulses because the impulses discharged by a neuron travel along its branches to activate all of its synapses. Thus, the central nervous system is made up of an almost numberless series of sources and routes for widespread or accessory neuronal activity. This accessory neuronal activity forms what may be considered neuronal pools of activity.

There is a complementary principle of convergence in the nervous system. This principle, also enumerated by Sherrington, implies that all neurons receive synaptic information from many other neurons, some of an excitatory nature and some of an inhibitory nature. The number of synapses on individual neurons is generally large, measured in hundreds or thousands, with the largest being about 80,000. Therefore, both excitation and inhibition play a large role in the nervous system.

The principles of divergence and convergence also suggest that, although individual neurons are neither excitatory nor inhibitory, certain neuronal systems act primarily as either excitatory or inhibitory mechanisms for effective overall neuronal functioning. An example is the large excitatory and inhibitory neuronal system in the reticular formation deep within the brain, which both activates and suppresses levels of consciousness during wakefulness and sleep, respectively.

The complexity of the neuronal firings and synaptic connections, particularly on the surface of the brain called the cerebral cortex, provides an intricate weaving of impulses into very complex spatial and temporal patterns. Sherrington has compared this neuronal activity to the weaving of an enchanted loom. No doubt these ever-changing neuronal designs are the basis for the integrative activity of the nervous system and are the foundations of emotion, thought, language, and action as well as that most human of behaviors—speaking.

It is sometimes difficult to grasp, and even harder to believe, that the rich range of behavior that we assume is specifically human, including the uniqueness of oral language, can ultimately be reduced to and equated with the mere ebb and flow of minute chemical and electrical changes in tiny, but intricate, synaptic mechanisms. This contemporary interpretation of neuronal function, reductionist as it appears, highlights the vast and mysterious frontier between mind and brain that faces the neuroscientist. Despite this great gulf between mind and matter, it is well for the speech-language pathologist to remember that this view of neuronal functioning provides the neurophysiologist with a basis for seeing the workings of the brain as a vast abstract complex of neuronal design on the enchanted loom of Sherrington. Despite our sophistication in studying neuronal function, the specifics of the neuronal patterns for understanding and producing language and speech in the brain are unknown.

Servomechanism Theory in Neuronal Function

Feedback

Several fruitful engineering concepts have been applied to neuronal transmission problems in the nervous system. These concepts have been particularly useful in explaining the possible control of neural impulses in the speech mechanism. The basic concept, known as the theory of servomechanism control systems, implies the concept of *feedback*. Feedback describes the functioning principle in self-regulating systems, either mechanical or biological. Feedback assumes that the output of any self-regulating system, such as a thermostat, is fed back into the system at some point so as to control or regulate the output of the system. This concept of self-monitoring is most appropriate for understanding the biologic system known as the speech motor control system. For instance, the questions of how a speaker monitors speech and what neuronal feedback mechanisms are available to control speech movements seem likely ones for explanation by servomechanism theory.

Open and Closed Control Systems

Two types of bioengineering control systems have been described as applicable to neuronal transmission in speech production: closed- and open-loop control systems. A *closed-loop system* employs *positive feedback* wherein output is returned as input to control further output. For example, if you are copying a complex and delicate drawing, the sensory input to your visual system guides the motor output of your hand. Similarly, hearing our own speech as we talk may at times serve to control the motor speech output as we continue to talk more. In these two examples, it is assumed that our motor output by hand or tongue is guided by the sensory input of vision or audition. We would further assume that if the sensory feedback were blocked, our drawing or speech would go awry.

In an *open-loop system*, the output is generally preprogrammed, and the performance of the system is not matched with the system. For instance, if you have learned a short poem by heart and practiced it over and over again, you may well be able to say the phonemes of the words in the poem without error even though your ears are stuffed with cotton. In an open-loop system the notion of *feedforward*, rather than feedback, is important. Once you have uttered a phrase of a well-learned poem, it will cue the next preprogrammed phrase of speech without the need to hear what was said through auditory feedback. An open-loop system thus typically generates another input via its output system. The term *negative feedback* is also used in control systems of the servomechanism type. It implies that when errors are fed back into the system, the error information will act to keep a given output activity within certain limits. Correcting an articulation error on hearing it is an example of utilization of negative feedback in speech activity.

Much speech research has viewed speech motor control as the product of a closed-loop feedback system with sensory monitoring from hearing, touch, and deep muscle sense guiding the movements of the speech muscles. Circumstantial evidence for this position has come from studies of sensory dysfunction in some speech disorders (see Chapter 6). Yet there is evidence that much of speech motor control is preprogrammed by the brain and that feedforward control is also important. It may well be that neurologic control of speech involves combinations of both open and closed loops in a multiple-pathway, hierarchical system that provides the necessary flexibility, speed, and precision to program and execute the everyday movements of speech with such complexity and ease.

Evoked Potentials in Speech and Language

Neurodiagnostic advances such as computerized tomography, magnetic resonance imaging, positron emission tomography (PET), and single photon emission tomography (SPECT) have increased our ability to understand the contribution of neuronal transmission to speech and language behavior. Another longtime diagnostic technique, electroencephalography (EEG), has been used for decades to diagnose lesions of the brain and to help clarify their nature. EEGs measures the electronic neuronal transmission in the brain with the use of noninvasive scalp electrodes. The EEG has been particularly helpful in diagnosing epilepsy and its subtypes. Epileptic syndromes range from mild abnormal electrical disturbances (petite mal seizures) to more serious abnormalities (grand mal seizures). Single (febrile) convulsions or a series of convulsions or seizures may occur. A series of seizures is called *epilepsy.*

The EEG has also been used to study what has been called *specific event—related electrical potential.* The method separates the electrical activity surrounding the specific event from the ongoing electrical background activity of the brain by use of an averaging computer. If a stimulus is repeated enough times and each repetition produces a circumscribed electrical response, it is possible through computer averaging to establish the onset of a response and its termination. This is called an *event-related potential* (ERP). It may be a response to internal or external stimulation of the nervous system.

Although this technique has been used widely by some speech and psychological researchers, it is not without problems (Caplan, 1987). Both its validity and reliability can be questioned. It is not always certain whether an electrical potential that occurs after a stimulus is of cerebral origin or is brought about by a motor act. When a language stimulus evokes a cerebral potential, it is not always clear that brain activity is present, nor does the absence of an electrical potential to a language stimulus mean there is no electrical activity. Many electrical currents simply do not reach the surface electrodes; some are too small and erratic. In addition, the waveforms derived from stimulation are highly complex, and it is often difficult to know what section of the waveform that was generated in response to the language stimulus has psychological meaning.

Despite these limitations, ERP has the capacity to measure events in the brain millisecond by millisecond. A research paradigm frequently used in language studies yields a *readiness potential*. The subject is asked to repeat a word or phrase or to speak freely with pauses of 3 or 4 seconds between portions of an utterance. The continuous EEG recording that precedes the onset of speech is analyzed by averaging waveforms across several utterances to discover the readiness potential.

Another measure that may be derived is called the *contingent negative variation* (CNV) or *expectancy waveform*. The subject is shown two separate visual stimuli. The interval between the stimuli is set, and the subject is required to say a particular word or phrase when the second visual stimulus arises. Under these conditions an electrical expectancy waveform occurs following the first stimulus.

Even with its many limitations, measurement of cerebral evoked potentials offers the hope of finding physiological correlates of psycholinguistic brain processes that occur so rapidly that they cannot be measured by other existing neurodiagnostic techniques. For instance, several attempts have been made to study the cerebral potential preceding speech. This is called the readiness potential.

In 1971, McAdam and Whitaker reported that a late negative potential occurred at Broca's area approximately 150 milliseconds before a subject uttered a polysyllabic word. As a control, the authors reported potentials from nonspeech acts such as coughing. They found that nonspeaking activities produced negative potentials in a symmetrical way over both hemispheres, and they interpreted their findings to indicate that Broca's area on the left was involved in speech planning. Grozinger et al. (1977) argued that McAdam and Whitaker's methodology was faulty; in addition, Grozinger et al. reported asymmetrical potentials over the two hemispheres as early as 2 to 3 seconds before the onset of speech, not just a few hundred milliseconds. They also reported early potentials that were related to respiration rather than onset of speech.

Other investigators (Szinles & Vaughan, 1977) argued that scalp electrodes were not free of contamination from sources of noncerebral origin and advocated direct cortical recordings from speech and language areas as the best approach to solving these technical problems. CNV studies claiming to find potentials that were larger over the dominant hemisphere were criticized on the grounds that hemispheric differences in CNV were not related to preparation in speech. Szinles and Vaughan suggested that asymmetrical CNVs in which a word is used as the first stimulus may be invalid.

In sum, the studies of electrical stimulation preceding speech are not conclusive, only suggestive, and certainly require a series of control studies to be considered valid. These studies do, however, suggest that very small electrical events occur within milliseconds after an auditory or visual event and that ERPs are one experimental method with which to measure language events as rapid as language. However, valid and reliable experimental paradigms need to be worked out.

Recent research with PET and SPECT scanning has served to answer some of the questions raised by evoked potential research with better reliability (Peterson et al., 1990). It should be noted that evoked potentials are used in audiological testing.

Myelin

Nerve fibers, or axons, may be classified as myelinated or unmyelinated. Large peripheral nerves as well as the large axons of the central nervous system acquire a white fatty sheath of wrapping as the brain develops. This is *myelin*. The myelin sheath is composed of *Schwann cells*. The Schwann sheet outside is called the *neurolemma*. Myelin is white, contrasting sharply with the gray unmyelinated nerve. The myelin sheet is thick and can be revealed by a special myelin stain. The thick insulation of myelin is interrupted at intervals by structures called the *nodes of Ranvier*. The design of myelin sheaths enhances rapid propagation of the electrical impulse along the nerve fiber. The impulse moves along the myelinated fiber by hopping from node to node, without any active contribution from the long internodal spaces. Action potentials develop only at the nodes (Figure 4–1). This mode of transmission is extremely efficient compared with the slow gliding along of the nerve impulses on unmyelinated fibers. The type of transmission in myelinated fibers is called *saltatory transmission*. The efficiency of saltatory transmission is achieved because of the insulation that prevents current flow between nodes; in addition, there is little leakage of current from the fibers. The conduction velocity of a myelinated fiber is directly proportional to the diameter of the fiber, whereas in an unmyelinated fiber the velocity is approximately proportional to the square root of the diameter. On average, transmission along a myelinated fiber is roughly 50 times as fast as one along an unmyelinated fiber.

Unmyelinated fibers are more common in the smaller nerve fibers of the peripheral nervous system, though the cranial nerves, which are part of the peripheral nervous system, are relatively large in diameter and are myelinated. Six of the cranial nerves innervate the speech muscles and provide neuromotor control for talking. The rapidity of transmission in these nerves helps supply neural innervation for the rapid muscular movements underlying speech.

Development of Myelin

Myelin is laid down in the nervous system as the brain develops. At birth, the human brain is relatively low in myelin. Most of the pathways that have been formed in prenatal life are unmyelinated, so the gray matter of the cortex is hard to distinguish from the white matter of the subcortical tissue at birth. The major increase in the laying down of the myelin lipid sheaths occurs during the first two years of life. The development of myelin parallels the development of *glia* in the brain. Glia are cells other than neurons that are found in the cortex of the brain. The term *glia* is from Latin and means "glue." The cells appear to stick together and seal up the available spaces in the cerebral cortex; they outnumber the neurons about 10 to one. Not all of the functions of the glial cells are clear, but one that is well-established is that of fabricating the myelin sheaths in which the myelinated axons are wrapped. The cells that make the myelin are called *oligodendroglia*. The other glial cells are known as *astrocytes*.

Since the infant brain shows a distinct lack of myelin at birth, its development has frequently been considered a significant index, among several others, of the maturation of the nervous system. Specific attempts have been made to relate major speech and language milestones, such as the appearance of babbling, first words, and word combinations, to the development of myelin in the nervous system. Although a case can be made for a positive relationship between communicative milestones and development of myelin, there is insufficient evidence to suggest that delays in the development of myelin are necessarily related to syndromes of speech and language delay. The area of neurologic developmental delays of myelin awaits further research.

Myelin Disorders

Multiple sclerosis is a disorder of myelin that produces a variety of neurologic symptoms, including a severe motor disturbance. It is caused by an autoimmune inflammatory response that damages the myelin sheath. If this inflammatory reaction is intense, the axons, too, may be damaged, producing irreversible neurologic deficits that show irregular fluctuating periods of exacerbation and remission.

About half of patients with multiple sclerosis have speech defects. A speech disorder resulting from involvement of the neuromuscular aspect of the nervous system is called *dysarthria*. Clinical symptoms of dysarthria are detailed in Chapter 8.

Summary

The neuron is the basic functional unit of the nervous system. Its primary property is excitability. The afferent processes of the neuron are called dendrites, and the efferent process is the axon. Neural transmission is a function basic to the nervous system, and the neuron with its processes serves as a basic conductive unit of the nervous system.

The synapse is a juncture point at which electrical impulses are transmitted from nerve to muscle, gland, or another neuron. Interneuron transmission occurs in the brain from nerve to nerve. Electrical transmission at the synapse is aided by the release of biochemical transmitters. Peripheral neuromuscular synapses release acetylcholine. Other neurotransmitters have been found in the brain. Firing at the synapse occurs as the result of the trigger of an action potential. This potential is influenced by the excitatory presynaptic potential and the inhibitory presynaptic potential.

Neuronal function at higher levels is accomplished in neuronal patterns and networks. The principles of network excitation and inhibition, as well as convergence and divergence and probabilistic selectivity of impulses at the synapse, are important in brain function. There remains a significant knowledge gap between understanding the electrical and biochemical properties in neuronal transmission and explaining the neuronal activity necessary for speech and language.

Myelin, an insulating covering on some nerves of the central and peripheral nervous system, allows rapid and efficient transmission of impulses. The six cranial nerves innervating the speech mechanism are myelinated, allowing the rapid muscular actions necessary for speech. Acquisition of myelin appears to be one index of nervous system maturation in the first 2 years of life, but there is no substantial evidence to suggest that speech and language delays in preschool children are associated with lack or delay of myelination.

Multiple sclerosis is a disorder of myelin that sometimes produces a motor speech disorder known as dysarthria. Currently there is no cure for the myelin deterioration in multiple sclerosis. Reduction of acetylcholine at the synapse as part of an autoimmune disease causes another neuromuscular disorder, myasthenia gravis, usually with an associated dysarthria. Myasthenia gravis is marked by extreme weakness of muscles on sustained effort. Drug therapy may alleviate the speech problems and weakness appreciably.

References and Further Reading

Caplan, D. (1987). Cerebral evoked potentials and language. In D. Caplan, *Neurolinguistics and linguistic aphasiology: An introduction*. New York: Cambridge University Press.

Eccles, J. C. (1973). *The understanding of the brain*. New York: McGraw-Hill.

Grillner, S., Lindblom, B., Lubker, J., & Persson, A. (1982). *Speech motor control*. Oxford: Pergamon Press.

Grozinger, B., Kornhuber, H., & Kriebel, J. (1977). Human cerebral potentials preceding speech production, phonation and movements of the mouth and tongue, with reference to respiratory, and extracerebral potentials. In J. E. Desmidt (Ed.), *Language and hemispheric specialization*. Basal: Krager.

Hebb, D. O. (1949). *The organization of behavior*. New York: John Wiley & Sons.

Jewett, D. L., & Rayner, M. D. (1984). *Basic concepts of neuronal function*. Boston: Little, Brown and Company.

Kandel, E. R. and Tauc, L. L. (1965). Mechanisms of heterosynaptic facilitation in the giant cell of the abdominal ganglion of a plysia depilans. *Journal of Physiology* (London) 181: 28–47.

McAdam, D. W., & Whitaker, H. A. (1971). Electrocortical localization of language production: Reply to Morrell and Huntington. *Science*, 174, 1360–1361.

Peterson, S. I., Fox, P. T., Snyder, A. Z., & Raichle, M. E. (1990). Activation of extrastriate and frontal cortical areas by visual words and word-like stimuli. *Science*, 249, 1041–1044.

Roland, P. E. (1993) *Brain Activation*. New York: John Wiley & Sons.

Szinles, J., & Vaughan, H. G. (1977). Characteristics of cranial and facial potential associated with speech production. In J. E. Desmidt (Ed.), *Language and hemispheric specialization*. Basal: Krager.

5 ▢▢▢
▢▢▢
▢▢▢

Neurosensory Organization of Speech and Hearing

"Speech is normally controlled by the ear."

—Raymond Carhart, *Hearing and Deafness*, 1947

Bodily Sensation

Classification

During the 19th century, neurophysiologists conceived of the execution of skilled motor acts primarily as the result of programming in the motor areas of the cerebral cortex, with some additional influences on the descending motor impulses from cerebellar and extrapyramidal mechanisms. This view of the nervous system has been modified during the 20th century to include the concept of sensory feedback control in motor acts. Audition, of course, plays a special and primary feedback role in the control of speech. Recently, specific efforts have been directed at determining the nature of other neurosensory controls exercised in speaking. Before we discuss sensory control in speech, it is necessary to understand in general the types of sensation mediated by the nervous system.

Sherrington's Scheme

Charles Sherrington (1926) proposed a classification of sensation that is in wide use today and has application for the sensory control of speech. He divided the sensory receptors into three broad classes: (1) exteroceptors, (2) proprioceptors, and (3) interoceptors. *Exteroceptors* mediate sight, sound, smell, and cutaneous sensation. Cutaneous superficial skin sensation includes touch, superficial pain, temperature, itching, and tickling. *Proprioceptors* mediate deep somatic sensation from receptors

beneath the skin, in muscles and joints, and in the inner ear. Proprioception includes the following senses: pressure, movement, vibration, position,
deep pain, and equilibrium. *Interoceptors* mediate sensation from the
viscera, as well as visceral pain and pressure or distension. Pain receptors,
either from cellular or tissue injury, are known as *nociceptive receptors*.

In addition, multisensory functions have been called the higher
sensations. The higher sensations include recognition of form, size, and
texture, as well as weight and two-point discrimination.

Neurophysiologists have classified the senses as special and general
senses. The term *special senses* reflects the traditional layperson's concept
that certain of the senses are primary. For the neurophysiologist, hearing,
vision, taste, smell, and balance are the special senses. The *general senses*,
in this classification scheme, include the remainder of the senses.

Anatomy of Sensation

The neuroanatomy of the senses is complex. The general
somatic sensory pathways—those dealing with bodily sensation—utilize
the spinal cord and spinal nerves. Sensation to the head and vocal
mechanism—larynx, pharynx, soft palate, and tongue—utilize the cranial
nerve pathways.

The pathways of somatic sensation are composed in general of a
three-neuron pathway from the periphery to the cerebral cortex. There is
some variation within this three-neuron organization for the sensations
of light touch, pain, temperature, and proprioception. The first-order, or
prime, neuron for sensation for any given spinal nerve is found on the dorsal
or posterior spinal root in a mass known as a *spinal ganglion*. For instance,
the superficial sensations of light touch and pain and temperature begin
in special receptors in the skin and are transmitted by spinal nerves to
the spinal cord through the spinal ganglion. From the first-order neuron,
an axon ascends or descends one or two spinal segments, traveling in a
tract called *Lissauer's tract* or the *dorsolateral fasciculus*. It then synapses
on the second-order neuron in the dorsal gray column of the spinal cord.
Fibers of the second-order neuron then cross the midline, and an axon
ascends to the third-order neuron in the ventral posterolateral nucleus of
the thalamus. A general name for the tract formed by the axon of the
second-order neuron is *lemniscus*.

Lateral Spinothalamic Tract

The crossed ascending sensory pathway in the spinal cord,
known as the *lateral spinothalamic tract*, transmits the sensations of pain
and temperature (Figure 5-1). The fibers enter the cord through the spinal

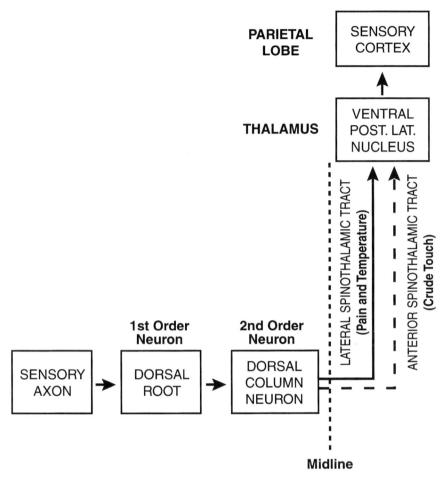

Figure 5–1 This flowchart depicts the lateral spinothalamic tract, which mediates pain and temperature, and the anterior spinothalamic tract, which mediates light or crude touch (POST., posterior; LAT., lateral).

root ganglion, travel up or down a few segments in Lissauer's tract, and end in the dorsal root of the gray matter. At this point the first-order neuron synapses with the second-order neuron and promptly crosses to the other side of the spinal cord. There, the fibers enter the lateral white column or the lateral spinothalamic tract and ascend to the ventral posterior lateral nucleus in the thalamus. The axons of the lateral spinothalamic tract synapse with a third-order neuron that leaves the thalamus, ascends in the internal capsule, and reaches the postcentral cortical gyri in the parietal lobe (areas 3, 1, and 2). This is the primary somatic sensory area of the brain, and pain and temperature sensations as well as pressure and touch are interpreted here.

Other fibers are given off as the lateral spinothalamic tract ascends. These terminate on the reticular nuclei in the brainstem; fibers from the nuclei then project to the thalamus, hypothalamus, and hippocampus. Somatic and visceral responses to pain, such as changes in respiration and heartbeat as well as nausea and fainting, are mediated through descending fibers from these structures.

Anterior Spinothalamic Tract

The *anterior* (or *ventral*) *spinothalamic tract* carries sensory information of light touch, including light pressure and touch and tactile location (Figure 5–1). The light touch fibers synapse within the dorsal gray horn cells in the spinal cord and ascend in the anterior spinothalamic tract to the brainstem and the posterior ventral nucleus of the midbrain. The tract also ends in the postcentral gyrus of the parietal lobe.

Proprioception Pathways

Proprioception, two-point discrimination, vibration, and form perception follow different pathways than those of the spinothalamic tracts. Proprioception is the sense that allows us to know exactly where our body parts are in space and in relation to one another. Two-point discrimination allows us to distinguish two adjacent points on the skin. Two-point sensitivity varies over the brain surface. The lips and fingertips are the most sensitive and the back the least sensitive. Vibratory sensation allows us to recognize vibrating objects. Form perception allows recognition of objects by touch alone.

Spinocerebellar Tract

Proprioception is conveyed by fibers from muscle tendons and joints and takes two major routes after entering the spinal cord. One of these major pathways is the spinocerebellar pathway, and the other is the dorsal column pathway. The spinocerebellar pathways are of lesser importance in human neurology because of the poor localizing information available about these tracts.

The spinocerebellar pathway has two tracts, dorsal and ventral. These tracts arise from the posterior and medial gray matter of the cord. The dorsal tract ascends ipsilaterally, but the ventral tract crosses in the cord. Both tracts terminate in the cerebellum and allow proprioceptive impulses from all parts of the body to be integrated in the cerebellum. It has been proposed that the spinocerebellar pathway functions in unconscious perception of already learned motor patterns.

Dorsal Columns

Conscious proprioception, two-point discrimination, and form perception have been called the sensory modalities of the dorsal, or posterior, columns of the spinal cord. The axons of the dorsal columns enter the cord after entering the peripheral nerves of the spinal cord with the first-order neuron at the dorsal root ganglion (Figure 5–2).The axons then ascend in the dorsal white columns to the medulla. Axons entering the cord at the sacral and lumbar regions, which mediate proprioception from the leg and lower body, are found in the medial dorsal columns, called the *fasciculus gracilis*. Axons from the more lateral dorsal columns, from the thoracic and cervical regions, are generally related to the arm and upper body. They are found in the *fasciculus cuneatus*. The second-order neurons leave the nucleus gracilis and nucleus cuneatus, cross over to the other side of the medulla, where they form a bundle called the *medial lemniscus*, which ascends to the third-order neuron at the thalamus and then proceeds to the parietal lobe.

Proprioceptive Deficits

Damage to the postcentral gyrus of the parietal lobe, the dorsal columns, or the dorsal root ganglion may produce a loss of proprioception, astereognosis, loss of vibratory sense, and loss of two-point discrimination in the trunk or extremities. If there is damage to those dorsal column fibers below the level of the medulla, the loss in proprioception is on the same side of the injury. Damage above the level of the medulla produces a loss in proprioception on the opposite side of the body. If the fibers of the spinocerebellar tract are damaged, proprioceptive loss occurs on the same side as the injury.

Damage to the spinothalamic tracts of pain and temperature usually result in loss to the opposite side of the body. The fibers of light touch take two routes, one ipsilateral and one contralateral. The ipsilateral fibers ascend with the proprioceptive fibers in the dorsal columns, and the crossed fibers ascend in the spinothalamic tract. The fibers of light touch branch extensively; because of this branching, touch is unlikely to be abolished by injury to a specific pathway in the spinal cord.

Sensory Examination

The neurologist employs several traditional and standard procedures for determining sensory loss. These are incorporated into the standard neurologic examination (see Appendix C).

The senses of light touch, pain, and temperature are mediated by the fibers of the dorsal root of the spinal cord, which come from a

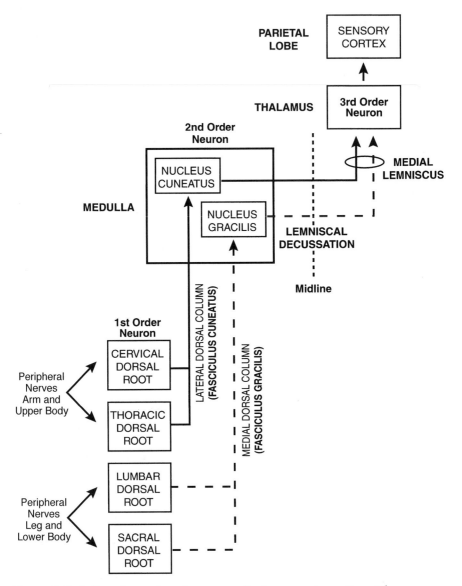

Figure 5–2 A flowchart of pathways mediating proprioception. The pathways are known as the *dorsal column modalities.*

circumscribed area of the skin known as a *dermatome.* In peripheral nerve injuries, impairment of touch corresponds to dermatomal zones; however, at the boundary of each segmental dermatome is an overlap area supplied by the adjacent segmental nerves. For instance, if the fifth thoracic nerve (T5) is severed, T3 and T6 will carry many of the pain and temperature sensations supplied by T5. This segmental overlap also is present in the spinal cord. Thus, overlap is greater for pain and temperature than for touch.

Light Touch

The sense of light touch is tested by determining the patient's ability to perceive light stroking of the skin with a wisp of cotton. Disorders of the sensory pathways from skin to cortex will show abnormal sensory reactions. Decreased tactile sensation is called *hypoesthesia*, and complete loss of sensation is called *anesthesia*. If tactile sensation is abnormally increased, it is known as *hyperesthesia*.

Inability to localize touch is called *atopognosis*. Topognosia is tested by touching the patient's body. With the eyes closed, the patient is asked to point to the spot where touch occurred. The neurologist compares similar areas of both sides of the body. Atopognosia is usually associated with a lesion of the parietal lobe.

Two-Point Discrimination

Two-point discrimination, or the ability to discriminate the shortest distance between two tactile points on the skin, is sometimes tested with points of a caliper. Right and left sides of the body are compared. Loss of discrimination suggests a parietal lobe lesion.

Double stimulation may also be utilized to determine a cortical sensory disorder. Two simultaneous tactile stimulations are presented to both sides of the body in similar areas, or to different areas. Lateralized sensory loss can then be determined. Frequently, sensory pathway or cortical sensory losses accompany lesions that produce cerebral language disorders.

Pain and Temperature

Pain and temperature disturbance are more likely to be sensory pathway disorders, and lesions of the ventral and lateral spinothalamic tracts may be present. Pain perception is lost on the side contralateral to the lesion. Pain is tested by the ability to perceive a pinprick or deep pressure. Increased pain, or tenderness, is called *hyperalgesia*. A diminished sense of pain is *hypoalgesia*, and a complete lack of pain sensibility is *analgesia*.

Temperature disturbances are tested by the ability to distinguish between warm and cold. For this test, the neurologist usually asks the patient to identify a test tube of warm water and one of cold water.

Dorsal Column Lesions

Dorsal column lesions produce disorders of proprioception, as well as astereognosis and related impairments. The following defects may be present with dorsal column lesions.

Inability to Recognize Limb Position

The patient cannot say, without looking, whether a joint is in flexion or extension, nor can the direction of displacement of limbs or digits—fingers and toes—be identified during movement.

Astereognosis

Astereognosis is the inability to recognize common objects, such as coins, keys, and small blocks, by touch. If this disorder is caused by a cortical sensory lesion rather than a dorsal column proprioceptive lesion, it is called *tactile agnosia*.

Two-Point Discrimination Disorder

Differentiating two tactile points from a single one is called two-point discrimination. Deficits are associated with a dorsal column lesion.

Vibratory Sensibility Disorder

The sensation evoked when a vibrating tuning fork is applied to the base of a bony prominence is lost with dorsal column problems. The patient cannot differentiate a vibrating tuning fork from a silent one on bony surfaces.

Body Sway Test

This test, called the *Romberg test*, requires the patient to stand with the feet together. The neurologist notes the amount of sway with the patient's eyes open and compares it with the amount of sway with the eyes closed. An abnormal accentuation of swaying with the eyes closed or actual loss of balance is called a *positive Romberg sign*. The visual sense can compensate for this loss of proprioception of muscle and joint position, if it is caused by a dorsal column disorder, so the patient may correct balance problems by opening his or her eyes. If the lesion is in the cerebellum rather than the dorsal columns, the *cerebellar ataxia* of balance will not be corrected by visual compensation as is the case in the *sensory ataxia* of the dorsal column.

Anatomy of Oral Sensation

The neuroanatomy of oral sensation is different from that of the trunk and extremities in that the cranial and oral sensations are mediated by the cranial nerves, as opposed to mediation by the spinal nerve and cord in bodily sensations. The sensory innervation of the speech mechanism is summarized in Table 5–1. Of particular importance to oral sensation is the trigeminal nerve (cranial nerve V). This cranial nerve is the primary somatic sensory nerve for the skin of the face, the anterior portion of the scalp, the anterior two thirds of the tongue, the teeth, and the outer surface of the eardrum. It mediates the sensations of pain, temperature, touch, pressure, and proprioception for the oral and cranial regions.

The glossopharyngeal nerve (cranial nerve IX), which is primarily sensory, also plays a role in mediating general somatic sensation in the cranial and oral regions. It mediates sensation from the posterior third of the tongue, the palatopharyngeal muscles, and the external ear.

Sensory Pathway of Cranial Nerve V

In studying the spinal pathways for sensation, it has been found that it is logical to separate the pathways for pain and temperature and the pathways for touch and pressure. This general model of the pathways for sensation is similar, with minor variations, for both the oral-cranial regions and the body and extremities. Pain and temperature receptors in the skin and mucous membranes in the face and muscles project to the neural cell bodies of the *Gasserian ganglion*. This ganglion in the face is analogous to the dorsal root ganglion of the spinal nerves. The Gasserian ganglia are called first-order neurons. Axons from the ganglion enter the pons and become a fiber bundle called the *descending tract of cranial nerve V*. The descending tract may sometimes reach the upper cervical region of the spinal cord. Fibers enter the adjacent spinal nucleus of cranial nerve V and synapse with second-order neurons. These cross over to the

Table 5–1   Sensory Innervation of the Speech Mechanism

Structure	*Cranial Nerve(s)*
Face	V: pain, temperature, touch to face
	VII: proprioception to face
Tongue	V: touch to anterior two thirds
	IX: touch to posterior third
Palate	IX: sensory to soft palate
Pharynx	IX: sensory to lateral and posterior pharyngeal walls
	X: sensory to lower two thirds of pharynx (forms pharyngeal plexus with cranial nerve IX)
Larynx	X: sensory to most of the laryngeal muscles

contralateral side on leaving the nucleus. Those contralateral fibers, called the *secondary trigeminothalamic tract*, then ascend to the level of the thalamus. From the thalamus, third-order neurons pass into the internal capsule and finally terminate in the primary somatosensory cortex in the postcentral gyrus of the parietal lobe.

The pressure and touch pathways of cranial nerve V have the same general organizational plan as the pain and temperature pathways. The first-order neurons are the cell bodies of the Gasserian ganglion. The axons of the cell bodies terminate in the main sensory nucleus of cranial nerve V. The second-order neurons reach the thalamus via the secondary ascending tract of cranial nerve V. Fibers travel both ipsilaterally and contralaterally, unlike the pain and temperature pathways of V. The third-order neurons are the relay fibers from the thalamus to the postcentral gyrus of the cerebrum.

The contralateral pathway organization of pain and temperature and the bilateral organization of pressure and touch can be observed clinically if a unilateral sensory cortex lesion is present. The patient suffers no major loss of touch or pressure from the face but loses pain and temperature sensations on the side of the face contralateral to the lesion.

Proprioceptive pathways of V are made up primarily of fibers from the muscles of mastication and the temporomandibular joint. The first-order neurons, the cell bodies of the mesencephalic nucleus, are located in the midbrain. The pathway from this point to the postcentral gyrus of the parietal lobe is not known.

The jaw reflex is mediated by the sensory input from the muscles of mastication and temporomandibular joint acting on the motor neuron of nerve VII, or the facial nerve. A hyperactive jaw reflex suggests a lesion in the corticobulbar fibers above the level of the pons.

Sensory Pathway of Cranial Nerve IX

The glossopharyngeal nerve has its first-order neuron in the ganglion of cranial nerve IX. Fibers pass to the nucleus solitarius from the ganglion. The route of the second-order neuron, the ascending central pathway to the thalamus, is not precisely known, but probably involves the reticular formation, with termination in the thalamus. The path of the third-order neuron to the cortex is likewise unknown.

In summary, the sensory pathway plan in the orofacial region and the body involves a sensory ganglion close to the primary sensory receptors. This is a first-order neuron. A second-order neuron is the pathway to the thalamus, and a third-order neuron projects from the thalamus to the sensory cortex.

Oral Sensory Receptors

Generally, sensory receptors in the oral region and respiratory system are excited by chemical or mechanical stimulation. Taste, of course, is based on chemical stimulation. Mechanicoreceptors respond when stimuli distort them. For instance, the tongue touching the teeth, alveolar ridge, or palate will compress mechanicoreceptors, and the receptors in turn will generate electrical impulses to the fibers.

The tongue mucosa and the tongue surface in particular are served by many different types of mechanicoreceptors. The endings in these receptors have been divided into diffuse, or free, endings and compact, or organized, endings. Some speech experts believe that free endings provide a general sense of touch in sensory control of speech articulation and that organized endings provide sensitive acuity in speech articulation.

Oral Proprioceptors

In addition to receptors in the mucosa of the oral region, there are receptors in the oral muscles themselves, in the joints of the jaw, and in the membranes of the teeth. The receptors in the temporomandibular muscles, the pterygoids, the masseter, and the temporalis, place stretch on the joint.

The periodontal receptors are fine filaments in the teeth that are responsive to extremely slight touch on the teeth. The pressure sense of these receptors is extremely sensitive and no doubt plays a role in sensory control of articulation.

Studying Oral Sensation

The role of the tactile receptors in the oral region has been widely studied in the speech science laboratory over the past two decades. Two-point discrimination for tactile sensation is assessed by speech scientists with an instrument called an *esthesiometer*. Subjects are asked to discriminate if they feel one or two points on the surface of the tongue. Normals can separate two points on the tongue tip when the points are only 1 to 2 millimeters apart. The sensitivity of the tongue tip is extremely delicate, but the back of the tongue and the lateral margins are less sensitive. Differences of less than 1 centimeter cannot be clearly distinguished at these points.

To determine the significance of tactile sensation in the sensory control of speech, the technique of *nerve block* has been used. An anesthetic, usually lidocaine, is injected into the branches of the trigeminal nerve. Tactile sensation of the tongue is mediated by the lingual branch of V (Figure 5–3). Nerve block techniques have resulted in some distortion of the articulation of speech, but for the most part speech remains intelligible. The consonants /s/ and /z/ are frequently distorted with tongue anesthetization.

Sensory Control Modalities

The sensory recognition abilities of the tongue raise the question of the relative significances of the various sensory control mechanisms in speech production. Intuitively, audition would appear to be the most powerful sensory mechanism controlling speech. If we misspeak, as in uttering a "slip of the tongue," we often hear our error and correct it. Additionally, congenitally deaf individuals, who do not hear their speech, show deviations in articulation and voice. Under certain conditions, as those cited, hearing our own speech provides a strong sensory control. But individuals who have developed normal speech and then lose their hearing do not immediately show articulation and vocal deviations. Persons with acquired deafness rely on sensory mechanisms other than audition to control most of their speech performance. For many speech sounds, the average auditory processes that provide feedback occur too late to be of help in ongoing speech. Where the tactile sensory receptors of the tongue have been interfered with by nerve block of the trigeminal nerve, it has been found that the addition of auditory masking does not increase the articulation error scores significantly. In brief, it seems that although audition, touch, and oral discrimination play roles in speech motor control, their exact significance is unclear.

Orosensory testing has not been widely used by neurologists or speech-language pathologists. More refined methodology is needed. Issues surrounding these aspects of speech physiology and their disorders are still relegated to laboratory studies.

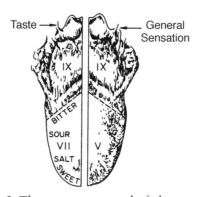

Figure 5–3 The sensory control of the tongue.

Speech Proprioception

According to Sherrington's classification (1926), proprioception refers to sensory receptors within the body itself. Most critical for speech are the *muscle spindles*, which are encapsulated structures within striated muscle, including muscles of the speech mechanism. The muscle spindle serves as the primary afferent proprioceptor within striated muscle. The distribution of muscle spindles varies considerably within the speech musculature. Muscle spindles are found in all intercostal muscles and all laryngeal muscles. The jaw muscles are also rich in spindles, but the facial muscles, including the lips, have very few. The tongue, the primary articulator for speech, assumes an intermediate position between the jaw and the face in a number of muscle spindles. A small number of spindle afferents have been found in the intrinsic tongue muscles. These afferents do not project to the lower motor neurons of the tongue muscle.

As a result of this distribution of spindles in the oral musculature, a stretch reflex can usually be elicited from the jaw but not from the facial muscles. In addition, the neural pathways for spindle information are not clear in the tongue. It has been suggested that the hypoglossal nerve (cranial nerve XII), generally considered to be a motor nerve, may carry some spindle afferents that enter the brainstem by the way of the dorsal cervical nerves, labeled Cl through C3. Other researchers have postulated that proprioceptive impulses from the tongue are conducted by the lingual nerve, a branch of the trigeminal nerve. At this point we do not have a clear picture of the proprioceptive pathways from the tongue.

In summary, it is apparent that the oromotor mechanism is richly endowed with exteroceptors and proprioceptors for control of the neuromuscular activity of speech but that no single type of sensory input is superior to another in the control of speech muscles. Different types of articulation probably demand different types of sensory feedback. Alveolar stops, for instance, may utilize primarily tactile sensation, while articulations with no contact, such as back vowels, may utilize auditory and proprioceptive feedback.

The Visual System

The Retina

The visual system processes and decodes a wealth of information, more than any other afferent system in the body. To begin this processing, the eye absorbs the light from an image and passes it through the pupil. The image is then inverted and reversed as it passes into the lens. The lens focuses and projects the light onto the retina, which is a light-sensitive 10-layer formation of nerve cells lining the inside of the eyeball. The retina is composed of two types of photoreceptors (*rods* and *cones*) and four types of neurons (*bipolar cells, ganglion cells, horizontal cells*, and *amacrine cells*). Rods play a special role in peripheral vision and in vision under low light. Cones, on the other hand, function under bright light and are responsible for discriminative vision and color detection. The rods and cones are first-order neurons and synapse with *bipolar cells*. These cells in turn synapse with the *ganglion cells*, which are third-order neurons. The axons of these cells converge to leave the eye within the *optic nerve*. After leaving the eye the axons acquire myelin sheaths.

This series of transmissions from first- to third-order sensory neurons is modified by horizontal cells and amacrine cells. They essentially "sharpen" the response of the ganglion cells to certain formations of light.

Path of the Optic Nerve

The point of exit for the optic nerve is called the *optic disk*, which can be seen through an ophthalmoscope. Since there are no rods or cones overlying the optic disk, it is essentially a small blind spot in each eye. The area on the retina for central fixated vision during good light is the *macula*. A small central pit in the macula called the *fovea centralis* is composed of closely packed cones, and vision here is sharpest and color vision most acute.

The optic nerve conveys visual impulses. It consists of about a million nerve fibers, which course through the optic canal of the skull to form the *optic chiasm* (Figure 5–4). The fibers from the retina of each eye originate from two different areas on each retina. The retinal fibers can be thought of as exiting either as *temporal fibers*—that is, as coming from the lateral half of the retina nearest the temple—or as *nasal fibers*, which originate from the lateral half nearest the nose. As Figure 5–4 shows, at the optic chiasm, the nasal fibers from each eye decussate while the temporal fibers continue ipsilaterally. This shift makes stereoscopic three-dimensional vision possible.

As you study Figure 5–4, you will see that the optics of the eye are such that the temporal half of one retina and the nasal half of the other retina receive information from the same half of the visual field. In other words, the temporal fibers of the left retina and the nasal fibers of the right retina carry information from the right half of the visual field, and the temporal fibers of the right retina and the nasal fibers of the left retina receive information from the left side of the visual field. Because of the

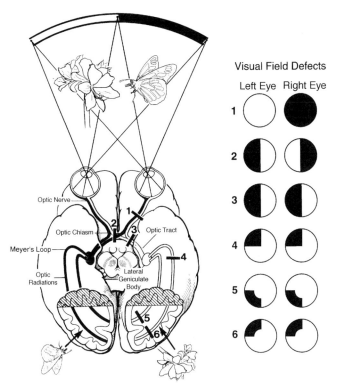

Figure 5–4 Visual pathways with lesion sites and resulting visual field defects. The occipital lobe has been cut away to show the medial aspect and the calcarine sulci.

decussation of the nasal fibers at the optic chiasm, all of the information from the contralateral side of the visual field travels in one pathway down the optic tract to the visual cortex. The visual cortex in the left hemisphere receives information about the contralateral right side of the visual field, while the right hemisphere processes information from the left visual field. This information is critical to understanding how a visual-field deficit occurs after brain injury.

After passing the point of the optic chiasm, most of the axons forming the optic tract course to the *lateral geniculate body*, which is a small swelling located under the pulvinar of the thalamus. They then pass through the internal capsule and around the lateral ventricle, curving posteriorly. Some fibers travel far over the temporal horn of the lateral ventricle and form what is called the *temporal loop* or *Meyer's loop* (Figure 5–4). These fibers terminate in the visual cortex below the calcarine sulcus. Meyer's loop carries fibers representing the upper part of the central visual field. Other optic fibers travel from the lateral geniculate body to the visual cortex above the calcarine sulcus. These fibers represent the lower part of the central visual field.

Some retinal ganglion cells terminate in the superior colliculus of the midbrain. The superior colliculus also receives synapses from the visual cortex. Fibers from the superior colliculus project to the spinal cord through the *tectospinal tracts*. These tracts control reflex movements of the head, neck, and eyes in response to visual stimuli.

Primary Visual Cortex

The characteristics of neurons in the visual cortex and the responses of individual cells have been studied in a wide variety of experimental animals. Scientists are interested in how patterns are perceived and recognized by the eye. It has been found by such experimenters as Hubel and Wiesel (1968) that there are many different types of receptive fields in the neurons of the visual cortex. These receptive fields are termed *simple, complex, hypercomplex,* and *higher order hypercomplex*. Simple receptive field cells respond to a slit of light of particular width, slant, or orientation and place on the retina. Complex receptive fields respond to slit-shaped stimuli over a large area of the retina rather than a specific place. For hypercomplex fields, the line stimulus must be of a certain length. Cells with higher order hypercomplex fields require more elaborate visual stimuli to respond.

The visual cortex is organized in columns of cells with similar properties. Some columns respond only to one eye and are monocular. Others respond to both eyes and are binocular. Since the eyes are located in different positions on the head, there is a difference of position on the retinas for a stimulus, giving binocular disparity to the columnar cells. This provides information about the depth of objects.

In addition to the primary visual pathways, two other major visual pathways can be distinguished: the *tectal*, or collicular, pathway and the *pretectal* nuclei pathway. Thus, fibers from the optic tracts do not all go to the lateral geniculate body. Some of them project to the subcortical pretectal nuclei and ascend to the thalamus and out from there to various regions of the cortex. This system seems to be important in the control of certain visual reflexes, such as the pupillary reflex, and certain eye movements.

The tectal, or collicular, pathway projects to the superior colliculi in the brainstem and to the thalamus and out to many regions of the cortex. The superior colliculi also receive input from somatosensory and auditory systems. The tectal pathway seems to be involved in a major way in our ability to orient toward and follow a visual stimulus.

The visual pathways do not operate independently of each other. They are interconnected at every level from retina to cortex, and each receives descending input from the cerebral cortex, providing for the richness of visual perception.

Visual Association Cortex

The area surrounding the striate cortex, the peristriate cortex (Brodmann's areas 18 and 19), is composed of neurons that have firing properties much like those of the primary visual cortex; however, these neurons also tend to show regional specialization for analyzing more complex aspects of visual stimuli such as motion, color, and form. Anatomists have been able to identify at least five different regions of this peristriate area, each with a different processing role.

The second major part of the visual association cortex is the temporal visual cortex located within the middle and inferior temporal areas. This association area receives input from the peristriate cortex and has four major cortical output pathways: (1) to the contralateral temporal visual areas; (2) to the prefrontal cortical area; (3) to the ipsilateral posterior association cortex of the superior temporal area; and (4) to the paralimbic and limbic areas of the medial temporal lobe. Like other neurons in primary and secondary visual cortex, neurons in the temporal visual association areas are sensitive to such properties of the visual stimulus as wavelength, size, length, and movement. These neurons, however, also seem to trigger in response to specific objects, including faces. Thus, this part of the visual system may extract complex features from visual stimuli so that neurons become responsive to individual patterns rather than to isolated stimulus features. This may provide the mechanism for object discrimination.

Visual Integration

As Mesulam (1985) points out, object recognition or identification requires interaction between the visual representation in the association areas and other components of mental operation, including integration with past experience. This process requires relay of information from these temporal visual association areas to paralimbic and limbic areas of the brain.

Damage to the association areas in the peristriate or temporal lobes or to their connections to other parts of the brain may have a number of different effects on visual processing. Mesulam lists the following consequences as possibilities: (1) impaired specialized visual processing and impaired formation of visual templates; (2) loss of visual templates previously formed; (3) disconnection of visual-auditory, visual-motor, visual-somatosensory, and visual-verbal pathways due to interruption of input from the visual association areas to the frontal and parietal association areas; and (4) interruption of pathways providing input to paralimbic and limbic structures from the visual association area.

Lesions in the peristriate areas have been noted to cause very specific disorders such as difficulty with color vision or movement perception, yet they cause no disturbance to other visual functions. Color and movement thus seem to have subregions in this cortex that are specialized for these functions. Ventrally situated lesions of the temporo-occipital cortex may cause disorders such as alexia and visual agnosias. These disorders are discussed further in Chapter 9.

Central Auditory Nervous System

A major aspect of speech and language function is dependent on audition. Audition is classified generally as one of the special senses and as an exteroceptive sense. The neurology of the central auditory pathways is crucial to an understanding of the mechanism of the communicative nervous system.

Receptor Level

The hair cells in the organ of Corti in the cochlea of the inner ear serve as the primary neural receptors for audition. The cell bodies of the primary neuron of the central auditory pathway are in the *spiral ganglion*. A distinction usually is made between the peripheral auditory system and the central auditory system. For the neurologist, the peripheral system includes the outer ear and cranial nerve VIII, and the central auditory system extends from the cochlear nucleus to the auditory cortex in the cerebrum. The otolaryngologist, on the other hand, considers the peripheral system as extending from the outer ear to the hair cells of the cochlea. The central system is from the auditory nerve to the cerebral cortex.

Cranial Nerve Level

The nerve of hearing, cranial nerve VIII, has two divisions: the *cochlear branch*, associated with hearing, and the *vestibular branch*, associated with balance. The cochlear nerve proceeds from the spiral ganglion through the internal auditory canal. It is accompanied by cranial nerve VII, the facial nerve, in the auditory canal. The two nerves enter the brainstem at the sulcus between the pons and the medulla.

Brainstem Level

The fibers of the cochlear division of cranial nerve VIII end in the dorsal and ventral cochlear nuclei, which are draped around the inferior cerebellar peduncle. The cochlear nuclei contain the secondary neurons of the auditory pathway. From the cochlear nuclei, most fibers of the auditory pathway proceed to the upper medulla and pons and cross the midline. Other fibers ascend in the brainstem ipsilaterally. Fibers course upward in the ascending central auditory pathway of the brainstem called the *lateral lemniscus*. The fibers take one of several routes, and synapses in the auditory system may occur at one or more of the following structures: the superior olives, the trapezoid body, the inferior colliculus, and the nucleus of the lateral lemniscus. All ascending auditory fibers terminate in the medial geniculate body, a thalamic nucleus.

Auditory Radiations and Cortex

The fibers arising from the medial geniculate body, coursing to the temporal cortex, are called *auditory radiations*. They pass through the internal capsule in their route to the bilateral primary auditory areas of the brain in the superior and transverse temporal gyri. These areas are numbered 41 and 42 and are known as *Heschl's gyrus*.

The nuclei of the auditory pathway—the trapezoid body, the superior olivary complex, the nucleus of the lateral lemniscus, and the inferior colliculi—serve as relay nuclei as well as reflex centers. The reflex centers make connections with the eyes, head, and trunk, where automatic reflex actions occur in response to sound.

Descending efferent fibers, in addition to the ascending afferent fibers, are present in all parts of the central auditory pathway. They probably serve as feedback loops within the pathways. Figure 5-5 shows a very simplified schema of connections along the auditory pathway.

Auditory Physiology

Sound is transmitted to the central auditory pathways by a traveling wave that is set up on the basilar membrane of the cochlea. The basilar membrane is narrower at the base of the cochlea than at its apex. The mechanics of the membrane on which the organ of Corti is located vary slightly from base to apex. The traveling pressure wave of a specific frequency causes the basilar membrane to vibrate maximally at a specific point along the length of the membrane. The vibration produces shearing forces in the hair cells that set up electrical charges in the dendrites of the spiral ganglion, in turn causing the nerve cells to fire.

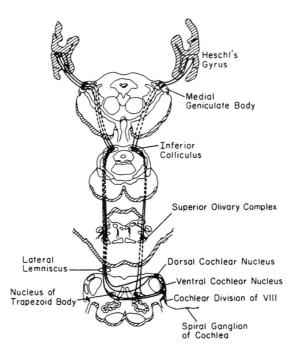

Figure 5–5 The central auditory pathways and the major auditory way stations. Source: Redrawn and reproduced with permission from S. Gilman and S. Winans, *Manter and Gatz's Essentials Of Clinical Neuroanatomy and Neurophysiology* (6th ed.) (Philadelphia: F. A. Davis, 1982).

Auditory nerve impulses ascend in the pathways of the central auditory nervous system. The organ of Corti serves as an analyzer of sound frequencies. It is *tonotopically* organized, meaning that the highest frequencies stimulate hair cells in the most basilar portion of the cochlea, where the basilar membrane is narrowest. The lowest frequencies stimulate the portions of the membrane at the apex. Frequency discrimination, therefore, is dependent on the frequency of the tone and the spatial response of the basilar membrane. Intensity discrimination depends on the length of the basilar membrane set in motion and the amplitude of the vibration. Displacement of a longer area of the membrane will activate more nerve fibers, and a greater amplitude of vibration will increase the frequency of the neural discharge.

Localizing the source of a sound depends on a comparison between the arrival time and the intensity of the sound at the two ears. Localization of sound occurs at higher levels in the auditory pathways. Central auditory structures, generally above the level of the inferior colliculus are capable of making appropriate comparisons for sound localization. Thus, in mammals and humans the temporal auditory cortex is not needed for simple sound recognition, but it is essential for sound localization and recognizing changes in the temporal sequencing of sounds. Temporal sequencing is a very crucial higher auditory function since it is a significant aspect of speech. Sound localization probably requires the inferior colliculus and auditory cortex, whereas temporal sequencing may require the cochlear nuclei, the medial geniculate nuclei, and the auditory cortex. There is a tonotopic organization in all of the central auditory nuclei, but the nuclei are used for analysis of several auditory properties of sound other than the recognition of tones or different frequencies.

Lesions of the Auditory System

Unilateral lesions of the central auditory system that completely destroy the receptors, auditory nerve, or cochlear nuclei will generally cause total deafness in that ear. However, unilateral lesions of the auditory cortex, medial geniculate body, or lateral lemniscus will produce impaired hearing, poorer in the contralateral ear, but will not result in total deafness because of the bilateral pathways and the abundance of fibers that cross over in the auditory system. Lesions in Heschl's gyrus bilaterally may cause either cortical deafness, nonverbal agnosia, or auditory agnosia. Unilateral cortical damage does not cause total deafness.

Summary

Three major pathways carry sensory impulses from the extremities and trunk to higher levels of the nervous system. One of these is the spinothalamic tract, which has two divisions. The lateral spinothalamic tract conveys impulses of pain and temperature. The anterior spinothalamic tract conveys impulses of light touch, light pressure, and tactile discrimination.

The second major pathway is known as the dorsal columns. The two tracts of the dorsal columns are the fasciculus gracilis and the fasciculus cuneatus. The fasciculus cuneatus is associated with sensation from the upper extremities and body, and the fasciculus gracilis is associated with the lower extremities and body. Both pathways convey proprioceptive sensations of movement and posture, vibration, stereognosis, and two-point discrimination. Lesions may produce specific sensory losses as well as a sensory ataxia of the dorsal columns.

The third major pathway includes the spinocerebellar tracts. The dorsal pathway ascends contralaterally. Both pathways end in the cerebellum and are thought to mediate conscious proprioception of movement. Cerebral lesions, marked by language loss, may have accompanying sensory loss involving the parietal lobe or subcortical pathway.

The oral cavity is very rich in sensory receptors. Tactile receptors of the mouth, tongue, pharynx, and teeth play a significant role in the articulation of speech. Tactile sensory receptors have been widely studied in the speech laboratory, but no standard clinical method for assessing the sensory integrity of the oral mechanism is widely accepted. Anesthetization of the tongue surface only distorts vowels and sibilants to a moderate degree.

Muscle spindles provide sensory control of muscle contraction through the gamma motor neuron system, jaw muscles, and laryngeal muscles. The tongue has fewer muscle spindles than these muscles do, and the facial and lip muscles have even fewer spindles than the tongue. Muscle spindles do not appear to exert a major influence on the highly precise and rapid control of the speech muscles.

Cranial nerve V supplies information to the lips, palate, and anterior two thirds of the tongue. Cranial nerve IX, the glossopharyngeal nerve, supplies sensation to the posterior third of the tongue.

The central auditory nervous system is complex. The primary auditory receptor is the spiral ganglion in the organ of Corti of the cochlea in the inner ear. The auditory nerve, cranial nerve VIII, enters the brainstem at the pontomedullary junction. Fibers go to the dorsal and ventral cochlear nuclei. From these nuclei, fibers proceed through complex contralateral and a few ipsilateral pathways to the medial geniculate bodies at the level of the thalamus. Auditory radiations ascend from the thalamus to Heschl's gyrus in each of the temporal lobes of the cerebrum. Bilateral cortical damage to Heschl's gyrus produces a spectrum of deficits including cortical deafness, nonverbal agnosia, and auditory agnosia. Unilateral cortical damage to Heschl's gyrus does not produce total deafness.

References and Further Readings

Barr, M. L., & Kiernan, J. A. (1993). *The human nervous system: An anatomical viewpoint.* Philadelphia: J. B. Lippincott.

Bess, F. H., & Humes, L. E. (1995). *Audiology: The fundamentals.* (2nd ed.). Baltimore: Williams & Wilkins.

Bordon, G. J., & Harris, K. S. (1984). *Speech science primer* (2nd ed.). Baltimore: Williams & Wilkins.

DeMyer, W. (1980). *Technique of the neurologic examination* (3rd ed.). New York: McGraw-Hill.

Gilman, S., & Winans, S. S. (1982). *Manter and Gatz's essentials of clinical neuroanatomy and neurophysiology* (6th ed.). Philadelphia: F. A. Davis.

Gregory, R. L. (1970). *The intelligent eye.* New York: McGraw-Hill.

Groves, P. M., Schlesinger, K. (1979). *Introduction to biological psychology.* Dubuque, IA: William C. Brown.

Hubel, D. H., & Wiesel, T. N. (1968). Receptive fields and functional architecture of the monkey striate cortex. *Journal of Physiology, 206,* 419–436.

Mesulam, M. M. (1985). *Principles of behavioral neurology.* Philadelphia: F. A. Davis.

Mountcastle, V. B. (1980). Central neural mechanisms in hearing. In V. B. Mountcastle (Ed.), *Medical physiology.* St. Louis: C. V. Mosby.

Sherrington, S. C. (1926). *The integrative action of the nervous system.* New Haven: Yale University Press.

Zeki, S. (1993). *A vision of the brain.* Boston: Blackwell Scientific Publications.

6

□ □ □
□ □ □
□ □ □

The Neuromotor
Control of Speech

*"We cannot state exactly the number of muscles that are
necessary for speech and that are active during speech.
But if we consider that ordinarily the muscles of the thoracic
and abdominal walls, the neck and the face, the larynx, and
pharynx and the oral cavity are all properly coordinated during
the act of speaking, it becomes obvious that over 100 muscles
must be controlled centrally."*

—Eric H. Lenneberg, *Biological Foundations of Language*, 1967

Speech is one of the most complex behaviors performed by
human beings. On average, a person will utter approximately 14 recogniz-
able speech sounds per second when asked to produce nonsense syllables
as rapidly as possible. This unusually brisk rate is maintained even when
one speaks conversationally or reads aloud. The number of separate neural
events supporting this complex coordination of the articulatory muscles
is, of course, very large, and the degree of neural integration in the motor
system for routine, everyday talk is truly amazing.

Speech requires the action of major mechanisms at every significant
motor integration level of the nervous system. Five major levels may be
identified: (1) cerebral cortex, (2) subcortical nuclei of the cerebrum, (3)
brainstem, (4) cerebellum, and (5) spinal cord. At each of these five levels of
the nervous system, there are components of the motor system that integrate
speech. For clinical purposes, the motor integration system of the brain for
speech may be divided into three great motor subsystems: (1) the pyramidal
system, (2) the extrapyramidal system, and (3) the cerebellar system.

The Pyramidal System

Voluntary movement of the muscles of speech is controlled
primarily by the pyramidal system. In fact, the pyramidal tract, itself, is
the major voluntary pathway for all movement. It is made up of the

corticospinal tract, the corticobulbar tract, and the corticopontine tract. The corticospinal tract controls the skilled movements in the distal muscles of the limbs and digits. The corticobulbar tract controls the cranial nerves, many of which directly innervate the muscles of speech. The corticopontine tract goes to the pontine nuclei, which in turn project to the cerebellum. The corticospinal, corticobulbar, and corticopontine tracts are called *corticofugal pathways* because they all descend from the cortex.

The Corticospinal Tract

The corticospinal tract descends from the cerebral cortex to different levels of the spinal cord. It begins in the motor cortex of the two cerebral hemispheres, primarily in the precentral gyrus of the cerebrum and to a lesser degree in the postcentral gyrus. The bilateral corticospinal fibers, therefore, begin in the frontal and parietal lobes of the brain. The fibers are considered the primary descending motor tracts because they course downward from the cortex to the spinal cord, where they synapse with the spinal nerves of the peripheral nervous system at various levels of the cord. The spinal nerves leave the neuraxis and innervate muscles of the trunk and limbs.

The fibers of the corticospinal tract are some of the longest motor axons in the nervous system. They provide a direct route for motor commands transmitted from the cortical motor areas and permit extremely rapid voluntary motor response in the nervous system (Figure 6–1).

Though we discuss at length the motor activation pathways of the pyramidal tract, it should not be overlooked that these are not purely motor pathways. Fibers are sent out at various points along the pathways to synapse on interneurons, influencing reflex arcs and nuclei in ascending sensory pathways. The most important example of this to the speech-language pathologist is the synapsing on the nucleus solitarius and on the trigeminal sensory nucleus. These interactions are important in the sensorimotor control of oral pharyngeal functions for speech and swallowing.

Descending Motor Pathways

The corticospinal tract descends from the bilateral motor cortices to the subcortical white matter in a fan-shaped distribution of fibers called the *corona radiata*, or radiating crown. The fibers converge to enter into an *L*-shaped subcortical structure called the *internal capsule*. Since all of the corticospinal fibers come together at this point, a small lesion in the internal capsule of one side can be devastating to the motor control of one half of the body.

The corticospinal fibers pass through the posterior limb of the internal capsule, and the corticobulbar fibers transverse the *genu*, or "bend," of the internal capsule. From that point both sets of fibers enter the cerebral peduncle of the mesencephalon, or midbrain. The fibers enter the pons and are intermingled with pontine fibers and nuclei, providing circuits from the motor cortex that reverberate through the cerebellum and return impulses to the cerebral cortex after cerebellar modulation. After the fibers cross the *basis pontis*, they reach the medulla, which is situated at the

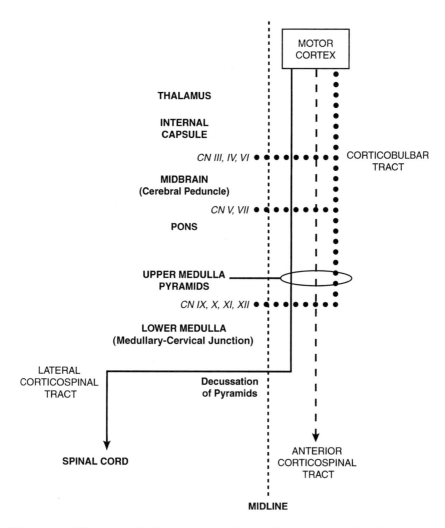

Figure 6–1 The pyramidal tract, including both corticospinal and corticobulbar fibers (CN, cranial nerve).

junction of this lower brainstem structure and the spinal cord. This is the medullary-cervical juncture. Here approximately 85 to 90 percent of the corticospinal fibers cross over to the other side of the neuraxis, providing contralateral motor control of the limbs. The corticospinal fibers into the medulla come together to form the *pyramids*, for which the pyramidal tract is named.

Decussation

The crossing of the right and left corticospinal tract is known as *decussation*. The few fibers, variable in number, that do not cross are known as the uncrossed *anterior corticospinal tract*. The primary corticospinal tract is the *lateral corticospinal tract*. The decussation means that a lesion interrupting the fibers above the crossing will have an effect on the side of the body opposite the site of the lesion. If the corticospinal tract is interrupted in the cerebrum, voluntary movement of the limbs is limited on the contralateral side of the body. By contrast, a lesion below the decussation impairs voluntary movement on the same, or ipsilateral, side.

Paralysis, Paresis, and Plegia

A gross limitation of movement is called *paralysis*, and an incomplete paralysis is known as *paresis*. A complete or near-complete paralysis of one side of the body is *hemiparalysis* or, more commonly a *hemiplegia*. The presence of a right-sided hemiplegia or *hemiparesis* is an extremely important sign for the speech-language pathologist. If the lesion is in the cerebrum, above the decussation, it suggests that the left hemisphere is involved. As noted earlier, the left hemisphere is the primary site of brain mechanisms for language, so right hemiplegia is often associated with language disorders. Lesions of the bilateral motor strip or the pyramidal tract alone may produce the motor speech disorder of dysarthria.

The Corticobulbar Tracts

The corticobulbar fibers of the pyramidal tract are the voluntary pathway for the movements of speech muscles, except those of respiration. They are the most important fibers of the pyramidal tract for the speech-language pathologist. Their course is not as direct as that of the corticospinal fibers. The corticobulbar fibers begin with the corticospinal fibers at the cortex and terminate at the motor nuclei of the cranial nerves.[1] Unlike the corticospinal fibers, the corticobulbars have many ipsilateral as well as contralateral fibers. The corticospinal and corticobulbar fibers separate at the upper brainstem level, with the corticobulbars decussating at various levels of the brainstem.

Bilateral Symmetry

The majority of the midline speech muscles work in bilateral symmetry. This is the result of the bilateral innervation that the corticobulbars provide. All of the paired muscles of the face, palate, vocal folds, and diaphragm work together in synchrony much of the time in wrinkling the forehead, smiling, chewing, swallowing, and talking. This bilateral innervation of the speech muscles has important implications for the degree of speech muscle involvement in cases of dysarthria.

In corticobulbar lesions, the bilateral innervation provides a safety valve for speech production. Assuming the left corticobulbar fibers to a cranial nerve are damaged, the motor nuclei of that nerve will still receive impulses via the intact right corticobulbar tract, and paralysis of the muscle will not be severe. However, the innervation of the limbs is primarily contralateral rather than bilateral, so lesions to the corticospinal fibers may produce severe unilateral limb paralysis. Lesions to corticobulbar fibers do not produce as severe weakness because of the bilateral innervation.

Contralateral and Unilateral Innervation

Each of the cranial nerve nuclei receives varying amounts of unilateral and contralateral innervation, even though the nuclei are bilaterally supplied. Those areas with a more unilateral supply will be more paralyzed after a unilateral lesion. The lower face and trapezius muscles are most affected. An intermediate paralytic effect is found in the tongue with a unilateral lesion. The diaphragm, ocular muscles, upper face, jaw, pharynx, and muscles of the larynx show little paralysis with a unilateral lesion.

---

[1]The corticobulbar fibers derive their name from their direction. At the longest point they extend from cortex to medulla. In older terminology the medulla was called the *bulb* because it appeared as a bulbous extension of the spinal cord. *Corticomedullar* would be a more consistent modern term, but *corticobulbar* is the term in common usage.

The nuclei for the facial nerve are complex. The facial nucleus combines bilateral innervation with contralateral innervation. The muscles of the upper half of the face are far more bilaterally innervated than the muscles of the lower half of the face, which receive more contralateral innervation. Some neuroscientists even hypothesize a cranial nerve nucleus for the upper half of the facial muscles and one for the lower half. In practical terms, this means that among the healthy population, most people can wrinkle their forehead or lift both eyebrows together. Only a few people, with more contralateral fibers, are able to lift their eyebrows one at a time. The muscles of the midface receive a more equal combination of bilateral and contralateral innervation. Most, but not all, people can wink one eye at a time because of the increase of contralateral fibers to eyelid muscles compared with forehead muscles.

In the lower face the innervation is primarily contralateral. Most people are able to retract one corner of the mouth alone when asked to do so because of the limited bilateral innervation of the lower face muscles. The principles of bilateral and contralateral innervation are practically applied when a speech cranial nerve examination is performed to determine if there are lesions affecting the corticobulbar fibers, bulbar nuclei, or the cranial nerves themselves. These principles are summarized for the cranial nerves in Table 6-1.

The concepts of bilateral symmetry and contralateral independence are of crucial practical clinical utility when analyzing and understanding muscle involvement in dysarthria. We will return to them when discussing the testing of the cranial nerves involved in speech in Chapter 7.

Table 6-1 Corticobulbar Innervation in the Cranial Nerves for Speech

Nerve	*Innervation*
Trigeminal (V)	Bilateral symmetry
Facial (VII)	Mixed bilateral symmetry and contralateral innervation
Glossopharyngeal (IX)*	Neither bilateral symmetry nor contralateral innervation
Vagus (X)	Bilateral symmetry
Spinal accessory (XI)	Contralateral innervation
Hypoglossal (XII)	Mixed bilateral symmetry and contralateral innervation

*The motor innervation of IX is only to a single muscle.

Lower and Upper Motor Neurons

A very useful concept in clinical neurology has been the notion of upper motor neurons and lower motor neurons. All of the neurons of the anterior and lateral corticospinal tracts, which send axons from the cerebral cortex to the anterior horn cells of the spinal cord, are considered upper motor neurons. The neurons of the corticobulbar tracts that send axons from the cerebral cortex to the nuclei in the brainstem are upper motor neurons as well. These long axons, part of one uninterrupted neuron, are also considered to be first-order neurons. No upper motor neurons leave the neuraxis. In other words, they are contained within the brain, brainstem, and spinal cord. The pyramidal tract with its upper motor neuron activation can be thought of as the *direct activation pathway*, or direct motor system, because of its direct connection and major activating influence on the lower motor neurons (Duffy, 1995).

Lower motor neurons are all the neurons that send motor axons into the peripheral nerves—the cranial and spinal nerves. They are designated second-order neurons. Charles Sherrington (1926) called the lower motor neuron the "final common pathway." By this he meant that the peripheral nerves—both cranial and spinal—serve as a final route for all the complex motor interactions that occur in the neuraxis above the level of the lower motor neuron. The final muscle contraction is the product of all the interactions that have occurred in the central nervous system.

Lesions of the upper and lower motor neurons produce wholly different sets of signs and symptoms. This distinction provides the neurologist with a powerful tool in neurologic examination for deciding where a lesion is located in the nervous system. The most striking sign of a lesion in both upper and lower motor neurons is paralysis. The type of paralysis, however, is quite different depending on the site of the lesion that produces the paralysis. Understanding the differences is a large step toward establishing a correct diagnosis of a neurologic disease involving motor disturbance.

Lower Motor Neuron Paralysis

If a lesion is in a cranial or peripheral nerve, or in the cell bodies of the anterior horn cell in the spinal cord, or in the cranial nerve axons in the brainstem before they leave the brainstem, neural impulses will not be transmitted to the muscles. This is called *denervation*. The result is that the muscles innervated by the cranial or spinal nerve become soft and flabby because of loss of muscle tone. This is a lower motor neuron paralysis.

The loss of muscle tone is called *hypotonia*. Hypotonia results in flaccid muscles. Thus, lower motor neuron paralysis is called *flaccid paralysis*. Lower motor neuron paralysis is also sometimes associated with loss of muscle bulk, a condition called *atrophy*. Muscles undergoing atrophy display some degree of degeneration because they become denervated. Signs of this degeneration can be observed clinically. Atrophic muscles will show *fibrillations* and *fasciculations*. These signs are caused by electrical disturbances in muscle fibers resulting from denervation. Fibrillations are fine twitches of single muscle fibers. Generally these can not be seen on clinical examination, except perhaps in the tongue, but must be detected by electromyographic examination. Fasciculations, on the other hand, are contractions of groups of muscle fibers that can be identified, with training, in skeletal muscles through the skin.

As muscle bulk is lost through atrophy in motor neuron disease, fasciculations may be seen in the muscles of the head and neck, as well as in other muscles of the body. These muscle twitches may be particularly observed in the relatively large muscle mass of the tongue if the bulbar muscles are involved.[2] Fasciculations have no direct effect on speech itself but serve only as a sign of lower motor neuron disease.

Interruption of a peripheral nerve by a lower motor neuron lesion also damages the reflex arc that is involved with that nerve. The result is that normal reflex responses mediated through the sensory and motor limbs of the arc become diminished. Reduced reflex response is called *hyporeflexia*. Complete lack of reflex is known as *areflexia*. Hyporeflexia and areflexia, however, are also associated with lower motor neuron disease.

A concept that will help you more fully understand the complexities of lower motor neuron disease is that of the *motor unit* (Figure 6–2). A motor unit is a structural and functional entity that may be defined as (1) a single anterior horn cell or cranial nerve neuron, (2) its peripheral axon and its branches, (3) each muscle fiber innervated by these branches, and (4) the myoneural juncture. Lesions may occur at many points within the motor unit and produce lower motor neuron signs. Figure 6-2 portrays a motor unit at the spinal cord level. The most obvious example of disorder is a lesion or cut in the spinal nerve (point 2). This damage will paralyze the muscle innervated by the nerve. In addition, the denervated muscle

---

[2]The term *bulbar muscles* refers to the muscles whose cranial motor nuclei are found in the medulla oblongata. These are cranial nerves IX (glossopharyngeal), X (vagus), XI (spinal accessory), and XII (hypoglossal).

Cell of Lower Motor Neuron

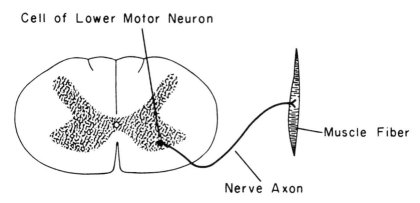

Muscle Fiber

Nerve Axon

Figure 6–2a The motor unit consists of the cell body of the lower motor neuron, the nerve axon, and the muscle fiber. Lesions at any point in the motor unit will produce signs of a lower motor neuron syndrome.

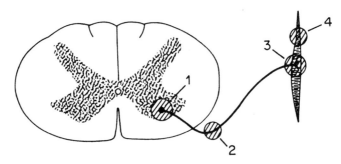

Figure 6–2b Lesion sites in the motor unit (and respective types of lower motor neuron disorders) include (1) cell body (motor neuron disease); (2) lower motor neuron denervation (motor neuropathy); (3) myoneural juncture (neuromyopathy); and (4) muscle fiber (myopathy or dystrophy).

will become hypotonic, areflexic, and atrophic. Finally, fasciculations will appear. If a cranial nerve is denervated, weakness of speech muscles results from hypotonia and loss of muscle bulk.

A lesion may also occur in the anterior horn cell in the spinal cord itself and produce paralysis and related lower motor neuron signs (point 1 on Figure 6–2). An example is acute bulbar poliomyelitis, which attacks the high cervical anterior horns as well as the cranial nerve nuclei of the bulbar muscles controlling speech. Speech muscles again may become weak and atrophic.

Lesions of the lower motor neuron type may also occur directly in muscles. An example of this type of lower motor neuron disorder is seen in *muscular dystrophy* (point 4). Speech muscles lose strength and show disturbances of muscle bulk. This lower motor neuron disease within a muscle is called a *myopathy*, as opposed to disease of the peripheral nerves, which is called a *neuropathy*. Lesions may also occur at the neuromuscular junction, as seen in *myasthenia gravis* (point 3). Speech muscles show fatigue and weakness in this myoneural disorder.

Upper Motor Neuron Paralysis

Types of Paralysis

Damage to the corticospinal tract anywhere along its course will produce a *spastic paralysis*. Spastic muscles display increased tone, or resistance to movement, a condition called *hypertonia*. Spastic hypertonicity can be identified by moving a limb through its full range of motion so that the joint is flexed or bent. The neurological examiner puts an increased stretch on the muscles during the range-of-motion testing. He or she thereby elicits a *muscle stretch reflex*, an increase in tone or tension that resists the flexion of the joint. The examiner can feel this increased resistance to movement. (The muscle stretch reflex controls the degree of contraction in a normal muscle and provides muscles with *tonus* or tone.)

A *clasp knife reaction* occurs in a spastic muscle when the neurologist feels increased tone or resistance to movement in the muscle after the joint has been briskly flexed and then feels the resistance fade. This reaction, which identifies spastic hypertonicity, is analogous to the resistance felt when a knife blade is first opened, followed by the reduction of resistance when the blade is straightened out. Thus we have the term *clasp knife spasticity*. Usually, this occurs more in extension than in flexion of the elbow. There is usually a short span of no tone, then a rapid buildup of tone, then a sudden release as the joint is moved—just as with opening a clasp knife.

Spasticity also is associated with exaggerated muscle stretch reflexes, resulting in *hyperreflexia*. Reflex action is tested at joints by putting stretch on tendons. This elicits the exaggerated muscle stretch reflex. Spastic paralysis, hypertonia, and hyperreflexia have most often been associated with pyramidal tract damage, particularly lesions of the corticospinal tract. However, the corticobulbar tracts are often also involved when a lesion interrupts the corticospinal tract, and signs of spasticity may be found in the midline speech muscles as well as in the distal limb muscles. Therefore, the clinical signs of spasticity, or upper motor neuron lesion, are of equal interest to the speech-language pathologist and the neurologist. Spastic speech muscles may be weak, slow, and limited in range or movement. Hypertonia may decrease muscle flexibility of the articulators and limit the ability to achieve a full range of motion of the speech muscles.

Confirmatory Signs

Several signs, in addition to a clinical demonstration of clasp knife spasticity, hypertonia, and hyperreflexia, are used by the neurologist to help verify the diagnosis of spasticity and localize the lesion to the pyramidal tract.

The *Babinski sign*, or extensor plantar sign, in particular, has been identified as an abnormal reflex sign that develops with corticospinal damage. It is the result of the release of cortical inhibition from a lesion. The sign has achieved considerable status in the diagnosis of upper motor neuron lesions because it is a highly reliable abnormal reflex, is new behavior released by the presence of a lesion, and is clearly associated with a relatively specific lesion site—the cortex or the corticospinal tract. The speech-language pathologist is not directly interested in it because it does not at all involve the midline speech muscles, but its presence as a confirmation of an upper motor neuron lesion of the spastic type is important to all who manage neurologic patients.

The Babinski sign is observed as a reflex toe sign. It is elicited by stimulating the sole of the foot in a strong scratching maneuver. The normal response to stimulation of the sole, or plantar portion of the foot, is a slight withdrawal of the foot and downward turning or curling under of the toes. With a corticospinal lesion, the great toe extends upward and the other toes fan as the foot withdraws slightly. Physicians will test this response several times to convince themselves that the upturning great toe sign can be repeatedly and automatically elicited. Automatic repetition of a given response such as this defines it as a reflex. The presence of a repeatable abnormal reflex sharply increases the probability of predicting with accuracy the possible site or sites of a neurologic lesion.

The Babinski sign is more reliable in adults than in infants and children. Normal infants are highly variable in display of the sign. The explanation usually given for this variability is that the immature nervous system and the damaged nervous system often show similar symptoms and signs. Damage to the nervous system often releases early reflex behavior that has become inhibited by development of higher centers, so signs of damage at that point in time are signs of immaturity at an earlier time. Clinical neurologists believe that the extensor plantar sign usually reaches stability by the age of 2 years. Other signs, such as a persisting *asymmetrical tonic neck reflex* and the *Moro reflex*, can be tested to suggest an upper motor neuron lesion in young children.

Another confirmatory sign of spasticity is *clonus.* Hyperactive muscle stretch reflexes associated with spasticity may show a sustained series of rhythmic beats or jerks when a neurological examiner maintains one tendon of a muscle in extension. To test for clonus, the Achilles tendon at the ankle is often put under extension. If there is an upper motor neuron lesion, the ankle and the calf will show sustained jerks. A few clonic jerks, called *abortive clonus,* are not clinically significant, but if the clonus is sustained over time, it is considered pathologic and an indicator of hyperreflexia. This sign is part of the clinical syndrome resulting from an upper motor neuron lesion.

Another set of reflex responses considered as confirmatory signs are the *superficial abdominal* and *cremasteric reflexes.* These reflexes, like the Babinski response, are called superficial reflexes because they are elicited by the cutaneous skin receptors, in contrast to the muscle stretch reflex, which is considered a deep reflex because it is elicited by receptor end organs deep within the tendons. The abdominal and cremasteric reflexes are elicited by stroking the abdominal quadrants and the inner surface of the thigh, respectively. The normal abdominal response is a twitching of the navel toward the quadrant stimulated. A normal cremasteric response in a male is the elevation of the ipsilateral testicle in response to thigh stimulation. No comparable reflex is found in the female. Absence of the reflexes indicates an upper motor neuron lesion. Sometimes, however, it is hard to find abdominal reflexes, especially if a person has had abdominal surgery (see Table 6–2 for a summary).

Table 6–2   Signs of Upper and Lower Motor Neuron Disorders

Upper Motor Neuron Disorders	*Lower Motor Neuron Disorders*
Spastic paralysis	Flaccid paralysis
Hypertonia	Hypotonia
Hyperreflexia	Hyporeflexia
Clonus	No clonus
Babinski sign	No Babinski sign
Little or no atrophy	Marked atrophy
No fasciculations	Fasciculations
Diminished abdominal and cremasteric reflexes	Normal abdominal and cremasteric reflexes

Alpha and Gamma Motor Neurons

In the final analysis, motor control of speech muscles, or any other musculature, is brought about by muscle contraction. At one time it was believed that the only route for control of voluntary muscle contraction was via the several descending motor pathways in the nervous system that end in nerve cells called *alpha motor neurons*. These motor neurons, called anterior horn cells, are in the largest cells in the anterior horns of the spinal cord. Homologous motor neurons are the cranial nerve neurons of the brainstem. Along with gamma motor neurons, the alpha motor neurons supply skeletal muscles. They discharge impulses through the spinal nerves to contract muscles of the trunk and limbs in the corticospinal system. One can assume that most motor commands for a given articulatory act are transmitted by the alpha motor neuron system through contraction of muscles innervated by cranial nerves.

The alpha motor neuron innervates fibers within the muscle called *extrafusal fibers*. The axon of each neuron branches to supply the fibers. An axon may supply only a few fibers, as in the case of a small muscle with precisely controlled contraction, or it may control several hundred fibers, as in the case of large muscles with strong crude movements.

There are two types of extrafusal fibers, type I and type II. Type I fibers contract slowly and are resistant to fatigue, while type II fibers contract faster but fatigue more rapidly. All muscle fibers in a motor unit are of the same type, which is determined by the trophic influences of the innervating neuron. The neuron supplies the trophic or nutritional factors that direct the differentiation of the fibers and keep the muscle healthy. These substances are called *myotrophic factors*. The motor neuron also supplies the acetylcholine that stimulates contraction of muscle.

Muscle Spindles

More recently, another level of neuromuscular control has been identified. This is at the level of the muscle spindle. Muscle spindles serve as sensory, or afferent, receptors within striated muscle. They provide sensory information on the status of the normal stretch mechanisms in muscle. The spindles are also innervated by efferent neurons, making them more complex sensory receptors than those found in the tendons and joints.

The muscle spindle is encapsulated, containing a limited number of short fibers that are parallel to other muscle fibers (Figure 6–3). Fibers of the muscle spindle are called *intrafusal fibers*, and the number of intrafusal fibers within a spindle varies.

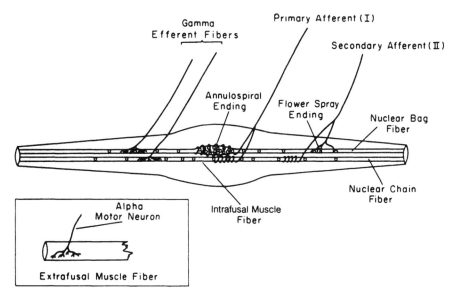

Figure 6-3 The muscle spindle. Source: Redrawn and reproduced with permission from W. Hardcastle, *The Physiology of Speech Production* (New York: Academic Press, 1978).

There are two types of intrafusal fibers: *nuclear bag fibers* and *nuclear chain fibers.* An aggregate of closely packed nuclei is found in the nuclear bag fibers, whereas the nuclei in the nuclear chain fibers are aligned single file. The nuclear bag and nuclear chain fibers are attached in parallel.

Two types of afferent axons arise from the intrafusal fibers. *Primary endings,* or *annulospiral endings,* are rapidly conducting afferent fibers that wrap around the center of the intrafusal fiber. *Secondary* or *flower spray endings* are more slowly conducting afferents and are found for the most part on the nuclear chain fibers.

Both primary and secondary afferents are stimulated by the lengthening of the intrafusal fibers and by the rate of change of their length. As the muscle fibers are stretched in response to the muscle contraction, the spindle afferents convey information to the alpha motor neurons, which control the neural discharge to extrafusal fibers. The primary afferents are large neurons with a rapid rate of conduction, up to 120 meters per second. The speed with which the spindles convey sensory feedback information to the central nervous system marks them as likely candidates for the neural mechanisms controlling the fine and rapid movements of speech muscles as well as other rapid motor activities.

Gamma Motor Neurons

The efferent innervation to the muscle spindle is supplied by *gamma efferents* or *gamma motor neurons*. Like the alpha motor neurons, these are part of a motor nerve. They are relatively small in size compared with the alpha efferents, but they make up approximately 30 percent of the motor neurons leaving the spinal cord.

The gamma motor neurons innervate the muscle spindle at each end. The firing of the gamma motor neuron causes the muscle spindle or intrafusal fibers to contract. This shortening of the fibers is detected by the annulospinal endings, and afferent impulses are sent to the spinal cord or brainstem where a synapse with an alpha motor neuron occurs. This synapse causes an efferent impulse to be sent to the extrafusal fibers of the muscle. A contraction of the fibers occurs until they are the same length as the fibers of the muscle spindles. Once this equalization takes place, the sensory receptor becomes "silent" and the process is terminated. This functional contractile process is known as the *gamma loop system*. Through this system, the gamma motor neurons form an important muscle stretch reflex mechanism that acts in conjunction with the alpha motor neurons. This sensitivity to stretch provides for fine compensations of muscle length and velocity and helps maintain muscle tone.

Speech muscles, which contain an abundance of spindles, have the potential for making compensations of movement if the specifications of a motor command are met. Evidence from the speech science laboratory indicates that rapid compensatory motor behavior is necessary for intelligible speech. Motor speech acts are rarely performed exactly the same way twice, but in most cases motor speech production meets the broad specifications of the motor commands in such a way that the listener can recognize an individual speech sound, or *phon*, as a member of a phoneme class.

The alpha motor neuron provides appropriate contraction of the extrafusal fibers innervated by the cranial nerves and the spinal nerves for articulatory acts, but local conditions produce variations in the way the actual articulatory movements are accomplished. The muscle spindle system, innervated by the gamma motor neuron system, with its sensory and motor servomechanism capabilities, makes the necessary muscle stretch reflex adjustments in the speech muscles for intelligible speech. This theory of muscle spindles provides an explanation for fine coordinated control at the level of the speech muscles. Thus, the muscle spindle mechanism offers a reasonable theoretical explanation for what is known as the problem of *motor equivalence* of speech movements.[3]

---

[3]*Motor equivalence* refers to the fact that the oral structures may be adjusted from several positions to achieve a target position for articulation.

Golgi Tendon Organs

Beyond the muscle spindle system, there are joint receptors and special tendon receptors called *Golgi tendon organs* that are involved in sensorimotor control of the speech muscles as well as other musculature of the body. The Golgi tendon organs are attached directly to the tendons of muscles. They respond when either stretching or contraction places tension on the tendon. The Golgi tendon organs serve to temper motor activity and inhibit activity in muscles when high levels of tension are placed on the tendon.

The Extrapyramidal System

We have identified the pyramidal system as the primary pathway for voluntary movement—that is, as the direct activation pathway. We have also indicated that a subdivision of that system, the corticobulbar tracts, is the primary pathway for the voluntary control of most speech muscles. Still another motor system, *the extrapyramidal system*, plays a significant role in speech and its disorders.

The extrapyramidal system is made up of subcortical nuclei called the *basal ganglia*, together with the subthalamic nucleus, substantia nigra, red nucleus, brainstem, reticular formation, and the complex pathways that interconnect these nuclei. We include in the extrapyramidal system, as some neuroanatomists do, the descending vestibulospinal, rubrospinal, tectospinal, and reticulospinal tracts.

The Indirect Activation Pathway

In his excellent summary of the anatomy of the motor pathways for speech production, Duffy (1995) discusses the concept of the *indirect activation pathway* of the extrapyramidal system and its contribution to the control of movement. He differentiates between these pathways and those of the "control circuits" of the basal ganglia and cerebellum. The basal ganglia and the cerebellum are not sources of input to the lower motor neurons, whereas the structures of the indirect activation pathways do have direct input to the lower motor neurons of the spinal cord and to some of the cranial nerve nuclei. The input of the indirect activation pathways to the cranial nerve nuclei, and thus to speech production, are poorly understood at this time, although projections to some of the nuclei have been documented.

According to Duffy (1995), the components of the indirect activation pathway consist of many short pathways and interconnections with structures between the origin of the pathway in the cortex and its termination at the lower motor neuron. The nuclei and tracts considered to be components of the indirect activation system are listed in Table 6–3.

The primary function of the indirect activation pathway is motor control to regulate reflexes and maintain posture and tone. The control is subconscious and requires integration of many muscles. Its effect seems to be *inhibitory*, whereas the direct activation system is *facilitory*. In speech, the indirect activation system probably inhibits interference with the movements of specific muscles so that appropriate speed, range, and direction of movement can be maintained. In general, damage to the indirect activation system affects muscle tone and reflexes. It usually is manifest in combination with damage to the direct activation system, the pyramidal tract.

Basal Ganglia

The term *extrapyramidal system* has clinical utility in that it is widely used to refer to a group of subcortical nuclei and related structures known as the *basal ganglia* (see Figure 2–11). Although the terminology used to describe the basal ganglia is not always agreed on and is generally confusing, there are three structures or major parts of the basal ganglia: (1) the *caudate nucleus*, (2) the *putamen*, and (3) the *globus pallidus* (Figure 6–4). Other structures include the subthalamic nucleus and substantia nigra (Weiner & Lang, 1989).

Table 6–3 Major Components of the Indirect Activation Pathway of the Extrapyramidal System

Components (Nuclei or Tracts)	Functional Role in Motor Control
Reticular formation or reticulospinal tracts	Excitation or inhibition of flexors and extensors; facilitation or inhibition of reflexes and ascending sensory information
Vestibular nuclei or vestibulospinal tract	Facilitation of reflex activity and spinal mechanisms controlling muscle tone
Red nucleus or rubrospinal tract	Facilitation of flexor and inhibition of extensor neurons

Source: Adapted with permission from J. R. Duffy, *Motor Speech Disorders: Substrates, Differential Diagnosis and Management.* (St. Louis: C. V. Mosby–Year Book, 1995).

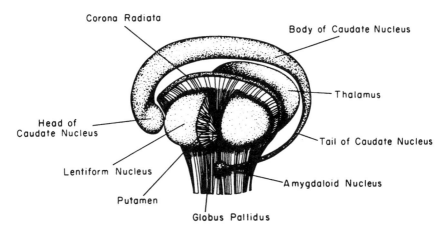

Corona Radiata

Body of Caudate Nucleus

Thalamus

Head of
Caudate Nucleus

Tail of Caudate Nucleus

Lentiform Nucleus

Amygdaloid Nucleus

Putamen

Globus Pallidus

Figure 6–4 A dissected view of the basal ganglia illustrating their relationship to the thalamus, amygdaloid nucleus, and corona radiata.

The caudate nucleus lies just medial to the anterior limb of the interior capsule. The putamen and globus pallidus lie anterior to the genu of the internal capsule. The caudate nucleus lies adjacent to the wall of the lateral ventricle, close to the thalamus, which is part of the diencephalon. The structure is divided into a head, body, and tail by some neurologists, but others divide the caudate into only a head and tail.

The putamen and globus pallidus together make up the *lentiform nucleus,* a thumb-sized structure wedged against the internal capsule. The lentiform nucleus is separated from the caudate nucleus except at the head of the caudate, where the two nuclear masses border on the anterior limb of the internal capsule. The putamen is the lateral portion of the lentiform nucleus, and the globus pallidus is in the medial region of the lentiform nucleus. The globus pallidus is crossed by myelinated fibers which give it a pale cast in its fresh state. The lentiform nucleus (that is, the putamen and the globus pallidus) combined with the caudate nucleus make up what is known as the corpus striatum (Table 6–4).

Other structures related in function to the basal ganglia are found near the reticular formation of the mesencephalon. These include the *subthalamus, substantia nigra,* and *red nucleus.* The *reticular formation* itself is also thought of as part of the subcortical extrapyramidal system. The extrapyramidal system is concerned with coarse stereotyped movements. It has more influence over proximal (midline) than over distal (peripheral) muscles. It maintains proper tone and posture. Even with destruction of the pyramidal tract, it can allow a person to eat and walk.

Table 6–4 Major Extrapyramidal Nuclei

Basal Ganglia		
Globus pallidus	Lentiform	Corpus
Putamen	nucleus	striatum
Caudate nucleus		

The extrapyramidal system is probably crucial in changing facial expression as we talk, whereas speech itself is probably primarily the result of pyramidal tract action.

Most of the efferent fibers from the basal ganglia leave the globus pallidus. In addition to the basal ganglia, the cerebellum and the cerebral cortex interact in a series of feedback loops, suggesting complex interaction of motor subsystems to coordinate everyday speech motor performance. The primary motor and sensory areas of the cortex project fibers particularly to the putamen. Fibers are projected to the caudate nucleus from the frontal, parietal, occipital, and temporal lobes. The neurons projecting from the cerebral cortex are *excitatory* and employ the neurotransmitter called *glutamate*. Neurons in the striatum project to the globus pallidus and are inhibitory in nature, using the neurotransmitter gamma-aminobutyric acid. Many of the interneurons of the striatum are excitatory and use the neurotransmitter acetylcholine.

Output from the basal ganglia comes primarily from the globus pallidus. Fibers from the globus pallidus ascend to the level of the internal capsule where they join cerebellothalamic fibers and synapse in the thalamus. Other fibers from the globus pallidus synapse in the subthalamic nucleus, while another set terminate in the midbrain. There is a series of circuits and feedback loops between the corpus striatum, globus pallidus, thalamus, and cerebral cortex as well as circuits and a feedback loop involving the corpus striatum, substantia nigra, thalamus, and cerebral cortex. These two circuits ensure that the basal ganglia interact with the cerebral cortex in all motor activity.

The functions of the basal ganglia are far from clear (Marsden, 1982), and it is difficult, from the results of lesions, to deduce these functions. Lesions of the basal ganglia generally produce two major types of movement disorders: (1) poverty of movement (*akinesia*) and (2) excessive involuntary movement (*dyskinesia*) (Weiner & Lang, 1989). Akinesia is often accompanied by muscular rigidity, as in Parkinson's disease. The symptoms of these movement disorders suggest that basal ganglia disorders result in deficits in the initiation of movement (akinesia), difficulty in continuing or stopping an ongoing movement (dyskinesia), abnormalities of muscle tone (*rigidity*), and the development of involuntary movements (*chorea, tremor, athetosis,* and *dystonia*). Thus, the basal ganglia are thought to participate heavily in motor control, particularly in the initiation of movement and also in the maintenance of ongoing movement. The basal ganglia particularly influence movements related to posture, automatic movements, and skilled voluntary movements.

Marsden (1982) argues that the basal ganglia are responsible for the automatic execution of learned motor plans. This involves subconscious selection, sequencing, and delivery of the motor programs of a learned or practiced motor strategy, such as playing an instrument or writing by hand. When the basal ganglia are damaged, it appears that the individual reverts to slower, less automatic, and less accurate cortical mechanisms for motor behavior.

Dyskinesias

The motor disturbances of the basal ganglia are usually classified as *involuntary movement disorders*. The most commonly used technical term for them is *dyskinesias* (*dys* = "disorder"; *kinesia* = "movement"). These disorders encompass a full range of bizarre postures and unusual movement patterns. The dyskinesias have long been described with such terms as tremor, writhing, fidgeting, flailing, restlessness, jerking, and flinging. Often the unusual movements that dominate the trunk and limbs of the dyskinetic patient are also reflected in the face and speech mechanism. The result is a serious and typical dysarthria. In general, the dysarthria reflects the specific symptoms of each specific type of dyskinesia.

The term *dyskinesia* is usually used to indicate movement disorders associated with extrapyramidal lesions, but the term may be used in a broader sense to include any excess of movement (*hyperkinesia*) or reduction in movement (*akinesia*). *Hyperkinesia* has been used to indicate those dyskinesias that present too much movement. *Hypokinesia* and *akinesia*, on the other hand, refer to too little movement and reduced movement, respectively. In actual clinical usage, the terms may not always be applied strictly to a person with extrapyramidal lesions. For instance, neurologists may apply *hyperkinesia* to the well-known extrapyramidally based twitching or fidgeting of chorea in Huntington's disease as well as to the abnormal hyperactivity of children in whom there may not be evidence of an organic lesion in the nervous system, let alone knowledge of a lesion localized to the extrapyramidal system.

Hypokinesia may be used to describe the reduced activity level of a depressive patient with no suspected neurologic lesion. By tradition, neurologists do not apply *hypokinesia* to limitations in movement resulting from lesions of the pyramidal tract or peripheral nerves. In other words, lesions that paralyze voluntary movement are not labeled *hypokinetic*. Thus, hemiplegia, quadriplegia, and paraplegia are not considered hypokinetic disorders.

Understanding of the underlying mechanism of several of the dyskinesias was greatly advanced when it was learned that the function of the neurotransmitter dopamine was disturbed. In certain cases of Parkinson's disease, the substantia nigra is damaged; either the activity of its cells is blocked or the cells die. The dark pigmented cells of the substantia nigra become depigmented by degeneration of the neurons in the area, and the synapses to pathways exiting from the basal ganglia are disrupted. Dopamine, which is released at these synapses, normally is greatly reduced in the brains of individuals with Parkinson's disease. Thus, the cause of this particular dyskinesia has been identified almost certainly as a lack of dopamine or dopamine action. This finding has led to the study of synaptic function and neurotransmitter action as a possible cause of other dyskinetic conditions. Dyskinesia symptoms can be produced by dopamine depletion in the laboratory animal and can be improved by the administration of L-dopa or similar drugs.

Dyskinetic Types

The responsibilities of speech-language pathologists do not extend to the identification of lesion sites in the complex circuitry of the extrapyramidal motor system, but such clinicians should attempt to recognize the standard dyskinesias of extrapyramidal origin and to determine the effect of the symptoms of specific dyskinesias on the dysarthria accompanying them. Undiagnosed cases of dyskinesia demand referral to a neurologist.

There are several distinct patterns of dyskinesia, but not all of them are related to the dysarthrias. We describe only those motor signs that produce motor speech symptoms.

Tremors

Tremors are defined as purposeless movements that are rhythmic, oscillatory, involuntary actions. Normal (or *physiologic*) and abnormal (or *pathologic*) tremors are usually distinguished. Tremors are pathologic if they occur in a disease and are characteristic of that disease.

Normal tremor is called *physiologic tremor*. There are several classifications of tremor in use today. The speech-language pathologist should be familiar with three types of tremor that are associated with vocal performance in normal and pathologic conditions.

Rest Tremor

Rest tremor designates a tremor that occurs in Parkinson's disease. A tremor of three to seven movements per second occurs in the patient's limbs and hands at rest. The tremor is temporarily suppressed when the limb is moved, and it sometimes can be inhibited by conscious effort. The voice may be affected by the tremor. Tremulous voice has been described in approximately 14 percent of a large sample of parkinsonian patients. It is a salient vocal deviation that is easily recognized among the other vocal deviations of the hypokinetic dysarthria of parkinsonism.

Physiologic or Action Tremor

Healthy people demonstrate a fine tremor of the hands on maintaining posture. The rate may vary with age but usually falls within the range of four to 12 cycles per second. An *action tremor* may affect the laryngeal muscles and produce an organic or essential vocal tremor, the mechanism for which is unknown. This normal tremor is distinguished from pathologic tremors associated with known neurologic diseases such as Parkinson's and cerebellar disorders.

Intention Tremor

This term refers to a tremor that occurs during movement and is intensified at the termination of the movement. Intention tremor has been associated with the ataxic dysarthria seen in cerebellar disease. It is often seen in cerebellar disorders but is not exclusive to cerebellar dysfunction.

Chorea

Chorea refers to quick, random, hyperkinetic movements simulating fragments of normal movements. Speech, facial, and respiratory movements, as well as movements of the extremities, are affected by choreic symptoms in this dyskinesia. The movement is close to what is popularly described as "fidgets." Chorea is one symptom of a hereditary disorder known as *Huntington's disease,* and it is seen in other extrapyramidal disorders as well.

Athetosis

The hyperkinesia of athetosis is a slow, irregular, coarse, writhing or squirming movement. It usually involves the extremities as well as the face, neck, and trunk. The movements directly interfere with the fine and controlled actions of the larynx, tongue, palate, pharynx, and respiratory mechanism. Like most other involuntary movements, the involuntary movements of athetosis disappear in sleep. In congenital athetosis, the most common type of spastic paralysis may also be observed, indicating involvement of both pyramidal and extrapyramidal systems. Lesion sites in pure athetosis are often in the putamen and the caudate nucleus. *Hypoxia*, or lack of oxygen at birth, is a common cause, producing death of brain cells before or during birth. *Choreoathetotic movements* have also been described; they appear to be a dyskinesia that lies somewhere between choreic and athetoid movements in terms of rate and rhythm of movement or that includes both types of movement. In fact, many of the involuntary movement disorders appear to blend one or more of the different clinical dyskinesias, as the term *choreoathetosis* implies.

Dystonia

In this disorder the limbs assume distorted static postures resulting from excess tone in selected parts of the body. The dyskinetic postures are slow, bizarre, and often grotesque, involving writhing, twisting, and turning. Dysarthria and obvious motor involvement of the speech mechanism are common. Often, differential motor involvement occurs in the speech muscles, and some dysarthrias have been observed that primarily affect the larynx. Others affect the face, tongue, lips, palate, and jaw. A rare dystonic disorder of childhood is called *dystonia musculorum deformans*. It may be accompanied by dysarthria in its later stages.

Fragmentary or focal dystonias have been described, and some neurologists assert that they contribute to *spastic* or *spasmodic dysphonia*, a bizarre voice disorder that mixes *aphonia* (lack of voice) with a strained, labored whisper. The etiology of spastic dysphonia is unclear. Injections of botulinum are effective in reducing the dystonia.

Myoclonus

Myoclonus has been used to describe differing motor abnormalities, but basically a myoclonic movement is an abrupt, brief, almost lightning-like contraction of muscle. An example of a normal or physiologic myoclonic reaction occurs when you are drifting off to sleep and are suddenly awakened by a rapid muscle jerk. This muscle jerk is myoclonus.

Pathologic myoclonus is most common in the limbs and trunk but also may involve the facial muscles, jaws, tongue, and pharynx. Repetitive myoclonus in these muscles, of course, may affect speech. Myoclonic movements in the muscles of speech have been described as having a rate of 10 to 50 per minute, but they can be more rapid. The pathology underlying these movements has been debated, but since they have been associated with degenerative brain disease, the cerebral cortex, brainstem, cerebellum, and extrapyramidal system have all been considered as possible lesion sites.

A special myoclonic syndrome involving speech muscles called *palatal myoclonus* has been described. It involves rapid movements of the soft palate and pharynx and sometimes includes the larynx, the diaphragm, and other muscles. The symptoms most often come on in later life and are characteristic of several diseases. This myoclonus has a specific pathology in the central tegmental tract of the brainstem, but the etiology can be varied. The most common cause is a stroke, or cerebrovascular accident, in the brainstem.

Orofacial Dyskinesia or Tardive Dyskinesia

In this syndrome, bizarre movements are limited to the mouth, face, jaw, and tongue. There is grimacing, pursing of the mouth and lips, and writhing of the tongue. These dyskinetic movements very often alter articulation of speech. The motor speech signs of orofacial dyskinesia usually develop after the prolonged use of powerful tranquilizing drugs, the most common class of which are the *phenothiazines*. Drug-induced dyskinesias associated with the phenothiazines and related medications may even produce athetoid movements or dystonic movements of the body. Parkinsonian signs and other symptoms associated with extrapyramidal disorders are also caused by these drugs. Orofacial dyskinesia also occurs in elderly patients without drug use. A rare disorder that includes dyskinesia of the eyelids, face, tongue, and refractory muscles is called *Meige syndrome*.

Other dyskinesias are included in the spectrum of extrapyramidal disorders but generally do not include motor involvement of the speech mechanism. These are defined in Table 6-5.

Table 6–5 Nonspeech Dyskinesias

Dyskinesias	*Definition*
Hemiballismus	Forceful, flinging movements that are continuous, wild, and unilateral and may involve half of the body
Akathisia	Motor restlessness or inability to sit still

The Cerebellar System

The third major subcomponent of the motor system that affects speech is the cerebellum. Interacting with the pyramidal and extrapyramidal systems, the cerebellum is known to provide significant coordination for motor speech. As noted, the cerebellum is located dorsal to the medulla and pons. The occipital lobes of the cerebral hemispheres overlap the top of the cerebellum. The anatomy of the cerebellum is complex, and the speech-language pathologist need only understand it in a gross sense to see the relationship of the cerebellum to speech performance.

Anatomy of the Cerebellum

The cerebellum can be divided into three parts. The thin middle portion is called the *vermis* because of its serpentine or worm-like shape. The vermis lies between two large lateral masses of the cerebellum, the cerebellar hemispheres (see Figure 6–5). The vermis connects these two hemispheres. The vermis and hemispheres are divided by fissures and sulci into *lobes* and also into smaller divisions called *lobules*. The division into lobes and lobules is helpful in clarifying the physiologic function of the cerebellum. Although the lobes and lobules have been classified differently by different investigators, we employ a classification system that divides the cerebellum into three lobes.

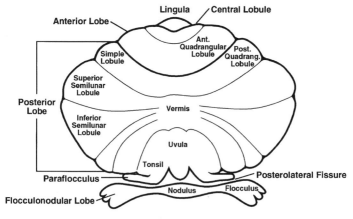

Figure 6–5 A schematic illustration of the cerebellum shows hemispheres, lobes, and lobules (Ant., anterior; Post., posterior; Quadrang., quadrangular).

The Three Cerebellar Lobes

The three cerebellar lobes are (1) the anterior lobe, (2) the posterior lobe, and (3) the flocculonodular lobe. The *anterior lobe*, which is modest in size, is that part of the cerebellum superior to the primary fissure. This part of the cerebellum corresponds roughly to what is known as the *paleocerebellum*, the second-oldest part of the cerebellum in a phylogenetic sense. The anterior lobe receives most of the proprioceptive impulses from the spinal cord and regulates posture.

The *posterior lobe*, the largest part of the cerebellum, is located between the other two lobes. It makes up the major portion of the cerebellar hemispheres. It is the newest part of the cerebellum and is therefore also known as the *neocerebellum*. The posterior lobe receives the cerebellar connections from the cerebrum and regulates coordination of muscle movement.

The *flocculonodular lobe* consists of two small wispy appendages, known as *flocculi*, in the posterior and inferior region of the cerebellum. The flocculi are separated by the *nodulus*, the inferior part of the vermis. The flocculonodular lobe, the oldest portion of the cerebellum, contains the fastigial nucleus, which is made up of fibers that travel from the nucleus to the four vestibular nuclei in the upper medulla. Via these fibers, the cerebellum mediates equilibrium.

Synergy and Asynergy

The connections that the cerebellum has with other parts of the central nervous system are important to its function. It is through these connections that the cerebellum sends and receives afferent and efferent impulses and executes its primary function—a synergistic coordination of muscles and muscle groups. *Synergy* is defined as the cooperative action of muscles. Assuring the smooth coordination of muscles is the prime task of the cerebellum. Specifically, the cerebellum, with other structures of the nervous system, maintains proper posture and balance in walking and in the sequential movements of eating, dressing, and writing. It also guides the production of rapid, alternating, repetitive movements such as those present in speaking and in smooth pursuit movements. Voluntary movement, without assistance from the cerebellum, is clumsy, uncoordinated, and disorganized. The motor defect of the cerebellar system has been called *asynergia* or *dyssynergia*. Asynergia is a lack of coordination in agonistic and antagonistic muscles.

Cerebellar Peduncles and Pathways

The cerebellum is connected to the rest of the nervous system by three pairs of *peduncles* or feet. The cerebellar peduncles anchor the cerebellum to the brainstem. All afferent and efferent fibers of the cerebellum pass through the three peduncles and the pons to the other levels of the nervous system. The *pons*, which means "bridge," is aptly named: it is literally a bridge from the cerebellum to the rest of the nervous system (Figure 6–6).

The *inferior cerebellar peduncle*, or *restiform body*, carries primary afferent fibers from the structures close to it; these are the medulla, spinal cord, and cranial nerve VIII. Thus, spinocerebellar, medullocerebellar, and vestibular fibers pass through the inferior peduncle.

The *middle cerebellar peduncle*, or *brachium pontis*, connects the cerebellum with the cerebral cortex by the pathways that transverse it. The middle peduncle is easily recognized: it is the largest of the three peduncles and also conveys the largest number of fibers to the cerebral cortex and pons. It carries pontocerebellar fibers as well as the majority

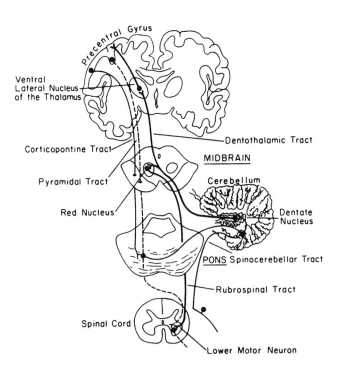

Figure 6–6 Major pathways of the cerebellum.

of the *corticopontocerebellar fibers*. These fibers convey afferent information from the temporal and frontal lobes of the cerebrum to the posterior lobe of the contralateral cerebellum.

The *superior cerebellar peduncle*, or *brachium conjunctivum*, conveys the bulk of efferent fibers that leave the cerebellum. The primary efferent fibers arise from an important nucleus deep in the cerebellum called the *dentate nucleus*. The *rubrospinal* and *dentatothalamic pathways*, along with several other tracts, leave via the superior peduncle and terminate in the *contralateral red nucleus* and *ventrolateral nucleus* of the thalamus. From here impulses are relayed to the cerebral cortex. The anatomy of the cerebellum is summarized in Table 6–6.

Cerebellar Role in Speech

We have outlined the major pathways and structures of the cerebellum to suggest a rough schematic of the feedback nature of the afferent and efferent connections of the structure. Sketchy as our presentation is, it still highlights the fact that the cerebellar motor subsystem significantly influences the function of the other motor systems in the production of motor speech. The fact that the cerebellum plays an important part in the synergy of rapid alternating movements and the fine coordination of muscles suggests that it interacts in a crucial way with the corticobulbar fibers to provide the specialized rapid and precise motor control needed for ongoing connected speech.

Auditory, tactile, and visual areas exist in the cerebellum. These motor, tactile, and auditory centers in the cerebellum, both cortical and subcortical, project to similar areas in the cerebrum, which in turn project back

Table 6–6   The Cerebellum and Its Pathways

Hemispheres	*Lobes*	*Peduncles*
Right	Anterior	Superior
Left	Posterior	Middle
	Flocculonodular	Inferior
Major afferent pathways and their lobes		
Vestibulocerebellar tracts		Flocculonodular lobe
Spinocerebellar tracts		Anterior lobe
Corticopontocerebellar tracts		Posterior lobe
Major efferent pathway and hemispheres		
Cerebrocerebellocerebral tracts		Right and left hemispheres

to corresponding cerebellar areas. The cerebellum, therefore, is neither completely vestibular, proprioceptive, nor motor in function, but serves to reinforce or diminish sensory and motor impulses, acting as a critical modulator of neuronal function. Through its afferent and efferent feedback circuits, the cerebellum ensures a desired level of neural activity in the motor parts of the nervous system.

Clinical Signs of Cerebellar Dysfunction

Cerebellar or cerebellar pathway lesions manifest themselves in incoordination of volitional movements and, often, in volitionally maintained postures. Clinical signs usually appear on the same side of the body as the cerebellar lesion. Upper motor neuron lesions of pyramidal pathways yield contralateral effects, whereas the cerebellum and its pathways manifest ipsilateral effects. Several classic signs of cerebral disorder follow.

Ataxia

Ataxia is the prime sign of a cerebellar lesion (*taxis* means "ordering in rank and file"). The term *ataxia* is often used in several senses. It may refer to the general incoordination of motor acts seen with cerebellar system lesions. In this sense it often describes a staggering or reeling gait and abnormal posture seen with cerebellar lesions. The patient compensates for the ataxic gait by standing and walking with feet wide apart in what is called a *broad-based gait*.

Decomposition of Movement

Decomposition of movement is also related to the ataxia. The patient will break a complex motor act into its components and execute the act movement by movement, so that the movement seems as if it were being performed by a robot. Decomposition of movement is considered an ataxic movement.

Dysmetria

Dysmetria is the inability to gauge the distance, speed, and power of movement. A patient may stop before the movement is performed or may overshoot the motor goal.

Adiadochokinesia or Dysdiadochokinesia

Adiadochokinesia or *dysdiadochokinesia* is the inability to perform rapid alternating muscle movements. Often the rate of alternating movement may be recorded in a neurologic examination. This measure is called an *alternate motion rate.* Diadochokinetic rate measures of the muscles of the oral mechanism during speech and nonspeech activities have long been used as an assessment task by the clinical speech-language pathologist. These rates, however, are used as measures of the integrity of the oral muscles in speech pathology and have not specifically been related to cerebellar function.

The neurologist may test alternating movements in many muscle groups in persons suspected of cerebellar disorders. Successive pronation or supination of the hands, rapid tapping of the fingers, and rapid opening and closing of the fists are all diadochokinetic diagnostic tests. During the testing of diadochokinesis or alternate motion rates, one may see awkwardness or clumsiness of alternate movements.

Rebound
The rebound phenomenon is the inability to check the contraction of the flexors and rapidly contract the extensor. It may account for the lack of smooth diadochokinetic movements.

Hypotonia
Hypotonia (or muscle flaccidity) with a decrease in resistance to passive movement, is seen in cerebellar dysfunction. The muscles of the body are flabby and lack normal tone.

Tremor
Tremor is seen as part of cerebellar disease. It is usually an intention or kinetic tremor not present at rest.

Nystagmus
Nystagmus is oscillatory abnormalities of the pupil of the eye, and it is often seen in cerebellar disorders. The rhythmic oscillations may be vertical, horizontal, or rotary.

Muscle Stretch Reflexes
Muscle stretch reflexes are normal or diminished. Often, *pendular reflexes* may be seen in cerebellar disease. When the knee jerk reflex is elicited, there is often a series of smooth to-and-fro movements of the limb before it comes to rest, as would be seen in a pendulum. This pendular reflex differs from a normal knee jerk response.

Ataxic Dysarthria
Ataxic dysarthria is present with some cerebellar lesions. The typical speech pattern in ataxic dysarthria results from asynergetic movement of the speech muscles. There are disturbances in the force,

speed, timing, and direction of the muscles used in speech performance. Articulation is generally imprecise, with distorted vowels and inaccurate consonant production. Articulatory control shows irregularity, and the prosody of speech is disturbed. Rate is slowed and timing of phonemes is abnormal. Stress on syllables is inappropriate, and loudness and pitch are deviant. Prosodic disturbances are obvious in the speech. Cerebellar signs and tests are summarized in Table 6–7.

Cerebellar Syndrome and Dysarthria

Some of the aforementioned signs of cerebellar disorder have been singled out as prominent in a *syndrome of cerebellar disorder*. This syndrome usually includes *ataxia, dysarthria, nystagmus,* and *hypotonia*. However, not all patients with cerebellar disease show all clinical signs of this syndrome, and dysarthria is not always seen in cerebellar disease. It may appear if the lesion is localized in the speech mechanisms that are found in the left cerebellar hemisphere (Lechtenberg & Gilman, 1978).

Summary

Traditionally, the neuromuscular control of speaking has been related to three classic motor systems—the pyramidal, extrapyramidal, and cerebellar systems. When the corticospinal tract of the pyramidal tract

Table 6–7   Cerebellar Dysfunction Signs and Tests

Abnormality	Signs and Tests
Gait ataxia	Broad-based gait seen on tandem walking test
Arm ataxia	Finger-to-nose test, hand pronation-to-supination test result in overshooting of nose and slowed pronation and supination
Overshooting	Rebound noted on arm-pulling test
Hypotonia	Flaccid muscle tone noted on passive movement testing; pendular reflexes elicited on reflex testing; rag doll postures observed
Nystagmus	Pupil oscillation seen when patient attempts to follow finger through field of gaze
Dysarthria	Articulation disorder is seen with disturbance in speech loudness, pitch, and/or stress; often associated with left cerebellar hemisphere lesion

is damaged by an upper motor neuron lesion, a contralateral hemiplegia (one-sided paralysis) may result. The corticobulbar tracts are the voluntary motor pathways (or direct activation pathways) for speech; they are part of the pyramidal system. Corticobulbar fibers innervate the cranial nuclei in the pons and medulla for the cranial nerves that control speech. The crossed and uncrossed fibers of the corticobulbar tracts are arranged so that the midline speech muscles function in bilateral synchrony for many tasks. Some speech muscles show mixed bilateral synchrony and contralateral independence.

Clinical lesions in the nervous system have been classically divided into upper and lower motor neuron lesions. Each type of lesion presents a different type of paralysis with its own associated signs. The hallmark of an upper motor neuron lesion is clasp knife spasticity (hypertonia), whereas the hallmark of a lower motor neuron lesion is a flaccid paralysis (hypotonia). Movement patterns are initiated by the motor cortex and transmitted to lower levels of the nervous system via descending pathways that end on the alpha motor neurons, the anterior horn cells, the spinal cord, or similar neurons of the cranial nuclei. Muscle spindles, which include sensory receptors (proprioceptors) deep within the muscle, aid in controlling movement patterns. An afferent-efferent feedback loop involving the gamma motor neuron and the muscle spindle influences the alpha motor neuron in the spinal cord and the cranial nerve nuclei. Although it is apparently important for speech, the loop's exact role is unknown.

The extrapyramidal system is an indirect motor pathway from the cortex. It involves structures and tracts such as the reticular formation, red nucleus, and vestibulospinal, tectospinal, and rubrospinal tracts, which are considered part of the indirect activation pathway for motor control because indirect input is provided to the lower motor neuron. The subcortical nuclei called the basal ganglia are also part of the extrapyramidal system. The basal ganglia, along with the cerebellum, make up the cortical control circuits; these circuits do not provide input into the lower motor neurons but make numerous connections with the cerebral cortex, cerebellum, brainstem, and spinal cord. Involuntary movement disorders, or dyskinesias, associated with special patterns of speech disturbance are tremor, tardive dyskinesia, chorea, athetosis, choreoathetosis, myoclonus, and orofacial dyskinesia. The speech disorders of the extrapyramidal system are dyskinetic dysarthrias; these may be hypokinetic or hyperkinetic. Disturbances of tone—as seen in the rigidity of Parkinson's disease and in dystonia—are also related to basal ganglia disorders.

The cerebellum is responsible for synergistic motor coordination and plays an important part in guiding the rapid, alternating, repetitive movements of speech. It provides afferent and efferent information to the corticobulbar fibers. The primary signs of cerebellar disorder are ataxia (incoordination) and asynergia (poor cooperative muscle actions). Dysdiadochokinesia is seen in the alternating movement rates of the oral musculature. Dysarthria, ataxia, hypotonia, and nystagmus (oscillating pupil) are often described as the classic cerebellar syndrome, but all four signs are not always present with cerebellar pathway lesions. Also, ataxic dysarthria is not seen in all cases of cerebellar disorder.

References and Further Readings

Pyramidal System

Feldman, R. G., Young, R. R., & Koella, W. P. (Eds.) (1980). *Spasticity: Disordered motor control.* Chicago: Year Book Publishers.

Kuypers, H. G. J. M. (1958). Corticobulbar connections to the pons and lower brainstem in man: An anatomical study. *Brain*, 81, 364–388.

Alpha and Gamma Neurons

Grillner, S., Lindbloom, B., Lubker, J., & Persson, A. (Eds.) (1982). *Speech motor control.* New York: Pergamon Press.

Hardcastle, W. J. (1976). *Physiology of speech production.* New York: Academic Press.

The Extrapyramidal System

Duffy, J. R. (1995). *Motor speech disorders: Substrates, differential diagnosis and management.* St. Louis: Mosby–Year Book, Inc.

Marsden, C. D. (1982). The mysterious function of the basal ganglia. *Neurology*, 32, 514–539.

Marsden, C. D. (1986). Movement disorders and the basal ganglia. *Trends in Neuroscience*, 9, 512–515.

Sherrington, C. S. *The integrative action of the nervous system.* New Haven: Yale University Press.

Weiner, W. J., & Lang, A. E. (1989). *Movement disorders: A comprehensive survey.* Mount Kisco, NY: Futura Publishing.

The Cerebellar System

Eccles, J. C. (1973). *The understanding of the brain.* New York: McGraw-Hill.

Lechtenberg, R., & Gilman, S. (1978). Speech disorders in cerebellar disease. *Annals of Neurology*, 3, 285–289.

7

□ □ □
□ □ □
□ □ □

The Cranial Nerves

*"To those I address, it is unnecessary to go further
than to indicate that the nerves treated in these
papers are the instruments of expression from
the smile of the infant's cheek to the last
agony of life."*

—Charles Bell, 1824

This chapter is intended to help the speech-language pathologist understand one of the most important parts of the nervous system with respect to the acts of speaking and swallowing. The cranial nerves make up a part of the peripheral nervous system that provides crucial sensory and motor information to the oral, pharyngeal, and laryngeal musculature. The speech-language pathologist should be very familiar with the names, structure, innervation, testing procedure, and signs of abnormal function of the cranial nerves. This information will be vital in working with the dysarthric and/or dysphagic adult and child.

The Origin of the Cranial Nerves

Names and Numbers

Twelve pairs of cranial nerves leave the brain and pass through the foramina of the skull. They are known both by their numbers, written in Roman numerals, and by their names. The names sometimes give a clue to the function of the nerves, but it is best to learn the number, the name, and concise descriptions of the various functions. Such descriptions are provided in Table 7–1. Many students use a mnemonic device to help them remember the cranial nerves—for example, *On Old Olympus' Towering Top A Finn And German Vend At Hops.* Of course, you can create your own device—an even more memorable one!

Table 7–1   The Cranial Nerves

Number	Name	Summary of Function
I	Olfactory	Smell
II	Optic	Vision
III	Oculomotor	Innervation of muscles to move eyeball, pupil, and upper lid
IV	Trochlear	Innervation of superior oblique muscle of eye
V	Trigeminal	Chewing and sensation to face
VI	Abducens	Abduction of eye
VII	Facial	Movement of facial muscles, taste, salivary glands
VIII	(Vestibular) Acoustic	Equilibrium and hearing
IX	Glossopharyngeal	Taste, swallowing, elevation of pharynx and larynx, parotid salivary gland, sensation to upper pharynx
X	Vagus	Taste, swallowing, elevation of palate, phonation, parasympathetic outflow to visceral organs
XI	Accessory	Turning of head and shrugging of shoulders
XII	Hypoglossal	Movement of tongue

Embryological Origin

The nuclei of the cranial nerves are of three different types. The motor nuclei are distinguished by the embryological origin of the muscles they innervate. The development of the body wall in the embryo is from blocks of mesoderm called *somites*. Cranial nerves III, IV, VI, and XII are derived from this somatic segmentation and thus are called the *somatomotor* or *somitic set*.

In the development of the embryo, the branchial (gill) arches are responsible for the structure, muscles, and nerves of the face and neck. Cranial nerves V, VII, IX, X, and XI are thus known as the *branchial set*.

The somites and branchial arches are transverse segments of the embryo. In contrast, the viscera, including the neuraxis, are developed from longitudinal tubes. The elaboration or diverticulation of the hollow tubes gives rise to three cranial nerves (I, II, and VIII) known as the *solely special sensory set*. There are branchial and somatic cranial nerves that have a visceral component—numbers III, VII, IX, and X. Cranial nerves V,

VII, IX, and X also have a general sensory component—that is, they participate in sensation of pain, pressure touch, vibration, and proprioception.

The Corticobulbar Tract and the Cranial Nerves

The cranial nerves consist of efferent motor fibers that arise
from nuclei in the brainstem and afferent sensory fibers that originate in
the peripheral ganglia. The motor or efferent parts are axons of the nerve
cells within the brain. These nerve cells with their processes are part of
the lower motor neurons. Groups of these nerve cells form the nuclei of
origin for the cranial nerves.

The motor nuclei of origin of the cranial nerves receive impulses from
the cerebral cortex through the corticobulbar tracts. The tracts begin in
the pyramidal cells in the inferior part of the precentral gyrus and also in
the adjacent part of the postcentral gyrus. The tracts then follow the path
illustrated in Figure 6–1: they descend through the corona radiata and the
genu of the internal capsule; they pass through the midbrain in the cerebral
peduncles; and they then synapse either with the lower motor neuron
directly or indirectly through internuncial neurons, a chain of neurons
situated between the primary efferent neuron and the final motor neuron.

The majority of the corticobulbar fibers to the motor cranial nerve nuclei
cross the midline, or decussate, before reaching the nuclei. There is bilateral
innervation for all of the cranial nerve motor nuclei except for portions of
the trigeminal, facial, and hypoglossal fibers. These are discussed later.

Whereas the motor parts of the cranial nerves are formed by axons of
nerve cells within the brain, the sensory or afferent parts of the cranial
nerves are formed by axons of nerve cells outside the brain. They are situated
on the nerve trunks or actually in the sensory organ itself—for example, in
the nose, ear, or eye. The central processes of these cells enter the brain
and terminate by synapsing with cells that are grouped together to form
the *nuclei of termination*. These cells have axons that cross the midline
and ascend and synapse on other sensory nuclei, such as the thalamus. The
axons of the resulting cells then terminate in the cerebral cortex.

The Cranial Nerves for Smell and Vision

Cranial nerve I, the *olfactory nerve,* is actually a plexus of thin
fibers that unite in about 20 small bundles called fila olfactoria. The olfactory
receptors are situated in the mucous membrane of the nasal cavity. The nerve
fibers synapse with other cells in the olfactory bulb and finally end in the

olfactory areas of the cerebral cortex, the periamygdaloid and prepiriform areas. Together, these are known as the primary olfactory cortex, and they also send fibers to many other centers within the brain to establish connections for automatic and emotional responses to olfactory stimulation.

Cranial nerves II, III, IV, and VI are concerned with vision. The *optic nerve* (II) is the primary nerve of sight. Its nerve fibers are axons that come from the retina, converge on the optic disc, and exit from the eye on both sides. The right nerve joins the left to form the optic chiasma. In the optic chiasma, fibers from the nasal half of the eye cross the midline, and fibers from the temporal half continue to run ipsilaterally. Most of the fibers synapse with nerve cells in the lateral geniculate body (of the thalamus) and then leave it, forming optic radiations. The optic radiations formed by these fibers terminate in the visual cortex and the visual association cortex.

Cranial nerve III is the *oculomotor nerve*, the nucleus of which is located at the level of the superior colliculus. Cranial nerve III has a somatomotor component that innervates the extraocular muscles to move the eyeball and a visceral component responsible for pupil constriction. Dysfunction of the third cranial nerve causes *ptosis* (drooping) of the eyelid. The eye may also be in abduction and turned down. If the visceral component is impaired, there is loss of the pupillary reflex and dilation of the pupil.

Cranial nerve IV is the *trochlear nerve*, the nucleus of which is at the level of the inferior colliculus. This nerve innervates the superior oblique muscle. Confirmed lesions cause diplopia (double vision).

Cranial nerve VI, the *abducens*, has its nucleus on the floor of the fourth ventricle. Dysfunction prevents lateral movements of the eyeball.

The remaining seven cranial nerves are vital for the production of normal speech and thus are given more attention, in the next part of this chapter, where we focus on the pathway, structures innervated, functional purpose, signs of dysfunction, and testing procedure for each nerve. Digest them one by one. Test yourself on them until you are firmly acquainted with each nerve. Refer to Figure 3–2 for attachment sites of the cranial nerves to the brainstem.

The Cranial Nerves for Speech and Hearing

Cranial Nerve V: Trigeminal

Anatomy

Both the motor and sensory roots of the trigeminal nerve are attached to the lateral edges of the pons. The motor nuclei are restricted to the pons, but the sensory nuclei extend from the mesencephalon to the spinal cord.

Innervation

The motor part of the trigeminal nerve innervates the following muscles: masseter, temporalis, lateral and medial pterygoids, tensor tympana, tensor veli palatine, mylohyoid, and the anterior belly of the digastric muscle.

The sensory fibers have three main branches:

1. The ophthalmic nerve, which is sensory to the forehead, eyes, and nose

2. The maxillary nerve, which is sensory to the upper lip mucosa, maxilla, upper teeth, cheeks, palate, and maxillary sinus

3. The mandibular nerve, which is sensory to the tongue, mandible, lower teeth, lower lip, part of the cheek, and part of the external ear

Function

Cranial nerve V is primarily responsible for mastication and for sensation to the face. Innervating the tensor velar palatine, it is partially responsible for flattening and tensing of the soft palate and for opening of the eustachian tube. Innervating an extrinsic laryngeal muscle (the anterior belly of the digastric), it also serves to assist in the upward and anterior movement of the larynx.

Testing

The jaw-closing and grinding lateral movements of chewing are the result of the function of the masseter and temporal, medial pterygoid, and lateral pterygoid muscles. The first three contribute to closure of the jaw, but only the masseter can be tested directly. To evaluate the masseter, palpate the area of the muscle (2 cm above and in front of the angle of the mandible) as the patient bites down as hard as possible and then relaxes. As the patient bites, you should feel the bulk of the muscle rise. Try this on yourself and many others to get the feel of it. The muscle body should feel very firm and bulky. The temporal muscle cannot be well-palpated; however, if it is atrophied (shrunken) from a lower motor neuron lesion, the temple of the face will be sunken.

You must also evaluate the strength of jaw closure. To do so, place your hand on the tip of the patient's mandible as the jaw is held open. Place the other hand on the forehead to prevent neck extension. Ask the patient to bite down hard against the resistance of your hand. She or he should be able to close the jaw against a moderate resistance.

The lateral pterygoids enable the jaw to lateralize in chewing. To evaluate them, ask the patient to open the jaw against resistance of your hand and note how the tip of the mandible lines up with the space between the upper medial incisors. Ask the patient to move the jaw from side to side and observe the facility of movement.

Finally, ask the patient to lateralize the jaw against resistance. Have him or her move the jaw to one side and hold it while you try to push it toward the center. Place your other hand against the opposite cheekbone so that the patient cannot use the neck to help.

The patient with a unilateral paralysis of cranial nerve V will show a deviation of the jaw to the side of the lesion and an inability to force the jaw to the side opposite the lesion. Atrophy may also be noted after a period of time. These problems result from lower motor neuron lesions. Upper motor neuron lesions that are unilateral do not affect cranial nerves as much, since the nuclei receive so many axons from the other hemisphere. Therefore, the paresis is usually transitory or mild unless there are bilateral upper motor neuron lesions.

In bilateral upper motor neuron lesions, there will be an observable limitation of jaw movements. Opening and closing movements of the jaw, though possible, are restricted. Gross chewing movements are seen, but chewing and biting may lack vigor and are performed slowly.

Neurologists may test for the jaw or masseter reflex when assessing the trigeminal nerve. A percussion hammer is used to strike a gentle blow to the examiner's finger while it is resting across the patient's chin and pressing down. The expected response in a patient with intact trigeminal function is often difficult to illicit; it is described as a bilateral contraction of the temporal and masseter muscles causing a sudden mandibular elevation. Because revealing results are difficult to elicit and thus must be very carefully interpreted, it is not recommended that this test be attempted by the speech-language pathologist.

To evaluate the sensory component of the trigeminal nerve, sensation to the face may be tested. The patient is asked to close the eyes, and a cotton swab is used to stroke the face in the three different distribution areas of the nerve. The examiner should stay in the central part of the face as there is considerable overlap on the periphery. Therefore, the ophthalmic division may be tested by stroking above the eyebrows; the maxillary division by stroking the upper lip in an upward movement toward the cheekbone; and the mandibular division by stroking between the lower lip and the chin in an upward movement toward the cheekbone. Left and right sides should be done separately and compared. Stroking should be done with firm pressure and kept consistent across all trials.

Cranial Nerve VII: Facial

Anatomy

The facial nerve is a complex nerve carrying two motor and two sensory components. It involves several different nuclei, all lying within the pons near the reticular formation.

The special sensory component of the facial nerve involves the taste fibers for the tongue and palate. These fibers have their primary sensory neurons in the geniculate ganglion. They enter the brainstem in the sensory root of the facial nerve, called the nervus intermedius. They run in a bundle, or fasciculus, called the *tractus solitarius*, and are joined in that bundle by the taste fibers from cranial nerves IX and X.

The taste fibers will split off from the facial nerve in the middle ear as the chorda tympani. This joins the lingual branch of cranial nerve V. The taste fibers then terminate in the nucleus of the tractus solitarius. The fibers are distributed to the taste buds of the anterior two thirds of the tongue. Some fibers also terminate in the taste buds in the hard and soft palates. Ascending fibers from the nucleus solitarius run to the ventro-posterior thalamus and then project to the cortical area for taste located at the lower end of the sensory strip in the parietal lobe.

The general sensory component of VII is a small cutaneous component whose nerve cells are found in the geniculate ganglion in the temporal bone. Impulses travel in the nervus intermedius, descending in the spinal tract of the trigeminal nerve and synapsing in the spinal nucleus of the trigeminal located in the upper medulla. This sensory component may supplement the mandibular portion of cranial nerve V, providing sensation from the wall of the acoustic meatus and the surface of the tympanic membrane.

The visceral motor component of cranial nerve VII is composed of cell bodies that are preganglionic autonomic motor neurons. These cell bodies are collectively called the *superior salivatory nucleus* and the *lacrimal nucleus*. The fibers from the nucleus travel in the nervus intermedius and divide in the facial canal, becoming the *greater petrosal nerve* and the *chorda tympani*. The petrosal nerve fibers follow a complicated path and join fibers of the trigeminal to reach the lacrimal and mucosal glands of the nasal and oral cavities, where they stimulate secretion.

The branchial motor component of the facial nerve is of critical importance to the speech-language pathologist. The fibers of the motor nucleus extend to the floor of the ventricle, curve around the nucleus of the abducens (cranial nerve VI), and exit the brainstem near the inferior margin of the pons. These fibers then join those from the nucleus of the tractus solitarius and the autonomic or parasympathetic nuclei and enter the internal auditory meatus as they extend through the facial canal of the petrosal bone. They leave the skull through the stylomastoid foramen. While coursing through the facial canal, the facial nerve travels through the tympanic cavity, innervating the stapedius muscle. Therefore, the facial nerve can be involved in pathologies related to the ear. Surgeons removing acoustic tumors must be mindful of the location of the facial nerve.

The part of the nucleus that innervates the lower part of the face receives most of the corticobulbar fibers from the opposite hemisphere; thus, innervation to these structures is primarily contralateral. The part that supplies the upper part of the face receives fibers from both cerebral hemispheres (that is, receives crossed and uncrossed fibers), and innervation is bilateral.

Innervation

The parasympathetic nuclei are also known as the superior salivatory and the lacrimal nuclei. The superior salivatory nucleus receives afferent information from the hypothalamus and olfactory system, as well as taste information from the mouth cavity. It supplies the submandibular sublingual salivary glands and the nasal and palatine glands.

The lacrimal nucleus solitarius receives information from afferent fibers from the trigeminal sensory nuclei for reflex response to corneal irritation. The sensory nucleus receives information concerning taste from fibers from the anterior two thirds of the tongue, the floor of the mouth, and the soft and hard palates.

The motor nucleus gives the face expression by innervation of the various facial muscles: that is, the orbicularis oculi, zygomatic, buccinator, orbicularis oris, and labial muscles. Other muscles innervated are the platysma, stylohyoid, and stapedius and the posterior belly of the digastric.

Function

Most important to the speech-language pathologist is the fact that the facial nerve is responsible for all movements of facial expression. All facial apertures are "guarded" by muscles innervated by the facial nerve: the eyes, the nose, the mouth, and the external auditory canal. Cranial nerve VII enables you to (1) wrinkle your forehead, (2) close your eyes tightly, (3) close your mouth tightly, (4) pull back the corners of your mouth and tense your cheeks, and (5) pull down the corners of your mouth and tense your anterior neck muscles.

Beyond these important movements in speech and swallowing, the facial nerve also assists in pulling the larynx up and back (through the belly of the digastric muscle). It provides motor innervation to the sublingual and submaxillary salivary glands, and it guards the middle ear by innervating the stapedius muscle, which dampens excessive movement of the ossicles in the presence of a loud noise. Finally, the facial nerve is partially responsible for taste.

Testing

Tests of facial expression are the primary tests for cranial nerve VII. Before you begin any motor testing, however, look closely at your patient's face at rest and note the symmetry. Then begin testing at the upper part of the face.

1. Ask the patient to wrinkle the forehead and look up at the ceiling. Note the symmetry of the wrinkling on both sides. Keep in mind that this ability or inability is diagnostic for localization. Since the upper part of the face is innervated bilaterally, only a lower motor neuron lesion would cause complete paralysis of this function. An upper motor neuron lesion causes some weakness on the opposite side, but it will not be nearly as perceptible because of the ipsilateral fiber innervation.
2. Next, ask the patient to close the eyes as tight as possible. Note the contraction of the orbicularis oculi and the consequent wrinkling around the eyes. Bilateral innervation is also present in this part of the face, though not to the degree that the forehead displays. The lower motor neuron–upper motor neuron difference holds true for dysfunction of this part of the face.
3. Finally, take a close look at mouth movements. First ask the patient to smile or pull back the corners of the lips. It helps to tell him or her to show the teeth when doing this, exaggerating the smile somewhat. Again, observe the symmetry of the two sides. Then ask the patient to pucker the lips, and observe the symmetry of constriction. Last, ask him or her to pull down the corners of the lips (as in pouting) or to try to wrinkle the skin of the neck. Inspect for symmetry. Test also for the strength of movement against resistance and compare the two sides of the mouth.

The patient with a lower motor neuron lesion of cranial nerve VII will have involvement of the entire side of the face on the side of the lesion (ipsilateral). See Figure 7–1 for an example of a unilateral facial paralysis. Though speech may be distorted, it is usually not significantly hindered by peripheral involvement of cranial nerve VII. The patient with an upper motor neuron lesion will show complete involvement of the lip and neck muscles, some degree of involvement of the area around the eyes, and little difficulty with the forehead or frontalis muscle. It should be noted

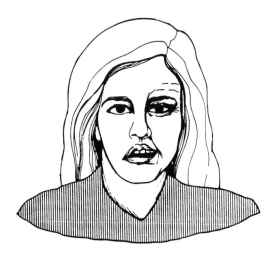

Figure 7–1 An illustration of a patient with a right lower motor neuron facial paralysis, which implicates involvement of the right VII nerve. Note the lack of contraction of orbicularis oculi, indicated by the lack of wrinkles around the eye. The patient lacks forehead wrinkles and has a flattened nasolabial fold on the right. The mouth also droops on the right.

that the paralysis is on voluntary movement. The patient may be seen to have almost normal movement for emotionally initiated movements such as a true smile, but will be unable to lateralize the lips when asked to do so voluntarily.

Since the facial nerve innervates the stapedius muscle, it may be paralyzed by a lesion. If this occurs, the patient may report that ordinary sounds seem uncomfortably loud.

The sensory component of the facial nerve may be assessed by testing the patient's sense of taste on the anterior two thirds of the tongue. Sensitivity of the two sides of the tongue should be compared. The patient should be able to identify the four primary tastes (salty, sour, bitter, and sweet) if the sensory pathways are intact.

Cranial Nerve VIII: Vestibular Acoustic or Vestibulocochlear

The following explanation assumes that you have completed a study of the anatomy of the ear and are well-versed in the structure and function of the cochlea and semicircular canals. It is imperative that you have a good working knowledge of the anatomy of the ear.

Anatomy

As you may ascertain from its name, the vestibulocochlear nerve consists of two distinct parts: the *vestibular nerve* and the *cochlear* or *acoustic nerve*. Both take afferent information from the internal ear to the nervous system, but, as their names imply, they carry different types of information.

The vestibular nerve consists of nerve cells and their fibers, which are in the vestibular ganglion located in the internal acoustic meatus. The fibers enter the brainstem in a groove between the lower border of the pons and the upper medulla oblongata. A few of the axons terminate in the flocculonodular lobe of the cerebellum. Most axons then enter the vestibular nuclear complex, which consists of a group of nuclei located in the floor of the fourth ventricle.

The cochlear nerve consists of nerve cells and fibers located in the *spiral ganglion* located around the *modiolus* of the cochlea. Nerve fibers wrap around each other in the modiolus, with a layering effect. Fibers from the apex, carrying low-frequency information, are found on the innermost part of the core, while fibers from the basal part of the cochlea, carrying high-frequency information, are found on the outermost layers. The nerve fibers from these cell bodies enter the brainstem at the lower border of the pons on the lateral side of the facial nerve. They are separated from the facial nerve fibers by the vestibular nerve.

When the cochlear fibers enter the pons, they divide into two branches. One branch enters the *dorsal cochlear nucleus* (high frequencies), and the other enters the ventral cochlear nucleus (low frequencies). Both nuclei are situated adjacent to the inferior cerebral peduncle.

From this point the axons take varied and complex paths. The system is largely contralateral. Most fibers decussate after the cochlear nuclei, though there are a few ipsilaterally projected fibers. The fibers form a tract called the *lateral lemniscus* as they ascend through the posterior portion of the pons and midbrain. All ascending fibers terminate in the medial geniculate body and from there project to the auditory cortex via the auditory radiations. Between the cochlear nuclei and the medial geniculate body, the fibers take one of several pathways including synapses at one or more of the following structures: the superior olives, the trapezoid body, the inferior colliculus, and the nucleus of the lateral lemniscus.

Innervation

Both portions of the vestibulocochlear nerve are primarily sensory in nature. The vestibular nerve receives afferent information from the utricle, saccule, and semicircular canal of the inner ear and from the cerebellum. The vestibular nerve also sends out efferent fibers that pass to the cerebellum through the inferior cerebral peduncles and also to the spinal cord, forming the *vestibulospinal tract*. In addition to these, efferent fibers are sent to the nuclei of cranial nerves III (oculomotor), IV (trochlear), and VI (abducens) through the medial longitudinal fasciculus. As outlined earlier, the cochlear nerve carries afferent fibers from the cochlea to the auditory cortex.

Function

Cranial nerve VIII takes afferent information from the internal ear to the nervous system. It is responsible for sound sensitivity, and it also innervates the utricle and the saccule of the inner ear, which are sensitive to static changes in equilibrium. In addition, innervation of the semicircular canals takes place through this nerve, controlling sensitivity to dynamic changes in equilibrium.

Testing

Although the speech-language pathologist may do hearing threshold screening or testing that may give information about the cochlear nerve, it is the audiologist who is usually responsible for thorough assessment of hearing and cochlear function. Neurologists often perform simple tuning fork tests for acuity and sound lateralization, while some prefer to use whispered words.

Testing the vestibular function is also not in the purview of the speech-language pathologist. Vestibular function is usually investigated with caloric tests that involve raising or lowering the temperature of the internal auditory meatus, thereby inducing current in the semicircular canals and stimulating the vestibular nerve for testing. Neurologists also use maneuvers of changing head position. Dynamic platform posturography is a technique developed in recent years to perform a functional assessment of how senses are used for balance.

The patient complaining of reduced hearing acuity, *tinnitus* (ringing in the ears), or dizziness should always be seen by an otologist and receive an audiological evaluation as well. The dizzy patient may be referred to a neurologist, who will usually also refer for audiological testing.

Cranial Nerve IX: Glossopharyngeal

Anatomy

The glossopharyngeal nerve carries two motor components and three sensory components. It can be found emerging from the medulla between the olive and the inferior cerebellar peduncle. The main trunk of the nerve exits the skull through the jugular foramen. There are three nuclei in the brainstem concerned with the functions of the glossopharyngeal nerve: the nucleus ambiguous, the inferior salivatory nucleus, and the nucleus solitarius.

Innervation

The *nucleus ambiguous* receives corticobulbar fibers from both hemispheres and is the efferent innervation to the stylopharyngeus muscle, which contributes toward the elevation of the pharynx and larynx. The inferior salivatory nucleus receives afferent information from the hypothalamus, from the olfactory system, and from the mouth cavity concerning taste. Efferent fibers supply the otic ganglion of the ear and the parotid salivary gland. The *nucleus solitarius* receives fibers arising from the inferior ganglia. Peripherally these visceral afferent fibers of cranial nerve IX mediate general sensation to the pharynx, soft palate, posterior third of the tongue, fauces, tonsils, ear canal, and tympanic cavity. The fibers decussate and travel upward to the opposite thalamic and some hypothalamic nuclei. From here the axons pass through the internal capsule and end in the lower postcentral gyrus.

Function

Cranial nerve IX is efferent to one muscle only—the *stylopharyngeus*. This muscle dilates the pharynx laterally and contributes to the elevation of the pharynx and larynx. It thereby serves to help clear the pharynx and larynx for swallowing. Secretomotor fibers are also provided for the parotid gland's production of saliva. Sensory fibers carry taste information from the posterior one third of the tongue. The glossopharyngeal nerve mediates the sensory portion of the pharyngeal gag.

Testing

Most of the functions of cranial nerve IX cannot be tested separately from those of cranial nerve X, as the vagus has the predominant control over laryngeal and pharyngeal sensory and motor function. However, testing the sensory portion of the pharyngeal gag does provide information about the integrity of cranial nerve IX. To do this, the examiner should use a cotton-tipped applicator with a long wooden end (as used in medical clinics). The examiner carefully puts the cotton tip back against one side of the posterior pharyngeal wall, avoiding any contact with the base of the tongue or the velum. With a gentle "poking" of the wall, a gag should be elicited. Both sides of the pharynx should be tested.

If a gag cannot be elicited, the examiner should ask if the patient feels the pressure of the touch. If the stimulus is felt and there is no gag, only the motor portion of the gag (mediated by the vagus) may be impaired.

This would be unusual. Since sensation precedes motor activity, the absence of sensation and of the gag implicates cranial nerve IX and gives the clinician information about the integrity of sensation to the upper pharynx, which can be important information in swallowing assessment.

Cranial Nerve X: Vagus

Anatomy

Like the glossopharyngeal nerve, the vagus also has three nuclei: the nucleus ambiguous, the dorsal nucleus, and the nucleus solitarius. These are also located in the medulla. The axon from the cell body of the nucleus ambiguous has a pharyngeal and a laryngeal branch. The laryngeal branch gives rise to the recurrent laryngeal nerve, which arises considerably below the larynx and ascends to terminate at the larynx. The right recurrent nerve runs in a loop behind the common carotid and subclavian arteries. The left recurrent nerve leaves the vagus at a lower level and loops under and behind the aortic arch. It then ascends to the larynx in a groove between the trachea and esophagus and enters through the cricothyroid membrane.

Innervation

The nucleus ambiguous receives an approximately equal number of corticobulbar fibers from both hemispheres; these fibers are efferent to the constrictor muscles of the pharynx and the intrinsic muscles of the larynx. The efferent fibers of the dorsal or parasympathetic nucleus innervate the involuntary muscles of the bronchi, esophagus, heart, stomach, small intestine, and a portion of the large intestine. The afferent fibers of the nucleus of the tractus solarius follow much the same path as those of the glossopharyngeal nerve and terminate in the postcentral gyrus.

Function

Vagus means "wanderer," and one can understand this name when considering the many functions of the vagus nerve. It is motor to the viscera (heart, respiratory system, and most of the digestive system). It supplies primary efferent innervation to the palatal muscles (except for innervation of the tensor palatine by the trigeminal). The vagus is also the primary efferent for the pharyngeal constrictors and is the afferent for the middle and inferior portions of the pharynx. In addition, it mediates sensation of the epiglottis. On its own, the vagus innervates the intrinsic muscles of the larynx, primarily through the recurrent laryngeal branch. The cricothyroid, however, is innervated by the superior laryngeal branch.

Testing

Remember that you are testing cranial nerves IX and X if you are evaluating swallowing function. Palatal function is controlled primarily by cranial nerve X with the tensor veli palatine innervated by V. Intrinsic laryngeal muscle function is covered solely by cranial nerve X.

Palatal function is tested by first observing the palate at rest as the patient opens the mouth to allow your view. Look at the palatal arches and observe their symmetry. Note if one arch hangs lower than the other. Next ask the patient to phonate an "ah" while you observe. The soft palate should elevate and move posteriorly and should do so symmetrically. If the palate does not elevate, the palatal gag reflex, innervated primarily by cranial nerve IX, should be tested by touching the tongue blade against the palatal arches. The gag is a reflex activity, and it is preserved in an upper motor neuron lesion since the reflex arc is still intact. As in all reflexes, it may be lost acutely after an upper motor neuron lesion; then it may become hyperactive. If both volitional and reflex activities of the palate are diminished, a lower motor neuron lesion is evidenced. Please bear in mind that palatal elevation is also reduced by a cleft palate, congenital oral malformations, and soft tissue palatal lesions. Do not overlook these vital facts in searching vigorously for an upper or lower motor neuron lesion.

Laryngeal function evaluation is adequately completed only by a direct or indirect laryngoscopy in which the vocal cords can be seen. A finer analysis of vocal cord movement patterns can be done utilizing laryngeal stroboscopy. Damage to the vagus nerve may cause paralysis or paresis of the vocal cord. There is bilateral innervation to the larynx, with the crossed and uncrossed fibers being approximately equal. Therefore, complete paralysis of a vocal cord from an upper motor neuron lesion is rare.

Preliminary assessment of laryngeal function is done through traditional clinical voice evaluation procedures. The patient is asked to phonate and prolong a vowel such as /a/. Maximum phonation time varies for normal adults. If the person can phonate for a 7 to 8 second duration, laryngeal and respiratory control is presumed acceptable. Perceptual analysis of the voice is done by the clinician during this phonation and during conversation. The patient may be asked to demonstrate laryngeal function and control by raising and lowering the pitch of a prolonged vowel or singing up and down the scale. Remember that the ability to change pitch depends on proper function of the cricothyroid muscle, which is innervated by the superior laryngeal nerve rather than the recurrent nerve. Estimate of the strength of laryngeal closure can be made perceptually by asking the patient to perform the *glottal coup*, which is essentially to make a short, sharp "grunting sound." A voluntary (as opposed to reflexive) cough should also be requested. The clinician is listening for the sound made at the larynx in these two maneuvers to be strong and sharp. Stress testing of the vocal mechanism is done by asking the patient to count to 300 or to keep talking for a prescribed length of time. More sophisticated analyses of the voice may be done employing instrumentation for acoustical analysis.

In spastic dysarthria cases from an upper motor neuron lesion, one will hear a rough, harsh quality on phonation. In bilateral upper motor neuron lesions (pseudobulbar palsy), there is a characteristic voice quality characterized by what Darley, Aronson, and Brown (1975) describe as "strain-strangle." This voice is harsh, with a very strained, tense quality as if the person is fighting to push the air flow through the larynx and supra-laryngeal areas.

A lower motor neuron lesion will cause complete paralysis of the ipsilateral vocal cord, resulting in a hoarse, breathy voice. In some lower motor neuron diseases, the voice will initially be strong; however, after the patient talks for a while, the voice becomes progressively weaker and more breathy. Transient hoarseness results sometimes from direct damage to the recurrent laryngeal nerve during carotid artery or thyroid surgery.

Cranial Nerve XI: Spinal Accessory

Anatomy
The accessory nerve consists of a cranial and a spinal root. The nucleus of the cranial root is found in the nucleus ambiguous of the medulla. It receives corticobulbar fibers from both cerebral hemispheres. These fibers then join the glossopharyngeal, vagus, and spinal accessory nerves.

The spinal root's nucleus is located in the spinal nucleus of the anterior gray column of the spinal cord. The fibers pass through the lateral white column and eventually form a nerve trunk, which joins the cranial root to pass through the foramen magnum. The spinal root then separates from the cranial root, however, to find its way to the sternocleidomastoid and trapezius muscles.

Innervation
The cranial root joins the vagus to innervate the uvula and the levator palatine. As mentioned earlier, the spinal root innervates the sternocleidomastoid and trapezius muscles.

Function
The accessory nerve's primary function is as motor to the muscles (including the sternocleidomastoid) that help turn, tilt, and thrust

forward the head or raise the sternum and clavicle if the head is in a fixed position and to the trapezius muscle, which is responsible for shrugging the shoulder.

Testing

When testing cranial nerve XI, we test the *spinal* part. The accessory part is accessory to the vagus and cannot be tested alone.

Initially, look at the size and symmetry of the sternocleidomastoids and palpate them. (Do this on yourself and others to get an idea of normal muscle size and firmness.) Ask the patient to turn the head to one side and hold it there while you try to push it back to the middle. Put one hand on the patient's cheek and the other on the shoulder to brace the patient. Gently push against the cheek and observe and palpate the sternocleidomastoid on the opposite side on the neck.

Next have the patient try to thrust the head forward while you resist the movement with your hand against the forehead. Again, observe and palpate the sternocleidomastoid muscle.

Finally, ask the patient to shrug his or her shoulders while you press down on the shoulders. You should feel the shoulders elevate against your gentle resistance.

Cranial Nerve XII: Hypoglossal

Anatomy

The hypoglossal nerve runs under the tongue and controls tongue movements. The nucleus, called the *hypoglossal nucleus*, is located in the medulla beneath the lower part of the fourth ventricle. It receives fibers from both cerebral hemispheres, with one exception. The cells serving the genioglossus muscle receive only contralateral fibers. The nerve fibers pass through the medulla and emerge in the groove between the pyramid and the olive. There are other apparent branches of the hypoglossal that are not connected with the hypoglossal nuclei but rather are derived from the ansa cervicalis of cervical vertebrae C1, C2, and C3. *Ansa* means "loop," and there are branches of these spinal nerves that form a loop and join the hypoglossal nerve to the sternothyroid, sternohyoid, and omohyoid muscles.

Innervation

The hypoglossal nerve innervates the intrinsic muscles of the tongue. It also innervates four extrinsic tongue muscles: the genioglossus, hyoglossus, chondroglossus, and styloglossus.

With the branches from the ansa cervicalis, cranial nerve XII contributes to the innervation of the sternothyroid, sternohyoid, and omohyoid muscles, thus contributing further to the elevation and depression of the larynx.

Function

The hypoglossal nerve innervates the muscles that are responsible for tongue movement. The four intrinsic muscles of the tongue control tongue shortening, concaving (turning the tip and lateral margins upward), narrowing, elongating, and flattening. The extrinsic muscles innervated account for tongue protrusion (genioglossus), drawing the tongue upward and backward (styloglossus), and retraction and depression of the tongue (hyoglossus). The hyoglossus also acts with the chondroglossus to elevate the hyoid bone, thus participating in phonation.

Testing

Initially, ask the patient to open the mouth and let you look at the tongue at rest. Inspect it for signs of atrophy. With a unilateral lower motor neuron lesion, one side of the tongue will look shrunken or atrophied. This atrophy occurs on the same side as the lower motor neuron lesion. With a lower motor neuron lesion, there may also be fasciculations or fibrillations, seen as tiny ripples under the surface of the tongue. Actually, authorities disagree whether these movements in the denervated tongue are fasciculations or fibrillations.

Normal tongues may also show some ripples when they are not completely relaxed. Therefore, if you think you see the fasciculations, ask the patient to move the tongue around and then relax it, and again observe the surface for fasciculation. Even in a normal tongue, however, you may continue to see the ripples. Therefore, as DeMyer (1980) points out, the clinician does better to rely on atrophy and weakness as signs of lower motor neuron damage. You should also observe the tongue for tremor or random movements at rest.

Next, ask the patient to protrude the tongue, and evaluate the symmetry of this posture. The tongue tip should be at midline. If the patient has weak lip musculature on one side, that side may be lower, causing the tongue to look as if it deviates to that side. Therefore, visually try to align the tip of the tongue with the midline of the jaw. You may also pull that side of the lip back so that it is symmetrical with the other side of the lip, and then ask the patient to protrude the tongue. If the cranial nerve is dysfunctional, the genioglossus will not be able to push its side out; the stronger side will overcome the weaker and the tongue will deviate to the weaker side (Figure 7–2).

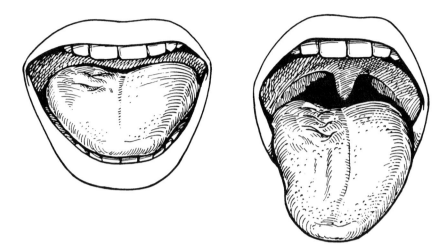

Figure 7–2 Unilateral paresis of the tongue. In the illustration on the left, the resting tongue shows a smaller weak side (atrophy) with a corrugated surface suggesting fasciculations and the effects of atrophy. These tongue signs suggest denervation. In the illustration on the right, the protruded tongue deviates to the weak side. In a lower motor neuron lesion, the deviated tongue points to the side of the lesion. Source: Redrawn and reproduced with permission from F. Darley et al., *Motor Speech Disorders* (Philadelphia: W. B. Saunders, 1975).

In lower motor neuron damage, the weakness is on the same side as the lesion. In upper motor neuron damage, because of the contralateral control, the tongue deviates to the side opposite to the lesion. For example, in many stroke patients with left hemisphere damage to the area of the motor strip, the tongue will show a characteristic deviation to the right on protrusion. This is usually less marked than in lower motor neuron tongue weakness.

The patient who has bilateral XII nerve damage will have weakness on both sides and will be unable to protrude the tongue beyond the lips. The clinician should try to assess the muscle tone of the tongue by moving the passive tongue with a tongue blade through the range of lateralization and elevation. Lower motor neuron lesions result in decreased tone or flaccidity. Upper motor neuron lesions result in increased tone or spasticity. Again, you must practice on many healthy people to be familiar with appropriate tonicity of the tongue musculature.

Strength of tongue protrusion may be tested by asking the patient to push against a tongue blade held immediately in front of the lips. You must try all of these tests for strength and rate of movement on yourself and your friends to familiarize yourself with the normal range of strength.

Other movements of the tongue must be evaluated to precisely document range, rate, and strength of the tongue for follow-up in treatment and for diagnostic purposes. Ask the patient to lateralize the tongue—that is, move it from one corner of the mouth to the other. The tongue should move the full range from corner to corner. Evaluate the strength of lateral movement by asking the patient to push the tongue against the inside of the cheek against your fingers placed for resistance on the outside of the cheek; ask the patient to make a ball in the cheek with the tongue. You may also put a tongue blade along the side of the tongue and have the person push against a light resistance.

The ability to elevate the tongue can be evaluated by having the person open the mouth to a moderate degree while you hold down the mandible with your finger on it. Ask the patient to try to touch the top lip and also the alveolar ridge with the tongue. This should be done with full range of movement and little effort.

Strength of elevation of the tip, blade, or back of tongue is difficult to assess with tongue blade resistance. Your hearing is the better assessor of strength of elevation. The tip of the tongue should be able to make firm contact to produce /t/, /d/, /tʃ/, (as in *ch*um), and /dʒ/ (as in *j*udge) and to elevate fully for /l/ and /n/. The blade of the tongue should elevate well to produce a distinct /i/ (e as in *ea*t) and /j/ (y as in *y*oung). Elevation of the back of the tongue is necessary for production of the velar consonants /k/ and /g/. Careful examination of the production of these consonants and vowels as well as others, in isolation and in context, will provide the most information regarding tongue elevation and strength.

Cranial Nerve Cooperation: The Act of Swallowing

The act of swallowing is highly complex and needs to be studied independently with respect to its cranial nerve innervation. Logemann (1984) describes normal deglutition as consisting of four phases: (1) the oral preparatory phase, (2) the oral phase, (3) the pharyngeal phase, and (4) the esophageal phase.

In the oral preparatory phase, the food is masticated and mixed with saliva, and it is formed into a cohesive bolus held against the hard palate. This stage is variable in duration depending on ease of mastication, oral motor efficiency, and whether one wishes to savor the taste. The oral stage begins when the lips seal and the back of the tongue begins moving the bolus posteriorly. The tongue forms a central groove that acts as a ramp or chute for the food. The oral stage is considered a voluntary part of the swallowing and typically takes less than 1 second. The pharyngeal phase, which also takes 1 second or less, begins with the triggering of the swallow response or pharyngeal response at the anterior faucial pillars. The triggering of the swallow causes several physiological activities to occur in the pharynx simultaneously: velopharyngeal closure; laryngeal elevation; inversion of the epiglottis; closure of all sphincters (aryepiglottic folds, false vocal folds, and true vocal folds); initiation of pharyngeal peristalsis (squeezing); and relaxation of the cricopharyngeal sphincter to allow material to pass from pharynx to esophagus. If the swallow is not triggered, this response does not occur, and none of these activities take place. The bolus may be pushed into the pharynx and come to rest in the valleculae or pyriform sinuses and spill over into the airway—that is, aspiration may occur.

Finally, in normal swallowing, the esophageal phase occurs as the bolus enters the esophagus through the cricopharyngeus and is passed through into the stomach. Normal esophageal transit time is 8 to 20 seconds.

Efficient swallowing demands cooperation and coordination of the cranial nerves that are also involved in speech production. Figure 7–3 is a simplified summary of the actions that take place in swallowing and the cranial nerves that are responsible. The trigeminal nerve (V) plays an important part because of the efferent control of the muscles of mastication and the afferent control for general sensation to the anterior two thirds of the tongue. Cranial nerve VII, the facial nerve, controls taste for the anterior two thirds of the tongue and controls the lip sphincter and the buccal muscles, allowing food to be held inside the mouth.

The hypoglossal nerve (XII) controls the movement of the tongue. Through research using pharyngeal manometry, it has been found that the tongue is the major force generating the driving pressure that pushes the bolus through the pharynx (Cerenko, McConnel, & Jackson, 1989). This action of the tongue has been compared with that of a plunger and is termed the *tongue driving force*. Pharyngeal constriction, controlled by the vagus nerve, has been found to be much less of a force than originally believed. A descending pharyngeal contraction was shown in the study by Cerenko et al. to be applied only to the residual bolus tail. This constriction serves to clear the bolus from the laryngeal vestibule. It is therefore termed the *pharyngeal clearing force*.

The vagus also mediates the action of the cricopharyngeus, which relaxes to allow the bolus to pass from the hypopharynx to the esophagus. The movement of the intrinsic muscles of the larynx to close the entrance to the airway is also innervated by the vagus. The elevation and anterior movement of the larynx is a significant mechanical force

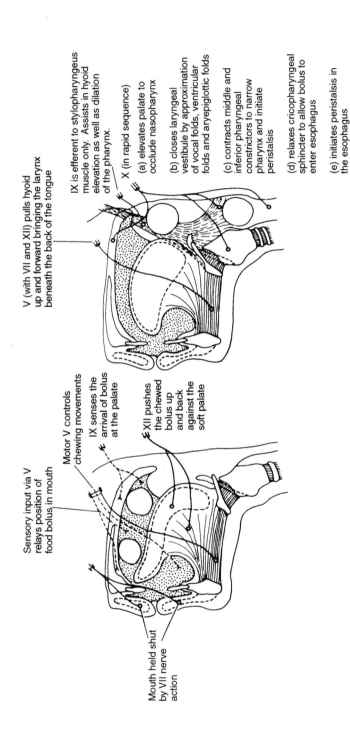

Figure 7–3 The neurology of swallowing. Redrawn and reproduced with permission from J. Patten, *Neurologic Differential Diagnosis* (London: H. Starke, Ltd., 1977).

contributing to the opening of the cricopharyngeus. Therefore, cranial nerves V, VII, IX, X, and XII, all with efferent innervation to one or more extrinsic muscles of the tongue and larynx, are important to this aspect of swallowing. The study by Cerenko et al. also indicated that the opening of the cricopharyngeus creates a negative pressure and, thus, a suction pump effect that significantly increases the rate of bolus flow and contributes to the elimination of the bolus before the larynx reopens.

The hypoglossal, glossopharyngeal, and vagus nerves therefore all contribute in a major way to clearing the bolus through the pharynx. The tongue driving force and the pharyngeal clearing force combined with the hypopharyngeal suction pump produce a rapid transit through the pharynx once the swallow response has been triggered.

The glossopharyngeal nerve is thought to be the primary afferent of the swallow response, and the vagus is thought to be the secondary afferent. The "swallowing center" is located in the medulla in the nucleus solitarius where the glossopharyngeus and vagus terminate. The sensory events stimulating the swallow response occur with stimulation to jaw, posterior tongue, faucial pillars, and upper pharynx. This stimulation is mediated through the glossopharyngeal, as well as the vagus nerves and trigeminal. These afferent fibers converge on the nucleus solatarius in the medulla. Via interneurons they communicate with neurons in the nucleus ambiguous, thereby stimulating the motor response. The medullary swallowing center is referred to as the *central pattern generator* (Larson, 1985). It is hypothesized that the triggering of the swallow response and the timing and sequence of the muscle contractions that follow are controlled by a network of neurons in the medulla. Sensory feedback may alter the detail of the central pattern generator to some extent (Miller, 1982).

If swallowing is inefficient and aspiration occurs, a reflexive cough should occur as one of the respiratory system's defenses against foreign matter. The cough reflex is induced by irritation of the afferent fibers of the pharyngeal distribution of the glossopharyngeal nerve along with the sensory endings of the vagus nerve in the larynx, trachea, and larger bronchi (Cherniack, Cherniack, & Naimark, 1972).

Assessment of Swallowing

The cranial nerve exam is critical to the assessment of swallowing. Careful evaluation of the sensory component of the cranial nerves is probably more important in the swallowing evaluation than when the examination is for a speech disorder alone.

Taste, carried by cranial nerves VII and IX, should be tested using some of the primary tastes (salt, sweet, bitter, and sour). Sour has been noted to be particularly stimulating to the swallow (Logemann et al., 1995) and should be one of the tastes used.

General sensation to the tongue, carried by cranial nerves V and IX (posterior one third), should be tested with the two sides and compared as to sensitivity to touch. As previously mentioned, the pharyngeal gag should be tested, if possible.

The motor examination for swallowing should consist of the same maneuvers as for the speech examination. The clinician will want to do an assessment of swallowing, observing the patient's attempt at swallowing a liquid, something of a pudding consistency, and a solid. This swallowing should only be done if the clinician's judgment is that it will be safe to try in the clinic setting. If there are concerns about patient safety or if the cranial nerve examination has pointed to a likely pharyngeal stage swallowing disorder, a modified barium swallow should be requested. This should be performed only by a speech-language pathologist or other professional with appropriate training and experience in the administration and interpretation of this radiological procedure. The purpose of the examination should be to document problems and to evaluate therapeutic alternatives that may improve oral intake. FEES, or Fiberoptic Endoscopic Examination for Swallowing (Langmore, Schatz, and Olsen, 1988) is another instrumental procedure that may be helpful when there is a pharyngeal stage disorder. Ultrasound has been used to examine the oral stage (Sonies, 1990) and manometry has been used to look at the pharyngeal and esophageal pressures (McConnel, Cerenko, Hersch, Weil, 1988).

Summary

The cranial nerves are vital for intact speech production, and the speech-language pathologist must be knowledgeable about their functions. There are 12 pairs of cranial nerves and seven of them are directly related to speech production: cranial nerves V (trigeminal), VII (facial), VIII (vestibular acoustic), IX (glossopharyngeal), X (vagus), XI (spinal accessory), and XII (hypoglossal). The five cranial nerves most involved in the oral musculature are summarized in Table 7–2. This chapter refers to the embryologic origin of the cranial nerves, explaining which are somitic or branchial in origin and which are the solely special sensory nerves. The anatomy, innervation, function, and testing of each of the nerves associated with speech is then discussed. The cooperation of several cranial nerves in the act of swallowing is also detailed.

Table 7-2 Summary of Cranial Nerve Function for the Oral Musculature

Cranial Nerve	Muscles Innervated	Movements and Sensation Innervated	Test Procedure	Signs of Lower Motor Neuron Damage	Signs of Upper Motor Neuron Damage
V: Trigeminal	Masseter, tensor tympani, tensor veli palatine, mylohyoid, digastric (anterior belly)	Jaw closing, lateral jaw movement	Palpation of masseter; closing and lateralization against resistance	Weakness, jaw deviation to lesion side, atrophy	Mild, transitory weakness
VII: Facial	Orbicularis oculi and oris, zygomatic, buccinator, platysma, stylohyoid, stapedius, portion of digastric (posterior belly)	Forehead wrinkling, closing eyes, closing mouth, smiling, tensing cheeks, pulling down corner of mouth, tensing anterior neck muscles, moving stapedius to dampen ossicles; taste from anterior two thirds of tongue and hard and soft palates	Observation of facial symmetry at rest; have patient wrinkle forehead, close eyes tightly, smile, pucker, and pull down lip corners; identification of tastes	Involvement of entire side of face, weakness, limited range of movement, decreased taste sensation	Complete involvement of lips and neck muscles, less involvement of eye area muscles, little difficulty with forehead muscles; weakness, limited range of movement of affected muscles; decreased taste sensation

Table 7-2 (continued)

Cranial Nerve	Muscles Innervated	Movements and Sensation Innervated	Test Procedure	Signs of Lower Motor Neuron Damage	Signs of Upper Motor Neuron Damage
IX: Glossopharyngeal	Stylopharyngeus, otic ganglion, parotid salivary gland, part of the middle pharyngeal constrictor	Elevation of pharynx and larynx, pharyngeal dilation, salivation; taste from posterior one third of tongue; sensation from posterior tongue and upper pharynx	Tested with cranial nerve X for motor; sensory test for pharyngeal gag		
X: Vagus	Inferior, middle, and superior pharyngeal constrictors; salpingopharyngeus glossopalatine, pharyngopalatine, levator veli palatine, uvular, cricothyroid, thyroarytenoid, posterior and lateral cricoarytenoid, interarytenoid, and transverse and oblique	Palatal elevation and depression, laryngeal movement, pharyngeal constriction, cricopharyngeal function	Observation of palatal movement, palatal gag reflex; laryngoscopic evaluation of vocal musculature; ability to change pitch; phonation time; assessment of swallowing	Absence of gag reflex, poor movement of palate or pharyngeal wall, absent or delayed swallow response, aspiration, breathy hoarse voice (may be	Poor palatal or pharyngeal wall movement, harshness or strained-strangled voice quality, delayed or absent swallow reflex, aspiration

				improved by pushing effort)	
	interarytenoid muscles; various muscles of the viscera, esophagus, and trachea				
XII: Hypoglossal	Superior longitudinal, inferior longitudinal, transverse, vertical, genioglossus, hyoglossus, and styloglossus	All tongue movements as well as some elevation of the hyoid bone	Observation for atrophy or fasciculations, as well as symmetry on protrusion; assessment for lateralization, protrusion, elevation, retraction (to observe range of movement); assessment of movement against resistance for strength testing on lateral, protrusion, and elevation movement; articulation testing	Atrophy, fasciculations, weakness, reduced range of movement, deviation of tongue to side of lesion, decreased tone, consonant imprecision	Weakness, reduced range of movement, deviation of tongue to contralateral side, increased tone, consonant imprecision

References and Further Readings

Barr, M. L., & Kiernan, J. A. (1983). *The human nervous system.* Philadelphia: Harper and Row.

Cerenko, D., McConnel, F. M. S., & Jackson, R. T. (1989). Quantitative assessment of pharyngeal bolus driving forces. *Otolaryngology Head and Neck Surgery*, 100, 1, 57–63.

Cherniack, R., Cherniack, L., & Naimark, A. (1972). *Respiration in health and disease* (2nd ed.). Philadelphia: W. B. Saunders.

Darley, F., Aronson, A., & Brown, J. (1975). *Motor speech disorders.* Philadelphia: W. B. Saunders.

DeMyer, W. (1980). *Technique of the neurologic examination: A programmed text* (3rd ed.). New York: McGraw-Hill.

Duffy, J. R. (1995) *Motor speech disorders: Substrates, differential diagnosis, and management.* St. Louis: Mosby–Year Book, Inc.

Langmore, S., Schatz, K., and Olsen, N. (1988). Fiberoptic endoscopic examination of swallowing safety: A new procedure. *Dysphagia*, 2, 216–219.

Larson, C. (1985). Neurophysiology of speech and swallowing. *Seminars in Speech and Language*, 6, 275–289.

Logemann, J. A. (1984). *Evaluation and treatment of swallowing disorders.* San Diego: College Hill Press.

Logemann, J. A., Pauloski, B. R., Colangelo, L., Lazarus, C., & Fujiu, M. (1995). Effects of a sour bolus on oropharyngeal swallowing measures in patients with neurogenic dysphagia. *Journal of Speech and Hearing Research*, 38, 556–563.

McConnel, F., Cerenko, D., Hersh, T., and Weil, L. (1988). Evaluation of pharyngeal dysphagia with manofluorography. *Dysphagia*, 2, 187–195.

Miller, A. J. (1982). Deglutition. *Physiology Reviews*, 62, 129–184.

Perlman, A. L. (1991). The neurology of swallowing. *Seminars in Speech and Language*, 12, 171–184.

Snell, R. S. (1980). *Clinical neuroanatomy for medical students.* Boston: Little, Brown and Company.

Sonies, B. (1990). Ultrasound imaging and swallowing. In M. Donner and B. Jones (Eds.), *Normal and abnormal swallowing: Imaging in diagnosis and therapy.* New York: Springer Verlag.

8 ⬜⬜⬜ ⬜⬜⬜ ⬜⬜⬜

Clinical Speech Syndromes of the Motor Systems

"Speech is deranged in a variety of ways by disease of the brain. The process of articulation is immediately affected by a mechanism of nerve nuclei situated in the pons and medulla, but these are excited to action by centers in the cerebral cortex. Thus there are higher and lower mechanisms; the former is cerebral, the latter is bulbar."

—William R. Gowers, *A Manual of Disease of the Nervous System*, 1888

The Dysarthrias

As a speech-language pathologist you will need an understanding of the function of the cranial nerves and the rest of the motor and sensory system for the treatment of the motor speech disorder known as *dysarthria*. In the Mayo Clinic study, Darley, Aronson, and Brown (1969a) define *dysarthria* as the speech disorder resulting from paralysis, weakness, or incoordination of the speech musculature that is of neurologic origin. Their definition encompasses any symptoms of motor disturbance of respiration, phonation, resonance, articulation, and prosody.

Damage to the motor system responsible for speech production may occur at any point along the pathway from the cerebrum to the muscle itself. In their classic studies of types of dysarthria resulting from certain sites of damage in the neural system, Darley, Aronson, and Brown (1969a, 1969b) identified six different dysarthrias based on neuroanatomical and acoustic-perceptual judgments of speech. In this chapter we describe the classic dysarthrias according to neuroanatomical site of dysfunction, associated disease processes, and the effects of these diseases on articulation, resonance, phonation, prosody, and swallowing. The following is not an exhaustive discussion of the diseases or of the types of dysarthrias resulting from neurological disease. Keep in mind that any disease or trauma that affects the movement, coordination, and timing of the oral musculature may produce a dysarthria.

Upper Motor Neuron Lesions

Recall that upper motor neuron damage may result in a spastic paralysis and hyperactive reflexes. The dysarthria associated with unilateral upper motor neuron lesions is called *unilateral upper motor neuron dysarthria*. The dysarthria associated with bilateral upper motor neuron lesions is known as *spastic dysarthria*.

Unilateral Upper Motor Neuron Dysarthria

As discussed by Duffy (1995), the dysarthria associated with unilateral upper motor neuron damage has been given scant attention in the literature probably because the symptoms are usually mild and sometimes transitory. This section on upper motor neuron lesions is devoted primarily to a discussion of spastic dysarthria for the same reasons. However, a brief review of unilateral upper motor neuron dysarthria, as it has been termed by Duffy, is warranted since it is as frequently encountered as the other types discussed in this chapter.

The primary etiology of unilateral upper motor neuron dysarthria is stroke. Many of the other etiologies of upper motor neuron damage cause more diffuse brain injury and will result more often in bilateral damage to the pyramidal pathways. Trauma and tumors can cause injury confined to a single hemisphere and can produce a unilateral upper motor neuron dysarthria. Unilateral upper motor neuron dysarthria can result from damage to either hemisphere.

Only a small number of studies have looked at the speech characteristics of unilateral upper motor neuron dysarthria (Duffy and Folger, 1986; Hartman and Abbs, 1992). The collective findings of these studies indicate that the most prominent deviant characteristic of speech is imprecise articulation. Slowed rate and irregular articulatory breakdown were also noted in a number of cases. Other characteristics present in some cases were harshness, reduced loudness, and hypernasality. Most characteristics were described as mild to moderate in severity, although some patients presented with more severe dysarthria. Though many patients demonstrated significant recovery during the spontaneous recovery period, some dysarthrias persisted and required speech therapy for the reduced intelligibility.

Swallowing in Patients With Unilateral Damage

Robbins' study (1989) of patients with left- and right-hemisphere strokes showed that the stroke patients differed from healthy patients by increased oral stage durations for liquid and semisolid swallows and by the occurrence of laryngeal vestibule penetration. This difficulty with oral stage transit was particularly true for left-hemisphere–damaged patients. Upon further analysis, Robbins also found that the right cerebrovascular accident (CVA) patients demonstrated laryngeal penetration and aspiration significantly more often than the left CVA patients. There was a much greater frequency of silent aspiration (that is, no coughing occurred reflexively) in the right CVA patients. More aspiration also occurred with anterior lesions than with posterior lesion sites.

Evatt et al. (1993) reported on a study of swallowing in 57 acute unilateral stroke patients. They found that aspiration in association with reduced pharyngeal clearance was present in 39 percent of the right-hemisphere–damaged patients and 57 percent of the left-hemisphere–damaged patients. The incidence of aspiration was also significantly greater in left-hemisphere–damaged patients than in right-hemisphere–damaged patients when analysis was done on individuals over the age of 65. A study by Alberts et al. (1992) using magnetic resonance imaging concluded that stroke patients should be individually evaluated for swallowing dysfunction regardless of the location or size of the lesion, since even small-vessel strokes were associated with aspiration in greater than 20 percent of patients.

Spastic Dysarthria

Etiology

Bilateral upper motor neuron damage may result from stroke, head trauma, tumor, infection, degenerative disease, and inflammatory or toxic-metabolic diseases. In most instances of spastic dysarthria, there is bilateral damage to both the direct activation pathway (corticobulbar or corticospinal tract) and the indirect activation pathway (extrapyramidal pathways from cortex to brainstem and spinal cord). This usually occurs because the pathways are in close proximity from cortex to the termination at the cranial nerve or spinal nerve. The resulting oral-motor disorder from bilateral upper motor neuron damage to both systems is sometimes called *pseudobulbar palsy*. This name is derived from the resemblance of the oral-motor and speech characteristics to lower motor neuron damage and flaccid dysarthria (bulbar palsy).

Associated Neurologic Characteristics

Direct activation pathway damage results in the characteristic loss of skilled movement, hyporeflexia, a positive Babinski sign, and muscle weakness and loss of tone.

Damage to the indirect activation pathway causes increased muscle tone (*spasticity*) and hyperactive stretch reflexes. This hypertonicity and hyperreflexia will dominate if both systems are damaged, which is usually the case. Although there is increased tone, the muscles are weak, range of movement is limited, and rate of movement is slow due to the direct activation motor system damage.

The Oral Musculature

In pseudobulbar palsy, the oral musculature usually shows severe impairment of range and rate of movement. The tongue may extend only to the lips on protrusion. The lips move slowly and excursion is limited. Palatal movement is severely reduced and very sluggish on phonation. The gag reflex may be absent in the acute stages but later returns and may be hyperactive. Chewing and swallowing are both frequently affected, and there is drooling in most cases.

Speech Characteristics

The patient usually demonstrates a classical spastic dysarthria. Speech characteristics are as follows.

Phonation

The voice of the patient with spastic dysarthria is described as harsh, and many have a characteristic strained-strangled quality. An effortful grunt is often heard at the end of vocalizations. Excessively low pitch is frequently found, with pitch breaks in some cases. Very little variation in loudness (*monoloudness*) and reduced stress are also noted. Occasionally heard in spastic dysarthria is excess and equal stress (that is, inappropriate stress on monosyllabic words and the usually unstressed syllables of polysyllabic words).

Resonance

Hypernasality is a frequent component of spastic dysarthria. Nasal emission is uncommon, however.

Articulation

As in most dysarthrias, imprecision of consonant production is a noticeable part of the speech disorder in spastic dysarthria. Vowel distortion has been noted in some cases. Zeigler and von Cramer's acoustic study (1986) of 10 patients with spastic dysarthria revealed a disproportionate impairment of the back of the tongue compared with the blade of the tongue. Impaired acceleration of the moving articulators also accounted for part of the distortion and the increase in production time often noted in these speakers.

Swallowing

Horner, Massey, and Brazer (1993) studied 70 patients with bilateral hemispheric strokes. Using videofluoroscopy, they found that 49 percent of the patients aspirated. The following symptoms associated with dysphagia are often observed in patients with bilateral upper motor neuron damage: reduced labial, lingual, and mandibular strength and sensation; delayed swallow response; reduced pharyngeal peristalsis; incomplete laryngeal elevation and closure; and cricopharyngeal dysfunction (Cherney, 1994). The dysphagia may be severe, and drooling may be noted. With mild dysphagia, the patient may unconsciously alter the eating pattern to eat more slowly and carefully, denying any difficulty (Duffy, 1995).

Lower Motor Neuron Lesions

Flaccid Dysarthria

Damage to the lower motor neuron system impairs the final common pathway for muscle contraction. The muscles become hypotonic or flaccid. Thus, every type of movement is affected; that is, voluntary, automatic, and reflexive movement are all impaired, and a flaccid dysarthria may be seen.

Etiology

Any disease that affects part of the motor unit—the cell body, its axon, the myoneural junction, or the muscle fibers themselves—may yield lower motor neuron symptoms. Thus, viral infections, tumors, trauma to the nerve itself, or a brainstem stroke with involvement of the nerve fibers may be the cause of the dysarthria. A disease known as *myasthenia gravis* (discussed in Chapter 4 and below) results from impairment of transmission across the myoneural junction or the synapse between the nerve and muscle. *Bulbar palsy* results from damage to the motor units of the cranial nerves. *Mobius syndrome (congenital facial diplegia)* involves bilateral sixth (abducens) and seventh (facial) nerve palsies of congenital origin. Mobius syndrome most commonly involves bilateral facial (VII) palsies and bilateral abducens (VI) palsies, rather than generalized bulbar palsy. Most patients with these palsies talk acceptably except for slurring. Direct muscle involvement is found in such diseases as muscular dystrophy, myotonia, and myositis.

Associated Neurologic Characteristics

Damage to the lower motor neuron system causes a flaccid paralysis. Reflexes are reduced; that is, there is hyporeflexia. The affected muscle usually becomes shrunken or atrophied over time. Many times the involved muscles, especially the tongue muscles, will be found to show *fasciculations*—tiny spontaneous muscle contractions of the motor unit or muscle fibers innervated by an axon. The fasciculations appear as spontaneous dimplings of the tongue, which may look as though there are tiny moving worms just beneath its surface.

The Oral Musculature

Since the cranial nerve nuclei are dispersed throughout the brainstem rather than being clustered together, the oral structures may be selectively impaired and should be evaluated carefully.

Muscle tone in lower motor neuron damage is flaccid or hypotonic. Muscles are weak. The affected side of the lips will sag, and in some cases drooling may be present. In bilateral weakness the whole mouth may sag, and the lower lip may be so weak that there is habitual open-mouth posture. The patient may have difficulty puckering the lips or pulling up the angles of the lips to smile.

Weakness of the mandibular muscles may not be readily evident in unilateral involvement. Careful observation will reveal that the jaw deviates to the side of weakness. With bilateral damage the jaw obviously sags. With damage to any component of the motor unit supplying the tongue, the muscles become atrophied and shrunken over time and the tongue is *atonic* or flabby. This tends to affect protrusion, lateralization, and elevation, particularly of the posterior portion of the tongue. Fasciculations are often observed after a period of time.

Palatal weakness or immobility may also be present, and there will be reduced or absent gag reflex. There may be pharyngeal involvement, causing swallowing difficulty and possibly nasal regurgitation of fluids.

Speech Characteristics

As a speech pathologist, you are most likely to be consulted concerning patients with a bulbar palsy resulting from vascular disease, head trauma, or diseases such as amyotrophic lateral sclerosis. These patients may exhibit a flaccid dysarthria and show some of the following characteristics on speech testing.

Phonation

Unilateral vocal fold paralysis is relatively unusual with those disease processes affecting the brainstem nuclei. If there is unilateral damage, the quality of phonation will depend on the position of the vocal fold. If it is paralyzed in an adducted position, the voice will be harsh and loudness will be reduced. If it is in the abducted position, more breathiness is heard with reduced loudness.

More likely is bilateral vocal cord involvement. The characteristics of this are a breathy voice, inspiratory stridor (or audible inhalation), and abnormally short phrases. Monotony of pitch and loudness are distinctive in many patients as well.

Resonance

Hypernasality is noted as an outstanding characteristic of the patients with flaccid dysarthria. Nasal emission of air is also found in a high percentage of patients.

Articulation

Imprecise consonant production may be present from mild to severe (unintelligible speech) degrees. The consonants requiring firm contact from tongue tip elevation are particularly vulnerable. *Plosives* such as /p/, /t/, and /k/, and *fricatives* such as /f/ and /s/ are frequently affected because of the lack of intraoral pressure that results from palatal dysfunction.

Swallowing

A brainstem CVA can cause a flaccid dysarthria with lesions affecting the motor nuclei. Robbins' study (1989) of 10 patients with brainstem CVAs found that these patients aspirated more frequently than did the patients with left or right cortical CVAs. Aspiration usually occurred during the swallow because of reduced airway protection or after the swallow because of large amounts of stasis in the pharyngeal recesses, particularly in the piriform sinuses. Incomplete as well as delayed relaxation of the cricopharyngeal sphincter was also noted in these patients.

Myasthenia Gravis

Speech Characteristics

Myasthenia gravis is a chronic autoimmune disease resulting from a reduction in available acetylcholine receptors at the neuromuscular junction. Usually, changes in the eyes such as ptosis (drooping of the eyelid) or double vision occur. The muscles may be weak, with the jaw sagging accompanied by weak chewing. Swallowing difficulty, or *dysphagia*, is not uncommon, and myasthenia especially should be considered with a history of difficulty with swallowing that worsens in use and improves with rest (Logemann, 1983).

Voice symptoms can exist without other signs of dysarthria. The flaccid dysphonia of myasthenia should be suspected when, despite normal laryngoscopic findings, the voice nevertheless becomes progressively more breathy and reduced in intensity as the client speaks. There may also be respiratory as well as extremity weakness, and it should be noted that myasthenia can occur with no oral motor involvement.

Mixed Upper and Lower Motor Neuron Lesions

Amyotrophic Lateral Sclerosis

In clinical practice one is very likely to find that a lesion or disease process has not confined itself to one motor system but, rather, has affected both upper and lower motor neuron systems. The most frequently encountered example of this damage is *amyotrophic lateral sclerosis* (also known as Lou Gehrig's disease). Amyotrophic lateral sclerosis, or ALS, causes progressive degeneration of the neurons of the upper and lower motor neuron systems and is of unknown etiology. Onset is typically in the fifth decade, although it may be earlier or later, and early symptoms depend on which motor neurons are affected initially. If brainstem nuclei are the first to be affected, the initial signs may be slurring of speech or difficulty swallowing. Often there is only a slight change in voice quality as the first sign. The bulbar or brainstem symptoms are particularly devastating, and verbal communication and oral feedings usually become impossible over time. The patient with this type of ALS has a variable life expectancy but typically may survive only 1 to 3 years after onset. Pneumonia is frequently the cause of death. There is no known effective treatment or cure for ALS, although there are many palliative treatments, including physical therapy, drugs for reduction of muscle pain, and speech therapy in some cases.

Associated Neurologic Characteristics

Signs may be present from damage to both upper and lower motor neuron systems. Muscles are weak but reflexes are hyperactive. Spasticity is usually present unless the lower motor neuron damage is well-advanced.

The Oral Musculature

The oral peripheral examination will yield indications of a pervasive weakness in lips, tongue, and palate. Range of movement will be reduced, and sometimes one side is slightly more affected than the other. The tongue may show fasciculations and, in more advanced cases, atrophy. The patient may report and demonstrate difficulty swallowing, especially liquids, and, with progression, difficulty handling oral secretions.

Speech Characteristics

Again, we face the signs of involvement of both upper and lower motor neuron systems. It is unpredictable as to which signs will predominate in a given case and what changes may occur through the course of the disease. The Mayo Clinic study (Darley, Aronson, & Brown, 1975) involved 30 patients with ALS. The characteristics of the speech of this group were as follows.

Phonation

Some patients showed symptoms similar to those shown by pseudobulbar palsy patients, with much harshness and a strain-strangle quality associated with low pitch. The harshness associated with ALS may often have a wet, gurgly quality. Other patients showed signs more like those of the bulbar group, with poor vocal fold adduction resulting in breathiness and short phrases. Audible inspiration was also noted. Monotony of pitch and loudness as well as reduction of stress were present in most patients.

Resonance

Hypernasality was frequent in these cases. Nasal emission, though noted, was not prominent.

Articulation

Imprecise consonant production was a principal characteristic. Vowels were often distorted, as were consonants. The slow rate and reduced range of movement of the articulators affected sound production greatly. Hypernasality also contributed to phoneme distortion, and precision of articulation was often so poor as to render speech unintelligible.

Swallowing

The degree of dysphagia in patients with ALS varies greatly depending on the extent of involvement of the oral musculature and the type of motor system involvement predominating. There is frequently evidence of poor lingual control with lingual stasis and aspiration before the swallow. A delayed swallow response may also be present, causing aspiration before the swallow. Poor tongue propulsion, weak pharyngeal contractions, and/or cricopharyngeal dysfunction may also result in pharyngeal stasis and aspiration after the swallow. Airway protection may be significantly better in patients with predominantly spastic (upper motor neuron) symptoms than in those with more lower motor neuron symptoms. The amount of aspiration may thus be reduced in these patients despite a severe dysarthria.

Dysphagia usually parallels or follows the loss of speech. Management of secretions and maintaining appropriate amounts of fluid intake are often huge challenges for ALS patients. Feeding tube placement is often necessary during the final course of the disease.

Basal Ganglia Lesions: Dyskinetic Dysarthrias

The basal ganglia control circuit contributes to complex movements by integrating and controlling the component parts of the movements and also helps to inhibit unplanned movement. Lesions produce dyskinetic movements and may yield two types of dysarthria, *hypokinetic* and *hyperkinetic.*

Hypokinetic Dysarthria: Parkinsonism

The most common disease associated with hypokinetic dysarthria is Parkinson's disease. In this disorder there are degenerative changes in the substantia nigra, which cause a deficiency in a chemical neural transmitter known as *dopamine* in the caudate nucleus and putamen. Parkinson's disease is usually idiopathic (that is, spontaneous, not caused by another disease), but parkinsonism (or parkinson-like symptoms) is caused by carbon monoxide poisoning, arteriosclerosis, manganese poisoning, and some tranquilizing drugs (for example, Compazine, Stelazine, and Haldol).

Associated Neurologic Characteristics

The major features of parkinsonism include one or more of the following (Capildeo, Haberman, & Rose, 1981). A tremor may be present at rest that tends to subside on movement and is absent during sleep. It is often called a *pill rolling tremor* because of the pattern of movement of the fingers, as if rolling a small pill between the thumb and the fingers. Rigidity is a common characteristic and is elicited by passive movement of the limb, which induces involuntary contractions in the muscle being stretched. The rigidity may be smooth or intermittent (referred to as *cogwheel rigidity*). *Bradykinesia*, also common in parkinsonism, is defined as reduced speed of movement of a muscle through its range. *Hypokinesia*, or reduced amplitude of movement, is a prime characteristic as well.

Dementia is a correlate of Parkinson's disease, with an incidence between 15 and 40 percent (Brown and Marsden, 1984). Language characteristics of this dementia include impaired receptive vocabulary, difficulty in comprehending the meanings of ambiguous sentences, impaired ability to describe objects verbally, and impaired ability to identify a speaker's intention.

Other features of parkinsonism are referred to as minor, but at least one of these features should be present for the diagnosis to be made. These include *micrographia*, or the tendency for the height of the handwritten letters to get smaller as the person writes. Excessive salivation and a dysphonia, described later, may be present. The parkinsonian facies is described as a *masked facies*, with very little movement used in facial expression. The parkinsonian posture is stooped and leaning slightly forward. There also may be a characteristic gait, called a *festinating gait*. This involves short, slow, shuffling steps.

Treatment for parkinsonism usually involves prescription of a drug that contains a chemical called L-dopa such as Sinemet or Parlodel. Physical therapy and speech therapy are also often prescribed.

Oral Musculature

Frequently the standard oral examination will yield only slow rate of movement of the lips and tongue as the major finding, with some reduced range of movement. Palatal movement may be sluggish.

Diadochokinetic rate testing may yield the most interesting information. When patients are asked to execute the syllable repetition for the diadochokinetic testing, reduction of range of movement becomes more evident. The patients also tend to show an accelerated or rapid rate of speaking. As repetition continues, constriction for consonant production may lessen, and syllables may seem to run together. Some patients may use so little movement, combined with a rapid rate, that there is no differentiation between syllables and more of a humming or whirring sound is heard.

Speech Characteristics

The speech of patients with Parkinson's disease varies tremendously depending on the stage of the disease and the effectiveness of medication. A study of the vocal tract characteristics of 200 Parkinson's patients helped to quantify and describe certain features in this disorder (Logemann, Fisher, Boshes, & Blonsky, 1978). Only 11 percent, or 22 of the patients, were found to have no vocal tract problems.

Phonation

Laryngeal disorders were found to be present in 89 percent of the patients in the Logemann et al. study. Hoarseness was the major perceived characteristic, occurring in 45 percent of the patients. Roughness, breathiness, and tremulousness also occurred. All patients, except one who had articulation problems, also showed laryngeal dysfunction.

Duffy (1995) notes that, even when not pervasive, a strained, whispered aphonia will occasionally be noted in the midst of a breathy, harsh voice quality; it occurs toward the end of a vowel-prolongation task and persists for several seconds. Dysphonia may, in fact, be the presenting and most debilitating speech feature in persons with hypokinetic dysarthria. Monopitch and monoloudness are also frequent characteristics of the vocal production of these patients. Maintaining adequate intensity is very difficult for most patients.

Articulation

A detailed analysis of the articulatory errors of the 200 Parkinson's patients in the Logemann et al. study showed that changes in the manner of articulation predominated over changes in the place of articulation (Logemann & Fisher, 1981). Stop plosives, affricates, and fricatives were most affected, as were the features of continuancy and stridency. Inadequate narrowing or constricting of the vocal tract as a result of inadequate tongue elevation appeared to be the reason for these changes. Netsell, Daniel, and Celesia (1975) have termed the result of this phenomena *articulatory undershoot*.

Resonance

Ten percent of the patients in the Logemann et al. study showed hypernasality. There was no regular pattern of hypernasality co-occurring with articulation or laryngeal disorders.

Prosody

Twenty percent of the patients in the Logemann et al. study showed what the authors called a *rate disorder*. Ten percent of the patients were judged as using syllables that were too short, whereas 6 percent used syllables that were too long. Abnormally long pauses occurred in 2 percent of those tested. In other descriptions of rate and prosody, variable rate, short rushes of speech, and inappropriate silences have been noted as characteristic. Patients with hypokinetic dysarthria are often described as showing *prosodic insufficiency*.

Compulsive repetition of phonemes and syllables, noted as dysfluency, has been observed frequently in Parkinson's patients. The presence of *palilalia* has also been noted with Parkinson's disease. Palilalia is characterized by repetitions that usually involve words, phrases, or sentences, and it is usually associated with bilateral subcortical damage.

In summary, the typical Parkinson's patient will be expected to have a phonatory disorder characterized by monopitch, monoloudness, and decreased intensity. Speech rate will likely be accelerated, especially during AMR (alternate motion rate) testing and within segments of conversational speech. Repeated phonemes as well as inappropriate silences will be noted.

Swallowing

Dysphagic symptoms have been identified in all four stages of the swallow in patients with Parkinson's disease. The exact nature of the disorder is still not well-understood (Logemann, 1988). The *oral stage* of the swallow may show a "rocking" pattern with the anterior tongue repetitively moving the bolus upward and backward while the posterior tongue remains elevated against the palate, preventing the bolus from entering the pharynx and preventing initiation of the swallow response. Though this may last for several seconds and significantly lengthen the oral preparatory and oral stages, many patients are unaware of the abnormality. Incoordination and tremulousness, with difficulty initiating tongue movement, are often a part of the oral stages in patients who do not demonstrate the rocking pattern.

Delay of the swallow response, causing aspiration before the swallow, is often noted in these patients. Other disorders include problems with soft palate function, poor laryngeal closure, and reduced pharyngeal peristalsis. Esophageal hypomotility or dysmotility may also be present.

Logemann (1988) notes that it is not unusual to find Parkinson patients who are aspirating chronically, as demonstrated by videofluoroscopy study, but who have very few indications of aspiration in their history or other examinations. These patients tend to aspirate silently, without cough or other external signs, and have not been diagnosed with an aspiration pneumonia. "The exact mechanism that permits this phenomenon is not well understood neurologically or in terms of pulmonary function" (Logemann, 1988, p. 313).

There is much variability among individuals with respect to onset and degree of dysphagia, but as the disease progresses, there is a greater tendency toward development or worsening of dysphagic symptoms. Medication can have a very positive effect and consideration should be given to timing its administration with meals. Over-medication can cause increased problems, however. The effect of medication should be considered (Robbins, Webb, & Kirshner, 1984).

Hyperkinetic Dysarthrias

Whereas hypokinetic dysarthria and hypokinesia are related to reduction of movement from extrapyramidal system damage, hyperkinetic dysarthria is related to increase in movement. The involuntary movement disorders of tremor, chorea, athetosis, and dystonia also result from extrapyramidal damage. The specific localization of the damage in these disorders is not well-understood.

Pathologic Tremor and Voice Disorders

Tremor can be classified as either normal or abnormal—that is, pathologic—depending on whether it is associated with a disease state. Both normal and pathologic tremor may occur at rest, in static postures, or with movement.

In speech pathology, we most often encounter *essential tremor* (also called *action, senile,* or *heredofamilial tremor*). Essential tremor of the voice is known in speech pathology as *organic voice tremor*. In this condition the extrinsic and intrinsic muscles of the larynx may show tremor either independently or along with tremor of other parts of the body, such as the hands, jaw, or head.

Speech Characteristics

In a pure organic voice tremor, articulatory and resonance characteristics are normal, and only phonation is affected. On prolongation of a vowel the mildly affected patient's voice will evidence a regular tremor of altering pitch and loudness. With the more severe disease, there may be complete voice stoppage, resembling the disorder known as *spastic dysphonia*. However, significant differences have been found between the two disorders in terms of regularity of voice arrest and accompanying characteristics. Organic voice tremor patients also demonstrate excessively low pitch and monopitch, intermittent or constant strained-strangled harshness, and pitch breaks.

Chorea

The two major diseases in this disorder group are *Sydenham's chorea* and *Huntington's chorea*. Huntington's chorea is autosomal dominantly inherited, and a child of a patient has a 50 percent chance of developing the disease. Onset is typically in the fifth decade, although there is a so-called juvenile variant as well as a senile variant. There is no known cause. The disease is progressive and fatal. Pathological changes documented usually include loss of neurons from the caudate nucleus, pallidum, and cerebral cortex, with less constant changes in other areas.

Sydenham's chorea (*Saint Vitus' dance* in ancient terminology) is a noninherited childhood disease that may follow strep throat, rheumatic fever, or scarlet fever. The symptoms usually clear up within 6 months.

Associated Neurologic Characteristics

Huntington's chorea is characterized by dementia and involuntary movements. Choreic movements are rapid and coordinated but purposeless movements. They occur unpredictably and may involve any group of muscles. Voluntary and automatic movements may be interrupted so that coordinated breathing and speech may be quite difficult. The limbs are hypotonic. Postures cannot be maintained.

The Oral Musculature

The presence of hypotonia and involuntary movement of the oral musculature is variable in chorea. It is very characteristic in Huntington's disease that the patient cannot keep the tongue protruded for more than a few seconds. Sydenham's chorea often involves involuntary movements of the mouth and larynx. Even if there is little involuntary movement of oral musculature, the speech will probably be affected by the movements of other parts of the body.

Speech Characteristics

In the Mayo Clinic study of 30 adults with chorea (Darley, Aronson, & Brown, 1975), the following problems were noted.

Phonation

A harsh voice quality and/or a strained-strangled sound were found in many patients. Transient breathiness also occurred. Excess loudness variations were prominent as a result of the poor control or ancillary movement. Lower than average pitch levels, voice stoppages, and pitch breaks were other characteristics noted in various patients. Sudden forced inspiration or expiration was observed in some patients.

Resonance

Forty-three percent of the patients in the Darley et al. study demonstrated hypernasality. The interference with resonance also contributed to articulatory problems, including imprecise consonants and short phrases.

Articulation

The difficulty of muscular adjustment yielded imprecise consonant production and, in 23 patients in the Darley et al. study, distorted vowels. Misdirection of movement resulted in a feature called *irregular articulatory breakdown.* Reduced stress and short phrases were also displayed by many of the chorea patients. Prolonged intervals and variable rates were very prominent and contributed to the perception of prosodic deviations.

Swallowing

Dysphagia is noted to be a frequent complaint in Huntington's disease (Leopold & Kagel, 1985). The severity of dysphagia varies from patient to patient primarily because of the constantly changing postures and interpatient variability inherent in the clinical population. The oral stages of the swallow are significantly affected by the irregular and uncoordinated tongue movements and changes in facial tone. Aspiration before the swallow may occur because these random movements push the bolus over the base of the tongue prematurely.

Irregular and uncoordinated movements of the vocal folds and the respiratory musculature as well as neck hyperextension may compromise airway protection. Pharyngeal peristalsis may be weak, and esophageal dysmotility has been reported.

Dystonia and Athetosis

Dystonia and athetosis are movement disorders classified as the *slow hyperkinesias.* Movements are characteristically unstable and sustained, suggesting possible conflicts between flexion and extension of the muscles.

Etiology

Most of these disorders do not have well-established etiologies or focal lesion sites. Encephalitis, vascular lesions, birth trauma, and degenerative neuronal disease are often precipitating diseases. Most hyperkinesias show localized damage to the confines of the basal ganglia. Involuntary movement disorders are sometimes due to the effects of drugs such as phenothiazine and related compounds, especially the more powerful tranquilizers.

Athetosis is a rare disorder that is usually seen as a form of congenital cerebral palsy. It is also seen as a rare progressive disease of adolescence, the cause of which is unknown, and as an accompanying residual deficit with hemiplegia after cerebral infarction. Localization of the lesion is difficult, but the putamen seems to be almost always involved.

Associated Neurologic Characteristics

Dystonia implies excess tone in selected parts of the body. Dystonia affects mainly the trunk, neck, and proximal parts of the limbs.

The slow movements are usually sustained for a prolonged period. The movements usually build up to a peak, are sustained, and then recede, although they occasionally begin with a jerk. Athetotic movements are slow and writhing and are predominantly of the arms, face, and tongue. The movements tend to be exaggerated by attempts at voluntary activity, which make voluntary movements clumsy and inaccurate.

Speech Characteristics

Phonation

The dystonic patient usually has a harsh or strained-strangled voice quality. Other patients, though fewer in number, may demonstrate intermittent breathiness and audible inspiration. Monopitch and monoloudness are also seen in these patients. Because of the involuntary movements, dystonic patients often experience voice stoppages and periods of inappropriate silence. Excess loudness variations accompany the excessive movement. Voice tremor is also found among dystonic patients.

Phonation in athetosis is often significantly affected. The patient often has poor respiratory reserve and respiratory patterns. Both dilator and constrictor spasms have been noted in laryngeal functioning. Voicing is often excessively loud or excessively breathy, and it is very unpredictable and frequently poorly coordinated with articulation.

Spastic or spasmodic dysphonia (SD) is a chronic phonation disorder of unknown etiology. It is included here because its symptoms are found to occur in disorders of movement, and some researchers have postulated that it may be a form of focal dystonia (Blitzer et al., 1985). Aronson and Hartman (1981) discussed differential diagnoses for patients with essential tremor who presented with SD. The signs of spastic dysphonia also occur in cases that appear to be psychogenic or idiopathic. No single cause has been identified.

Spastic dysphonia is characterized by a strained voice quality with voice arrests due to laryngeal adductor spasm. It is frequently associated with pain in the laryngeal area. Though it is assumed that the interruptions to phonatory airflow are due to hyperadduction of the vocal folds, indirect laryngoscopy usually reveals normal vocal fold movements.

Abductor laryngospasms also occur in some patients, as does a mixture of adductor and abductor spasms. These spasms may be different forms of spastic dysphonia. Rosenfield (1988) postulates that voice production in SD can be viewed as a primary problem resulting from abnormal movements in the speech motor system. Further, it may also be considered as resulting from an attempt to cope with the underlying movement disturbance. SD can also be a focal laryngeal dystonia.

Treatment of SD is controversial, and while various treatments have been shown to be successful, no single treatment has been discovered. Psychogenic spastic dysphonia necessitates careful differential diagnosis and may respond to behavioral therapy (Aronson, 1985). Recurrent laryngeal nerve resection (Dedo, 1976) has had varying success according to published clinical reports. Patients must be carefully selected (Ludlow, Naunton, & Bassich, 1984), and symptoms may reappear following the procedure (Rosenfield et al., 1984; Wilson, Oldring, & Mueller, 1980). There is ongoing active investigation and a clinical trial of the use of botulinum, a toxin injection, which has been found to improve voice production dramatically for some SD patients (Brin et al., 1989; Ludlow et al., 1990).

Articulation

As might be predicted, the articulation of patients with these involuntary movement disorders is highly variable, with a range of severity from slight distortion to unintelligible. The dystonic patients of the Mayo Clinic study were found to demonstrate prominent articulation imprecision of consonant production. They also showed vowel distortion and irregular breakdown of articulation. Short phrases were noted with prolonged intervals. Prolongation of phonemes and variability of rate were also frequently observed. Reduction of stress was a relatively prominent characteristic of speech production.

Kent and Netsell (1978) and Platt, Andrews, and Howie (1980) have investigated the articulation of athetoid adults using cinefluorographic and intelligibility measures. The studies found that athetoid speech is frequently reduced in intelligibility as a result of articulation problems. Kent and Netsell found large ranges of jaw movement, inappropriate tongue positioning, prolonged transition time, and retruding of the lower lip. Platt and colleagues found particular difficulty with accuracy of anterior tongue placement, reduced precision of fricatives and affricatives, and inability to achieve extreme positions in vowel formation. They found place and voicing errors to be predominant, particularly in final consonants.

Resonance

Of the 30 dystonic patients studied by the Mayo Clinic, 11 were found to show hypernasality. In the Kent and Netsell (1978) cinefluorographic study of athetoid adults, all subjects had trouble achieving velopharyngeal closure. The most severe problem, however, was velar control. Instability of velar position was noted frequently. The velum sometimes moved inappropriately, causing a loss of closure, or in some cases, the velum showed repetitive movements that were not related to respiration.

Swallowing

Dysphagia in dystonic patients has been described on a limited basis in the literature. Bosma et al. (1982) describe difficulty with lip control and lingual coordination in a patient with drug-induced bulbar and cervical dystonia. The patient had difficulty holding food in the mouth and controlling it to prevent premature entrance into the pharynx. The pharyngeal stage was normal in patients studied by Bosma et al.

Pharyngeal stage efficiency may depend on the posturing of the head and neck. Often, there is a pulling of the neck to the side or a hyperextension, and this may cause stasis and perhaps aspiration if the airway cannot be protected during the prolonged posturing.

Tardive Dyskinesia

Another movement disorder resulting from extrapyramidal damage is tardive dyskinesia, which is attributable to the long-term use of phenothiazine and similar drugs. Symptoms include choreiform, myoclonic, and peculiar rhythmical movements, with a high incidence of abnormal movements in the oral region. Constant random movements of the lips and tongue may be found with a frequent "fly catcher's" movement of the tongue in which the tongue involuntarily moves in and out of the mouth. There may also be palatal involvement. Intelligibility is affected variably, with some patients becoming unintelligible because of the random movements. Most patients, however, have only a mild speech disorder.

The random movements may result in poor coordination in any of the four stages of swallowing. Pocketing of food, pharyngeal stasis, and aspiration before, during, or after the swallow may be found on study of the dysphagia. Reflux of food may be a result of esophageal discoordination. Decreased sensation may also result in lack of reflexive cough or "silent" aspiration.

The Cerebellum and the Cerebellar Pathway Lesions

Ataxic Dysarthria

As noted, the cerebellum serves as an important center for the integration or coordination of sensory and motor activities. It receives fibers from the motor and sensory cortex either directly or through intervening nuclei. Damage to the cerebellum and/or its pathways causes a disorder called *ataxia*, and the motor speech symptoms yield an *ataxic dysarthria*.

Etiology

In ataxic dysarthria there has been damage at some point in the cerebellar control circuit. Damage may occur localized to the cerebellum alone or may be part of more generalized damage affecting several systems. Etiologies include degenerative diseases (Friedreich's ataxia, olivopontocerebellar atrophy, and multiple sclerosis), stroke, trauma, tumors, alcohol toxicity, drug-induced neurotoxicity (from such drugs as Dilantin, Tegretol, lithium, or Valium), encephalitis, lung cancer, and severe hypothyroidism.

Associated Neurologic Characteristics

Ataxia is a disruption in the smooth coordination of movement with failure to coordinate sensory data with motor performance. The hand may overshoot its target when reaching for an object. If the outstretched arm is pushed aside, it swings past its former position and overcorrects. Abnormalities like these are shown when the patient is asked to touch his or her nose or run the heel down the shin. Rapid alternating movements may be affected. Equilibrium is affected and gait may be impaired. Movement is slow to be initiated and slow through the range. Repetitive movements may be irregular and poorly timed, a condition called *dysdiadochokinesia*. Muscle tone is hypotonic. Intention or kinetic tremor (tremor during purposeful movement) is also present.

Speech Characteristics

Dysarthria with localized damage to the cerebellum has the following characteristics.

Phonation

Voice may be approximately normal or may occasionally show excessive loudness variations. Harshness similar to a coarse voice tremor may also be noted.

Resonance

Velopharyngeal functioning is usually intact, with normal resonance characteristics. Occasionally, hypernasal resonance is found. Less frequently, nasal emission is demonstrated.

Articulation

Imprecise consonant production, vowel distortion, and irregular articulatory breakdown mark the speech of ataxic dysarthria. Rate is usually slow, although some patients use normal rate.

Prosody

Prosodic changes are usually readily observable in ataxic dysarthria. A speech prosody characteristic termed "excess and equal stress" by Darley, Aronson, and Brown (1969a) is a predominant feature, although it is not found in all speakers with ataxic dysarthria. This description refers to the tendency to put excessive vocal emphasis on usually unstressed syllables and words, using a slow, metered pattern. Duffy (1995) postulates that in some patients the irregular articulatory breakdown may predominate, giving the speech an "intoxicated" irregular character that overrides the measured aspect of excess and equal stress patterns.

Also contributing to the prosodic changes is the prolongation of phonemes and of normal intervals in speech. You may read or hear the term *scanning speech* in connection with ataxic dysarthria. This term was originated by Charcot in 1877 to describe the speech of a multiple sclerosis patient. Charcot described the speech as being very slow, with a pause after each syllable as if the words were being measured or scanned. This seems to be almost equivalent to what Darley, Aronson, and Brown (1969a) described as excess and equal stress. Others have used the term *scanning speech* to describe a different set of characteristics; therefore, the term has not been found useful and is not recommended.

The term *explosive speech* has also been used to describe ataxic production. The Mayo Clinic study noted excess loudness variations with excessive effort in 10 of 30 ataxic speakers. This forceful effort and increase in intensity, especially noted after pauses, gives the impression of explosiveness.

Other Mixed Dysarthrias With Diverse Lesions

Multiple Sclerosis

Etiology

The etiology of multiple sclerosis (MS) has not been discovered, although evidence suggests that a viral agent may initiate demyelination (Rodriguez, 1989). MS is a complex disease causing demyelination in various tracts of mainly white matter. The lesions involve the entire central nervous system, but the peripheral nervous system is seldom involved.

Associated Neurologic Characteristics

Early signs are often mild or unnoticed. They may include transient parathesias of the extremities, transient diplopia or blurring of vision, mild weakness or clumsiness, and mild vertigo. More severe signs of MS include marked difficulty with gait, dysarthria, significant weakness, visual disturbances, nystagmus, bladder disturbance, and personality change due to frontal lobe involvement. Van den Burg et al. (1987) also noted impairments in perceptual motor functioning and mild deficiencies in intelligence, specifically in memory, in a group of 40 mildly disabled MS patients.

MS may take different forms. Some patients show a relapsing-remitting course in which they have attacks (or exacerbations) from which they recover completely, especially in the early stages of the disease. In the later stages, these patients may accumulate disabilities with each new attack. Other patients may show a chronic progressive course, which usually involves progressive spinal cord dysfunction. This form may evolve from the relapsing form or be present from the onset of the disease (Weiner & Levitt, 1994).

Speech Characteristics
Duffy (1995) cautions that a mixed spastic-ataxic dysarthria may be the most common type of dysarthria associated with MS but should not be considered the only type found in MS. Because of the variable sites of damage in the disease, many different dysarthrias are possible. Spastic, ataxic, or a mixture of these dysarthrias occurs more frequently.

In the Mayo Clinic's study of 168 patients diagnosed with MS (Darley, Aronson, & Brown, 1975), 59 percent were judged as having normal overall speech performance. Twenty-eight percent showed minimal impairment, and 13 percent had more severe impairment. Darley and colleagues labeled the dysarthria that they most often found as a *mixed spastic-ataxic dysarthria*. The primary speech deviations were as follows.

Phonation
The most frequently encountered deviation was impairment of loudness control. Harsh voice quality was also seen frequently. Breathiness was noted in 37 patients. Pitch control and inappropriate pitch levels were also found.

Articulation
About half of the patients were judged to have defective articulation. Although the cerebellar system is frequently involved in MS, only 9 percent of patients showed the irregular articulatory breakdowns characteristic of ataxic dysarthria.

Resonance
One quarter of MS patients demonstrated some degree of hypernasality.

Prosody

A characteristic called *impaired emphasis* ranked high in the speech of these subjects. Impaired features included judgments of rate, appropriateness of phrasing, pitch and loudness variation for emphasis, and increased stress on usually unstressed words and syllables. Only 14 percent of patients demonstrated the ataxic characteristic called *excess and equal stress.*

Shy-Drager Syndrome

Etiology

This syndrome was first described by Shy and Drager in 1960. It appears usually after the fourth decade of life and affects males more often than females by a ratio of 3 to 2. It is a degenerative disease of the autonomic nervous system and may also affect several components of the central nervous system. Prognosis is usually poor, though progression is slow.

Associated Neurologic Characteristics

With this disease, involvement may include the pyramidal, extrapyramidal, or cerebellar system or some combination of the three systems. Early signs usually involve autonomic nervous system disorders including bowel and bladder incontinence, impotence, reduction of perspiration, and difficulty maintaining blood pressure when standing (known as *orthostatic hypotension*). Later symptoms include a gait disturbance, weakness, tremor of the limbs, and dysphagia and dysarthria.

Speech Characteristics

A study by Ludlow and Bassich (1983) comparing acoustic and perceptual analyses of Parkinson's disease and Shy-Drager syndrome documented the following characteristics for the speech of seven patients diagnosed as having Shy-Drager syndrome.

Phonation

Strained-strangled voice quality and breathiness were noted in the voice quality of these patients. A "wet hoarseness" was also identified in many cases. The voice was often judged too soft, and mean intensity level was below normal.

Resonance

Hypernasality may occur if the involvement of the pyramidal system produces elements of a spastic dysarthria.

Articulation

Imprecise consonants are a predominant part of this dysarthria. A variable rate was also ranked high in the deficiency ratings.

Prosody

Although the Shy-Drager patients were shown to have poorer-than-normal ability to change fundamental frequency, their ability was better than that of Parkinson's patients. Acoustic analysis showed, however, that the Shy-Drager patients use their retained ability to change pitch very poorly. The results are acoustically perceived as monopitch and reduced stress.

Summary

Paralysis, weakness, and/or incoordination of the oral musculature may result in the clinical entity known as dysarthria. The classic study by Darley, Aronson, and Brown (1969a, 1969b) identified six different types of dysarthria based on perceptual analyses: spastic, flaccid, ataxic, hypokinetic, hyperkinetic, and mixed. Further research using perceptual and acoustic analysis has added to the detailed knowledge about the speech characteristics associated with diseases, trauma, and injuries to the neuromuscular aspect of the speech mechanism. Table 8–1 lists other diseases or syndromes that are usually accompanied by dysarthria.

Table 8–1 Other Neurological Diseases Associated with Dysarthria

Name	Etiology	Speech Symptoms
Bell's palsy	Inflammation or lesion of cranial nerve VII	Slurring due to unilateral weakness of labial muscles
Polyneuritis	Follows infections or may be due to diabetes or alcohol abuse	Flaccid dysarthria
Hemiballismus	Lesions of subthalamic nucleus	Hyperkinetic dysarthria
Palatopharyngola-ryngeal myoclonus	Brainstem lesions producing rhythmic myoclonic movements of the palate, pharynx, and/or larynx	Hyperkinetic dysarthria, which is sometimes only noted on vowel prolongation
Gilles de la Tourette's syndrome	No known etiology	Hyperkinetic dysarthria with spontaneous, uncontrolled vocalizations such as barking, grunting, throat clearing, snorting;

Table 8–1 *(continued)*

Name	Etiology	Speech Symptoms
		echolalia and coprolalia (obscene language without provocation) may be present
Olivoponto-cerebellar atrophy	Degeneration of olivary, pontine, and cerebellar nuclei	Mixed dysarthria, which may include ataxic, spastic, hypokinetic, and/or flaccid types
Wilson's disease	Hereditary; associated with poor processing of dietary copper	Mixed dysarthria of hypo-kinetic, spastic, and ataxic types
Progressive supra-nuclear palsy	Neuronal atrophy in brainstem and cerebellar structures	Mixed dysarthria, which may include hypokinetic, spastic, and ataxic types

References and Further Readings

Alberts, M. J., Horner, J., Gray, L., Brazer, S. R. (1992). Aspiration after stroke: Lesion analysis by brain MRI. *Dysphagia, 7,* 170–173.

Aronson, A. E. (1985). *Clinical voice disorders* (2nd ed.). New York: Theime-Stratton.

Aronson, A. E., & Hartman, D. E. (1981). Adductor spastic dysphonia as a sign of essential (voice) tremor. *Journal of Speech and Hearing Disorders, 46,* 52–58,

Blitzer, A., Lovelace, R. E., Brin, M. F., Fahn, S., & Fink, M. E. (1985). Electromyographic findings in focal laryngeal dystonia (spastic dyspho-nia). *Annals of Otology, Rhinology and Laryngology, 94,* 592–594.

Bosma, J., Geoffrey, V., Thach, B., Weiffenbach, J., Kavanagh, I., & Orr, W. (1982). A pattern of medication induced persistent bulbar and cervical dystonia. *International Journal of Orofacial Myology, 8,* 5–19.

Brin, M. F., Blitzer, A., Fahn, S., Gould, W., & Lovelace, R. E. (1989). Adductor laryngeal dystonia (spastic dysphonia): Treatment with local injections of botulinum toxin (Botox). *Movement Disorders, 4,* 287–296.

Brown, R. G. & Marsden, C. D. (1984). How common is dementia in Parkin-son's Disease? *Lancet,* ii, 1262–1265.

Capildeo, R., Haberman, S., & Rose, F. C. (1981). The classification of Parkinsonism. In F. C. Rose & R. Capildeo (Eds.), *Research progress in Parkinson's disease.* Kent, England: Pitman Medical Limited.

Charcot, J. M. (1877). Lectures on the diseases of the nervous system. Vol. 1 London: The New Sydenham Society.

Cherney, L. R. (1994). *Clinical management of dysphagia in adults and children.* Gaithersburg, MD: Aspen Publishers.

Darley, F., Aronson, A., & Brown, J. (1969a). Differential diagnostic patterns of dysarthria. *Journal of Speech and Hearing Research, 12,* 246–269.

Darley, F., Aronson, A., & Brown, J. (1969b). Clusters of deviant speech dimensions in the dysarthrias. *Journal of Speech and Hearing Research, 12,* 462–496.

Darley, F., Aronson, A., & Brown, J. (1975). *Motor speech disorders.* Philadelphia: W. B. Saunders.

Dedo, H. H. (1976). Recurrent laryngeal nerve surgery for spastic dysphonia. *Annals of Otology, Rhinology and Laryngology, 85,* 451–459.

Duffy, J. R. (1995). *Motor speech disorders: Substrates, differential diagnosis, and management.* St. Louis: Mosby–Year Book, Inc.

Duffy, J. R. & Folger, W. N. (1986). Dysarthria in unilateral nervous system lesions. Paper presented at the annual convention of the American Speech–Language–Hearing Association, Detroit, MI.

Evatt, M. L., Reus, C. M., Brazer, S. R., Massey, E. W., & Horner, J. (1993). Dysphagia following unilateral ischemic stroke. *Neurology, 43* (supplement), A159 (Abstract).

Hartman, D. E. & Abbs, J. H. Dysarthria associated with focal unilateral upper mottor neuron lesions. *European Journal of Disorders of Communication, 27:* 187, 1992.

Horner, J., Massey, E. W., & Brazer, S. R. (1993). Aspiration in bilateral stroke patients: A validation study. *Neurology, 43,* 430–433.

Kent, R., & Netsell, R. (1978). Articulatory abnormalities in athetoid cerebral palsy. *Journal of Speech and Hearing Disorders, 43,* 353–374.

Leopold, N. A., & Kagel, M. C. (1985). Dysphagia in Huntington's disease. *Archives of Neurology, 42,* 57–60.

Logemann, J. A. (1983). *Evaluation and treatment of swallowing disorders.* San Diego: College Hill Press.

Logemann, J. A. (1988). Dysphagia in movement disorders. In J. Janokovic & E. Tolosa (Eds.), *Advances in neurology: Vol. 49. Facial dyskinesias.* New York: Raven Press.

Logemann, J. A., & Fisher, H. B. (1981). Vocal tract control in Parkinson's disease: Phonetic feature analysis of misarticulations. *Journal of Speech and Hearing Disorders, 46,* 348–352.

Logemann, J. A., Fisher, H. B., Boshes, B., & Blonsky, E. R. (1978). Frequency and co-occurrence of vocal tract dysfunction in the speech of a large sample of Parkinson patients. *Journal of Speech and Hearing Disorders, 43,* 47–57.

Ludlow, C., & Bassich, C. J. (1983). The results of acoustic and perceptual assessment of two types of dysarthria. In W. R. Berry (Ed.), *Clinical dysarthria*. San Diego: College Hill Press.

Ludlow, C. L., Naunton, R. F., & Bassich, C. J. (1984). Procedures for the selection of spastic dysphonia patients for recurrent laryngeal nerve section. *Otolaryngology Head and Neck Surgery*, 92, 24–31.

Ludlow, C. L., Naunton, R. F., Fujita, M., & Sedory, S. E. (1990). Spasmodic dysphonia: Botulinum toxin injection after recurrent nerve surgery. *Otolaryngology Head and Neck Surgery*, 102, 122–131.

Netsell, R. (1984). A neurobiological view of the dysarthrias. In M. McNeil, J. Rosenbek, & A. Aronson (Eds.), *The dysarthrias: Physiology, acoustics, perception, management*. San Diego: College Hill Press.

Netsell, R., Daniel, G., & Celesia, G. G. (1975). Acceleration and weakness in parkinsonian dysarthria. *Journal of Speech and Hearing Disorders*, 40, 467–480.

Platt, L. J., Andrews, G., & Howie, P. M. (1980). Dysarthria of adult cerebral palsy: II. Phonemic analysis of articulation errors. *Journal of Speech and Hearing Disorders*, 23, 41–55.

Robbins, J. (1989). Swallowing and brain imagery in asymptomatic normals and stroke patients. Paper presented at Swallowing and Swallowing Disorders: From Clinic to Laboratory, Northwestern University, Evanston, IL.

Robbins, J., Logemann, J. A., & Kirshner, H. S. (1986). Swallowing and speech production in Parkinson's disease. *Annals of Neurology*, 19, 283–287.

Robbins, J., Webb, W. G., & Kirshner, H. S. (1984). Effects of Sinemet on speech and swallowing in Parkinsonism. Paper presented at American Speech-Language-Hearing Association Convention, San Francisco, CA.

Rodriguez, M. (1989). Multiple sclerosis: Basic concepts and hypothesis. *Mayo Clinic Proceedings*, 64, 570.

Rosenfield, D. B. (1988). Spasmodic dysphonia. In J. Jankovic & E. Tolosa (Eds.), *Advances in neurology: Vol. 49. Facial dyskinesias*. New York: Raven Press.

Rosenfield, D. B., Miller, R. H., Jankovic, J., & Nudelman, H. (1984). Persistence of spasmodic dysphonia symptoms following recurrent laryngeal nerve surgery: An electrodiagnostic evaluation. *Neurology*, 34 (supplement 1), 291 (Abstract).

Shy, G., & Drager, G. (1960). A neurological syndrome associated with orthostatic hypotension: A clinical pathologic study. *Archives of Neurology*, 2, 511–527.

van den Burg, W., van Zomeren, A. H., Minderhoud, J. M., Prange, A. J. A., & Meifer, N. S. A. (1987). Cognitive impairment in patients with MS and mild physical disability. *Archives of Neurology*, 44, 494–501.

Weiner, H. L., & Levitt, L. P. (1994). *House officer series: Neurology* (5th ed.). Baltimore: Williams & Wilkins.

Wilson, F. B., Oldring, D. I., & Mueller, K. (1980). Recurrent laryngeal dissection: A case report involving return of spastic dysphonia after initial surgery. *Journal of Speech and Hearing Disorders*, 45, 112–118.

Yorkston, D. M., & Beukelman, D. R. (1981). Ataxic dysarthria: Treatment sequences based on intelligibility and prosodic considerations. *Journal of Speech and Hearing Disorders*, 46, 398–404.

Yorkston, K. M., & Beukelman, D. R. (1989). *Recent advances in clinical dysarthria*. Boston: Little, Brown.

Yorkston, K. M., Beukelman, D. R., & Bell, K. R. (1986). *Clinical management of dysarthric speakers*. Boston: Little, Brown.

Zeigler, W., & von Cramer, D. (1986). Spastic dysarthria after acquired brain injury: An acoustic study. *British Journal of Communication Disorders*, 21, 173–187.

9 The Central Language Mechanism and Its Disorders

". . . it was Wernicke's paper which made the first searching attempt to link the facts of anatomy with the facts of behavior in a way that permitted prediction of syndromes and the organized test of hypothesis. Like Meynert he gave the brain life."

—Norman Geschwind, *Cortex*, 1967

Broca's discovery of a specific speech-language area in the left hemisphere of the brain had dramatic consequences for neurology. It prompted European neurologists to formulate numerous hypothetical models of the central language mechanism. Several of these models were highly speculative and were based on limited evidence of the correlation between behavioral deficits and brain lesions. Even today the central mechanism for language is not completely understood, and it remains risky to attempt to formulate a model for normal and abnormal communication. However, it is generally conceded that the model formulated by Carl Wernicke is the most valid and powerful model of the central language mechanism (Buckingham, 1982). The model presented here is based on Wernicke's conception and its modern variations (Eggert, 1977).

A Model for Language and Its Disorders

Perisylvian Zone

The major neurologic components of language are situated in the area of the dominant hemisphere known as the perisylvian speech area. Table 9–1 summarizes the components of the language model. This zone contains Broca's area, Wernicke's area, the supramarginal gyrus, and the angular gyrus, as well as the major long association tracts that connect the many language centers.

Table 9–1   Major Components of the Central Language Mechanism Model

Broca's area	Motor programming for articulation
Motor strip	Activation of muscles for articulation
Arcuate fasciculus	Transmission of linguistic information to anterior areas from posterior areas
Wernicke's area	Comprehension of oral language
Angular gyrus	Integrates visual, auditory, and tactile information and carries out symbolic integration for reading
Supramarginal gyrus	Symbolic integration for writing
Corpus callosum	Transmission of information between hemispheres
Subcortical areas	Thalamic naming and memory mechanisms; insular, capsular, and striatal language and speech mechanisms

Broca's and Wernicke's Areas

The location and limits of Broca's area in the frontal lobe are well-defined by research from several sources, and there is considerable documentation that the area functions primarily as a center for the motor programming of speech articulation movement. Wernicke's area, found in the temporal lobe, rivals Broca's area as a major component in a model of neurologic language functioning. The function of the center is well-agreed-on, although its borders are sometimes disputed. In contrast to Broca's area, which serves the expressive aspects of motor speech, Wernicke's area is devoted to another major aspect of language—reception of speech. It is assumed that neural structures in Wernicke's area not only allow for comprehension of oral language, but also, in some as-yet-undefined manner, underlie the formulation of internal linguistic concepts. During speaking these concepts are transmitted anteriorly in the brain, traveling forward to Broca's area for the motor programming and expression of language. Little is actually known about the neural correlates of this internal aspect of language, and major advances in knowledge await future research.

Arcuate Fasciculus

Wernicke must be given credit for developing a language model that highlights the connective association pathways between the frontal and temporal speech-language areas. In fact, he postulated in addition to a motor (Broca's) and a sensory (Wernicke's) aphasia, an aphasia involving these connective association tracts, called *conduction aphasia*. The fiber connections between Broca's area and Wernicke's area are now generally agreed on to be the *arcuate fasciculus*. The fibers, as described earlier in Chapter 2, leave the auditory association area in the temporal lobe, arch around and under the supramarginal gyrus, and pass through the parietal operculum. They travel forward as part of the long association tract known as the *superior longitudinal fasciculus*, finally ending in Broca's area.

Angular Gyrus

Included as a significant component of the language model is the angular gyrus in the left parietal lobe. Joseph J. Dejerine (1849–1917) suggested that this area was one of two sites associated with the reading disorder called *alexia*. Alexia can also be associated with a lesion of the left occipital lobe accompanied by a lesion of the splenium of the corpus callosum. The left occipital lobe lesion produces a right hemianopsia. The lesion in the splenium prevents the right occipital cortex from transmitting information to the left angular gyrus. The hemianopsia compounded by this disconnection syndrome produces severe alexia (Dejerine, 1891, 1892).

Inferior Frontal Gyrus

D. Frank Benson has described a third alexia, known as *frontal alexia* (Benson, 1977). The lesion is in the inferior frontal gyrus and extends to the subcortical tissue in the anterior insula of the dominant hemisphere. This third type of alexia is often seen in cases of Broca's aphasia. It may be considered an *aphasic alexia*—an alexia associated with a major aphasic syndrome.

Supramarginal Gyrus

Anterior to the angular gyrus is the supramarginal gyrus, curving around the posterior end of the Sylvian fissure. Together with the angular gyrus, it is known as the *inferior parietal lobule*. Lesions of the supramarginal gyrus are associated with *agraphia*, or writing disorders (see Figures 9–1 and 9–2 for current models of the cortical language mechanisms).

Subcortical Mechanisms

The model displayed in Figure 9–1 suggests that neural mechanisms for language are limited to the cerebral cortex, but evidence from several sources indicates that subcortical mechanisms also play a

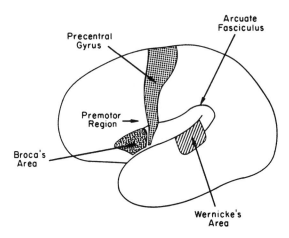

Figure 9–1 A model of the central language mechanism on the dominant cerebral hemisphere. Geschwind (1975) labeled the components of the brain mechanisms for language. Source: Reprinted with permission from N. Geschwind, "The Apraxias: Neural Mechanisms of Disorders of Learned Movements" (*American Scientist*, 63, 189–195, 1975).

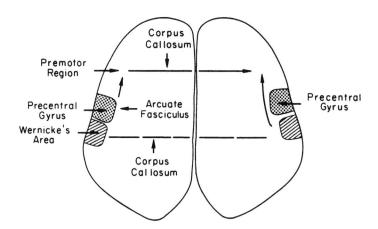

Figure 9–2 A superior view of the model of the central language mechanism showing the corpus callosum and the interhemispheric motor pathways that may be involved in apraxia. Source: Reprinted with permission from N. Geschwind, "The Apraxias: Neural Mechanisms of Disorders of Learned Movements." (*American Scientist*, 63, 188–195, 1975).

role. Wilder G. Penfield and Lamar Roberts were among the first investigators to present evidence for possible subcortical mechanisms for language and speech (Penfield & Roberts, 1959). They suggested that the pulvinar and ventrolateral nucleus of the thalamus serve as relay stations between Broca's and Wernicke's areas. They demonstrated massive fiber tracts to and from the thalamus and the major cortical speech areas. In addition, direct electrical stimulation of the left pulvinar and ventrolateral nucleus have produced naming problems.

Subcortical aphasias have been reported since the last century, but their existence has remained controversial. In recent years, however, several cases of thalamic hemorrhage in the dominant lobe, verified by computerized tomographic brain scan, have indicated that aphasia can result from subcortical lesion alone, without cortical damage (Crosson, 1984). These cases of hemorrhage frequently involved the pulvinar. Aphasia after thalamic infarction has also been reported and appears to occur most frequently if the infarction is in the territory of the tuberothalamic artery, which supplies the ventral anterior thalamus (Crosson, 1992).

In addition to thalamic aphasia, lesions in the internal capsule, striatum, and globus pallidus appear to give rise to speech and possibly language disturbances. The function of the basal ganglia does not appear to be limited to motor programming. Normal language and cognition may depend to a limited extent on the integrity of the thalamus and the basal ganglia.

Recent theories concerning the function of the subcortical structures in language vary as to the mechanism and extent of involvement. Alexander, Naeser, and Palumbo (1987) believe that lesions of the basal ganglia and surrounding structures are most likely to produce dysarthric and dysphonic symptoms rather than language deficit. Other theorists propose that cortical-striatal-pallidal-thalamic-cortical loops are involved in language (Crosson, 1992). Wallesch and Papagno (1988) suggest that the structures in this loop serve to monitor and select lexical input, which is then sent forward to the anterior language cortex in a modular fashion. The lexical alternatives from which the loop selects information originate in the posterior language cortex of the left hemisphere. Crosson (1992) suggests that the loop triggers the release of language segments at the appropriate time after semantic monitoring, thus serving more of a regulatory than an information-processing function. Crosson has also theorized that the thalamus arouses the anterior language cortex and transmits semantic segments from the anterior to the posterior cortex for monitoring.

Subcortical language mechanisms are not completely understood, and it is apparent that they play a less significant role than cortical mechanisms do, but their existence appears to be well-confirmed. Newer imaging methods will probably provide better information about subcortical activity. For example, Metter and his colleagues (1983, 1988) have found that subcortical lesion is accompanied by remote hypometabolism, indirectly affecting

the left perisylvian area. This was found to be related to language functioning in the patients studied. Further research on brain activation and blood
flow should continue to shed light on the true functioning of these areas
as a part of the language mechanism.

Model Functioning

Experts who accept this model describe its function in the
following manner. Neural motor plans for speech sounds and their sequence
in syllables and words are formulated in Broca's area, area 44. Motor
commands are projected to the adjacent premotor cortex (area 6) and to
the lower portion of the motor cortex (area 4), and the actual movement
commands for articulation are projected to the muscles of the vocal
mechanism via the corticobulbar tracts and the cranial nerves.

Speech perception of oral language is a function of Wernicke's area,
which is composed of the superior and middle temporal gyri. *Neologistic jargon aphasia* results from damage to both these gyri. Neologistic
jargon aphasia is characterized by unintelligible fluent speech performance.
The neologisms noted in the speech refer to coined words that normally
do not appear in the language. Neologistic jargon aphasia with severe
semantic and syntactic disturbances is associated with damage at the
temporal-parietal juncture, including the supramarginal gyrus and parietal
operculum. The disorders suggest that the processing of sentences at the
syntactic and semantic levels may involve the auditory association areas
of the left temporal lobe (areas 22 and 42), the supramarginal gyrus (area
40), and the parietal operculum in Wernicke's area. The utterance, in a
manner as yet unknown, is transmitted via the arcuate fasciculus to Broca's
area, where the detailed plans for articulation and vocalization are evoked.
A neurolinguistic model such as this, which indicates that Wernicke's
area is primarily responsible for auditory comprehension as well as part
of the mechanism for initiating plans for the deep structure of sentences,
is found in the work of the linguist Harry Whitaker (1971).

The calling up of words is a critical function in any model of the
language mechanism. The angular gyrus is important for word recall as
well as for reading and writing. Word recall defects are associated with
lesions in the perisylvian zone. Such defects are also present in generalized brain syndromes such as encephalitis. The fact that neurologists
view word recall disorders, or *anomia*, as nonlocalizing symptoms has
been interpreted to mean that the lexical store required for semantic
concepts in sentences has broad representation throughout the brain.

Collosal fibers convey auditory information received at the right
Heschl's gyrus to the left hemisphere for processing in the major central

language system of the perisylvian zone. Split-brain studies indicate that the right hemisphere participates in language processing to a limited degree only. The right hemisphere comprehends sentences at a low level, recognizing noun and verb categories equally well, but does not process syntax as well as the left hemisphere does (Springer & Deutsch, 1989).

Although the primary cortical brain mechanisms for language are encompassed in the perisylvian zone, disturbances of language can be produced by lesions outside the primary speech-language zones. *Transcortical* or *border zone aphasic syndromes* have been identified as occurring in these zones. These syndromes are associated with lesions falling beyond the perisylvian area (Figure 9–3). Characterized by aphasia without repetition disturbance, these syndromes are thought to involve cortical areas in a vascular border zone between the territory of the middle cerebral artery and that of the anterior and posterior cerebral arteries. In *transcortical motor aphasia*, the lesion is anterior or superior to Broca's area. In *transcortical sensory aphasia*, the lesions are at the posterior temporal juncture of the dominant hemisphere. The implication that can be drawn from these clinical data is that language is supported by wide territories in the left hemisphere, with a focus on brain mechanisms in the central portion of the hemisphere devoted to language.

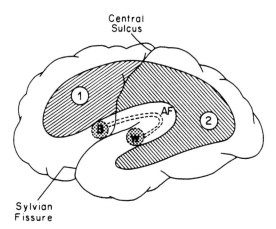

Figure 9–3 The transcortical border zone. Around the perisylvian speech zone is a large area (shown striped on this diagram) that is the site of the transcortical aphasias (B, Broca's area; W, Wernicke's area; AF, arcuate fasciculus; 1, area of transcortical motor aphasia; 2, area of transcortical sensory aphasia). Source: Redrawn and reproduced with permission from M. Espir and F. Rose, *Basic Neurology of Speech and Language* (3rd ed.) (Blackwell Scientific Publications, 1983).

Model Usefulness

The model described had its strongest advocate in a contemporary neurologist, Norman Geschwind (1926–1984). The Geschwind model is a connectionist conception of the higher mental functions of speech and language, and as such it gives importance to the classic language and speech centers and highlights the significance of the interconnection of the association fibers between major centers. The model has been of significant use to the clinical neurologist because it allows a high degree of predictability of symptoms associated with specific lesion sites. In addition, the model also predicts possible aphasic syndromes not yet described. It does this by postulating possible lesion sites for these syndromes. In general the model has been confirmed by clinical studies. The classic language centers have been established through computerized tomography and other current objective neurodiagnostic procedures.

Geschwind (1969), however, pointed out that there are some conditions under which the model has not always fulfilled its promise. First, certain features of aphasic syndromes are not readily explained by the model. Second, aphasic cases occasionally occur whose existence is not predicted by the model. Third, in a few cases the expected symptoms do not appear when there is an adequate lesion. Despite these limitations, the model has been extremely useful for neurologists, linguists, and speech-language pathologists.

Whitaker (1971) correlated the neurologic model with a form of generative transformational grammar. His linguistic analyses of Broca's and Wernicke's aphasia provided evidence for neurologic sites for several linguistic mechanisms. He also suggested that the classic linguistic distinction between *competence* and *performance* in language plays a special role in aphasia. Contrary to the beliefs of many neurolinguists who hold that competence—the tacit knowledge of language—is retained intact in aphasia while only performance is disturbed, Whitaker believes that both competence and performance are compromised after cerebral injury.

New Approaches to Models

In recent years research in aphasia has felt the impact of the field of cognitive neuropsychology as experimental psychologists test and develop their information-processing models of cognition in aphasic and other brain-damaged individuals. Much of the initial work was done in Britain, mainly with investigations of reading (Coltheart et al., 1980). These models are testimony to the belief in cognitive neuropsychology that investigations of individual patients from a particular theoretical stance are preferable to comparisons of groups of patients categorized by the classical syndrome models (Code, 1990).

Many cognitivists believe that attempting to map brain structure to cognitive function is not a useful task at this time because current definitions of what constitutes a "function," such as naming or reading, are too broad. For example, Rothi and Moss (1985) have demonstrated that failure to read a word aloud correctly may result from a breakdown in any number of processes involved in the task. Thus, information-processing models require that one fractionate a task into its different components. Individuals are then studied in such a manner as to identify where during the process the breakdown may occur, resulting in inaccurate or inefficient performance.

These models usually represent the brain as a specialized computer that has domain-specific modules associated with defined neural structures with input and output routes mapped as the model becomes more specific to function. The modules are usually represented as boxes with the input and output routes as arrows (see Coltheart, 1987; Marshall, 1985; Roeltgen & Heilman, 1985). These models appeal to clinicians because techniques for assessment and treatment may be adapted from them.

The development and use of such models is well-established in both speech-language pathology and neuropsychology. Their acceptance is variable, however, as much controversy exists regarding the independence of language from other psychological operations. It is also argued that no model, as yet, can deal with the complexity of human language. Marin (1982) points out that the organism strives mainly to understand or express meaning in all communication and that a model is needed where meaning is the primary emphasis.

The cognitivists' models of language functioning are, in one sense, a reaction against the dominant connectionist model advocated by Geschwind and others. Caplan (1992) argues that connection theory provides an inadequate functional analysis of patient's deficits in terms of indicators of specific processing deficits, although it does give information about the location of classic aphasia syndromes. Many of the specific processing deficits have been analyzed with grammatic concepts that have been generated by a rule-based grammar, as posited by Chomsky, that has been espoused by speech-language pathology for the last 30 years (see Chapter 1). Other critics (Churchland, 1995) have pointed out that this innate rule-based grammar has not yet truly been validated. Pinker (1994), who believes that the rule-based generative grammar posited by Chomsky is gene-based, argues that our present neuroimaging techniques are not yet sensitive enough to reveal the specific microneuronal circuitry that will provide us with information about how noun phrases and verb phrases are created and modified (see Chapter 1). Thus, linguistic operations cannot be viewed neuronally to validate the theory of productivity and creativity underlying a generative transformational grammar.

Churchland (1995) believes that a rule-based grammar as proposed by Chomsky need not be the only method for verifying how a grammar may be generated in humans. He points to the artificial intelligence work on neural networks by Ellman (1992). Recursive neural networks, which generate language without a rule base, appear to produce acceptable sentences with a low level of productivity. Obviously higher levels of productivity and creativity in language must be developed if artificial intelligence technology is to challenge the standards of use and creativity implied in Chomsky's theory of language. With the type of genetic evidence now available from the work of Gopnik (1990), which implies that specific language defects are gene related, Chomsky's claims of innate rules may have a degree of validity that has not yet been successfully challenged; however, all of this intensive research may soon give the speech-language pathologist a clearer insight into how the brain really processes language.

Aphasia Classification

The aphasia literature is characterized by a proliferation of clinical classification schemes. The history of aphasia is peopled by students of the disorder who either communicated poorly to each other about the disorder or were in clear disagreement about the nature of the syndromes. Syndromes were often named or classified in terms of personal bias. This situation has resulted in a number of confusing classification systems. Similar names in two classification systems might be used to describe radically different language syndromes, each with strikingly different lesion sites.

Speech-language pathologists who have devised classification systems have generally disregarded the site of lesion in their systems, basing their classifications on patterns of performance on standardized language tests. Tests that use classification systems based on performance alone, rather than extensive neurologic data, are Wepman and Jones' *Language Modalities Test for Aphasia* (Wepman & Jones, 1961), Schuell's *Minnesota Test for Differential Diagnosis of Aphasia* (Schuell, 1965), and the *Porch Index of Communicative Ability* (Porch, 1967, 1971). The approach to classification based on language performance alone has further complicated the issue of classification.

Dichotomous Classification

It is common to classify patients broadly into one of two categories based on the general locus of the presumed lesion, before specific syndromes are identified. The dichotomous classification of *receptive* and *expressive* aphasia, introduced in 1935 by the neurologist Theodore Weisenburg and the psychologist Katherine McBride, has been one of the most widely used modern divisions. Expressive aphasia is generally associated with anterior lesions and receptive aphasia with posterior lesions.

The *motor* and *sensory* division of aphasia introduced by Wernicke has been widely employed. Motor aphasia usually implies anterior cortical pathology, usually located in the frontal lobe. Sensory aphasia implies a posterior lesion in the temporal lobe. Some experts have done away with the classic terms *motor* and *sensory* and directly classify the aphasias as *anterior* and *posterior*, referring to lesion site.

A recent and widely used dichotomy for spontaneous language in aphasia is *fluent* versus *nonfluent*. All aphasics show some degree of expressive involvement in conversational language, and it has been argued that the expressive language of an aphasic can be appropriately described as fluent or nonfluent. This dichotomy is often considered to be better than expressive versus receptive because it recognizes that practically all aphasics demonstrate some expressive difficulty.

Classification Agreement

Much of the supposed confusion in classification is artificial. There is generally more agreement on the critical features that distinguish various aphasia syndromes than on the names applied to them. The syndromes of the *speech area*, or perisylvian zone, are the most widely accepted of the aphasic syndromes. These include Broca's, Wernicke's, and global aphasia, generally considered the most common aphasic syndromes. Conduction aphasia is a less common perisylvian syndrome. The transcortical aphasias and various alexic syndromes have their lesion sites outside the perisylvian zone, and they are even less common.

Broca's Aphasia

This aphasia is marked by nonfluent conversation, decreased verbal output, increased effort in speaking, shorted sentence length, dysprosody, and *agrammatism* (reduction of syntactic filler words with retention of nouns, verbs, and adjectives). There are often accompanying motor speech disorders such as apraxia of speech and dysarthria. Some neurologists believe that what are known as speech apraxic symptoms by speech-language pathologists are merely a form of transient nonfluent aphasia. Lesions limited to Broca's area alone produce speech apraxia or this form of transient aphasia. More widespread lesions produce a chronic and classic clinical picture.

Comprehension of spoken language is always qualitatively better in Broca's aphasia than is production of language. There is much variation in language production, from near normal to clearly abnormal. Broca's aphasics often have difficulty in understanding syntactic relationships and show difficulty in comprehending those syntactical items that they have difficulty expressing. Repetition is always abnormal, and *confrontation naming* (naming objects and pictures) is poor. Oral reading and reading comprehension are usually poor, although some patients do well. Writing is poor, marked by misspellings and letter omission. In addition, the patient usually has a right hemiparesis and uses the left hand for writing. Some patients cannot write at all because of paresis (Figure 9–4).

Wernicke's Aphasia

Wernicke's aphasia is a fluent aphasia characterized by difficulty in understanding language as well as difficulty in repetition of language. The speech is fluent but paraphasic. *Paraphasia* includes the omission of parts of words, incorrect use of correct words, use of neologisms, and substitution of incorrect phonemes for correct ones. *Verbal paraphasia* is the incorrect use of words; *literal paraphasia* is the substitution of incorrect phonemes for correct phonemes.

The fluent verbal output may be excessive, a condition called *logorrhea*. Phrase length is normal, and in most cases syntactic structure is acceptable. Articulation and prosody are usually not abnormal. The speech often lacks meaningful and substantive words and is described clinically as *empty speech*. Use of jargon is common, and some patients whose language is unintelligible because of excessive jargon and neologistic terms are called *neologistic jargon aphasics*.

Comprehension of language is poor, and some patients appear to understand no spoken language at all. Others understand only some words, and certain patients have distinct problems in discriminating phonemes. Repetition of spoken language is poor, and failure and paraphasic errors characterize confrontation naming tasks. Reading is generally disturbed, often paralleling the disturbance in comprehension of spoken language.

Conduction Aphasia

This is a fluent aphasia characterized by intact comprehension and articulation. Repetition is poor and phoneme substitutions are frequent because of the inability to match acoustic information with motor

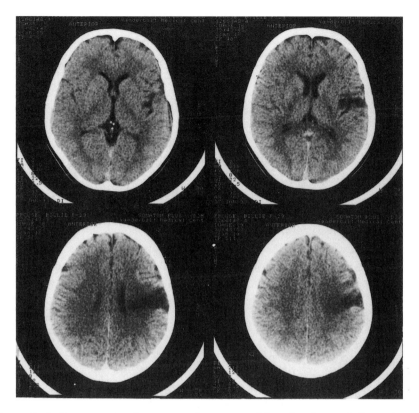

Figure 9–4 Computerized tomography scans of four horizontal slices from a patient with Broca's aphasia and a right hemiparesis. Note the darkened area in the left hemisphere, which defines the infarction. Source: Courtesy of Howard S. Kirshner, M.D. (Department of Neurology, Vanderbilt University School of Medicine, Nashville, Tennessee).

plans for the output of phonemes. Wernicke postulated a lesion in the connection between Broca's and Wernicke's area for conduction aphasia. Conduction aphasia is less well-accepted as a diagnosis than Broca's or Wernicke's aphasia because of questions about the site of lesion. The lesion is not always in the arcuate fasciculus as Wernicke postulated, but the language syndrome has been described repeatedly and can be diagnosed from symptoms alone without neuropathologic evidence. Two distinct locations of pathology have been demonstrated in conduction aphasia. One involves the arcuate fasciculus in the dominant hemisphere, usually deep in the supramarginal gyrus. Some experts argue that the supramarginal cortex itself rather than deep white matter is the critical site. The other major site is said to be in the left temporal lobe in the auditory association area.

Conversational speech is fluent and paraphasic, but generally the speech quantity is reduced compared with that of a Wernicke's aphasic. Pauses, hesitation, and incidents of word-finding difficulties are common, so the speech is dysprosodic. Literal paraphasia is often present. Articulation is good. Comprehension of spoken language is also adequate in most cases. If comprehension is disturbed, the diagnosis of conduction aphasia should be questioned.

Repetition of language presents a serious problem to the conduction aphasic, and the dramatic difference between comprehension and repetition is a clue to correct diagnosis. Repetition is much poorer than the ability to produce words in conversational speech, and paraphasic substitutions of words are often present in repetition attempts. Errors are also present in confrontation naming.

Reading disturbance is usually seen in conduction aphasia. Oral reading is paraphasic, whereas silent reading for comprehension is adequate. Writing disturbance or dysgraphia is present. Spelling is poor, with omissions, reversals, and substitutions of letters. Words in sentences may be reversed, omitted, or misplaced.

Global Aphasia

This aphasic disorder, also known as *total aphasia*, is accepted by many neurologists and speech-language pathologists. Global aphasia is marked by severe impairment of both understanding and expression of language. The person is usually mute or uses repetitive vocalization. This aphasia is usually associated with a large lesion in the perisylvian area. The lesion does not serve as a localizing one for the neurologist, except when it's in the left perisylvian area.

Expressive language is always limited, although true mutism rarely appears other than initially. The patient can often use inflected phonation and sometimes can use simple words, such as expletives, repetitively. Comprehension is often reported to be better than production in the global aphasic, who may also become adept at interpreting nonverbal communication through gestures and facial and body language. This nonverbal comprehension may be mistaken for comprehension of the spoken word.

The global aphasic does not repeat. If a patient who appears to have global aphasia repeats adequately, the speech-language pathologist and neurologist should suspect that one of the transcortical aphasic syndromes, described later in this chapter, is present instead of a true global aphasia. Confrontation naming is severely or completely impaired, and reading and writing are also severely or totally impaired. Many of the language dysfunctions are not reversible with treatment.

Transcortical Aphasias

These language disturbances are a set of aphasic syndromes whose lesions fall outside the perisylvian area. They have been given various names, but Wernicke identified them as transcortical aphasias, and they are probably identified most commonly by this name. Benson (1979) called them border zone aphasic syndromes since the lesions are usually found in a vascular border zone between the field of the middle cerebral artery and the area supplied by the anterior or posterior cerebral arteries. A hallmark of the transcortical aphasias is the retention of the ability to repeat with good accuracy. In contrast, the aphasias of the perisylvian area present a repetition defect.

Three transcortical aphasias are generally recognized: *transcortical motor aphasia, transcortical sensory aphasia,* and *mixed transcortical aphasia.* This last type has also been called a syndrome of *isolation of the speech area.*

Transcortical motor aphasia is a nonfluent aphasia marked by more dysfluency and effort in conversation than is usually seen in Broca's aphasia. Serial speech, repetition, and comprehension appear surprisingly adequate. The lesion is anterior or superior to Broca's area in the dominant hemisphere.

A transcortical sensory aphasia is fluent and marked by paraphasias with semantic and neologistic substitutions. Comprehension is poor, in sharp contrast to repetition, which is surprisingly good. Reading, writing, and naming are poor. The site of the lesion is controversial. It is usually found deep to and posterior to Wernicke's area in either the temporal or the parietal border zone, or it may be located in both of these sites.

Mixed transcortical aphasia is rare. The most striking feature is severely disordered language except in one area—repetition. Patients do not speak unless they are spoken to, and answer only in repetition. The most striking feature is *echolalia,* the repetition of heard phrases. Examples of echolalia may be incorporated into the patient's speech. The articulation of phonemes is good, but the expressive language as a whole is nonfluent. Comprehension is defective, with little or no demonstrable understanding of spoken language. Visual-field defects and other neurologic signs are common. The pathologies are mixed but generally appear to involve the vascular border zones of the left hemisphere.

Anomic Aphasia

Word-finding difficulties, known as *anomia,* are common in many types of aphasia as well as in nonaphasic medical conditions. In fact, many neurologists believe it is inappropriate to consider a diagnosis of aphasia without evidence of some anomia. Further, anomia occurs in most types of dementia and is a clear diagnostic feature of Alzheimer's syndrome, a major dementia. Anomia often is the only major language residual following recovery from aphasia of any clinical type, and it remains a long-lasting problem in the recovered aphasic.

Clearly, anomia is not a good localizing symptom for the neurologist. Rather, it is a common symptom in what is called *nonfocal brain disease.* In those neurologic conditions in which the whole brain is generally affected, anomia is a common language symptom. It occurs in many brain conditions, including encephalitis, increased intracranial pressure, subarachnoid hemorrhage, concussion, and toxic-metabolic encephalopathy.

When anomia is the most prominent symptom in the aphasic syndrome, the condition is known as *anomic aphasia.* The clinical picture generally includes only limited receptive or expressive difficulty, but on occasion a disorder of confrontation naming may take an extreme form in these patients, and given patients may be unable to produce virtually any appropriate names. Spontaneous speech is usually fluent but interrupted by word-finding difficulties. Nonspecific words may be substituted for precise lexical items. These verbal paraphasias are usually semantic rather than phonemic errors. Usually, the patient exhibits good expressive syntax except for pauses for word recall. *Circumlocution,* the utterance of circuitous and wordy descriptions for unrecalled words, is common in anomic aphasia. Comprehension is normal or near normal and repetition is generally intact. Reading and writing are more variable, and word-finding difficulties are obvious in written language.

Anomic aphasia may appear as an isolated syndrome or may be the final stage of recovery from other syndromes, such as Wernicke's, conduction, and transcortical aphasia. Some controversy exists regarding whether a recovered aphasic who becomes anomic at the endpoint of recovery should be classified as an anomic aphasic or according to the primary syndrome at the onset of the aphasia.

Associated neurologic defects are variable. The site of the lesion causing anomia is also variable, but anomic symptoms in and of themselves are less variable than in other classic aphasic syndromes. In severe and isolated anomia, a possible focal lesion may be found in the left hemisphere. A prominent site for a lesion is in the left angular gyrus. Anomia is a common early sign in a recently described syndrome called *progressive aphasia.*

Progressive Aphasia

Slowly progressive aphasia without generalized dementia is a newly described aphasia syndrome. It is defined as an adult-onset, degenerative, language disorder syndrome that selectively affects the language areas of the dominant hemisphere. Language symptoms may show a slow dissolution over an extended period of time, but intellectual functions other than language are spared. Anomia is often an early sign, but poor auditory comprehension, stuttering, deteriorating verbal memory, and reading and spelling difficulties have been reported. Other intellectual functions remain intact and psychometric testing reveals overall intelligence quotients within the normal range.

In progressive aphasia, neurodiagnostic testing fails to demonstrate contralateral or global brain abnormalities of the type reported on positron emission tomography scans of individuals with Alzheimer's disease. Some cases of progressive aphasia have been reported as presenile in onset, but other reports have suggested that onset beyond age 65 may also occur. Pathologic evidence of progressive aphasia is limited as yet. Structural lesions have been demonstrated, but reports of hypometabolism in language areas without evidence of structural abnormality have also been reported.

Subcortical Aphasia

An emerging category of aphasia, based on recent evidence of lesions, is known as *subcortical aphasia*. Although many aphasia experts have hypothesized the existence of subcortical speech and language disturbance over the years, it was not until the advent of modern neuroimaging techniques that documented evidence of such lesions became available. The reports of several investigators suggest that basal ganglia and thalamic lesions are primarily responsible for subcortical aphasia. Subcortical aphasia associated with thalamic hemorrhage without involvement of the cerebral cortex clearly establishes the disorder. Aphasia associated with left thalamic lesions is characterized by a relatively consistent clinical picture of fluent expressive speech marked by verbal paraphasias and neologisms. Repetition is typically intact. Auditory and reading comprehension remains at relatively high levels. Some researchers have noted additional characteristics as usually being present: reduced vocal volume, aspontaneity in oral expression, and word-finding deficits with frequent perseveration.

Subcortical aphasias associated with basal ganglia lesions have sometimes been classified by anatomic sites. Each site is said to be associated with a different cluster of speech and language symptoms. Several speech and language syndromes affecting the basal ganglia have been described. The syndromes vary widely, and no general clinical descriptions are associated with basal ganglia lesions. Kirshner (1995) identified the head of the caudate nucleus, anterior limb of internal capsule, and anterior putamen as the most commonly reported lesion sites causing an aphasia (Figure 9–5). These lesions result in the *anterior subcortical aphasia syndrome*, which is characterized by dysarthria and decreased fluency but has a longer phrase length than in a Broca's aphasia. Paraphasias are also noted.

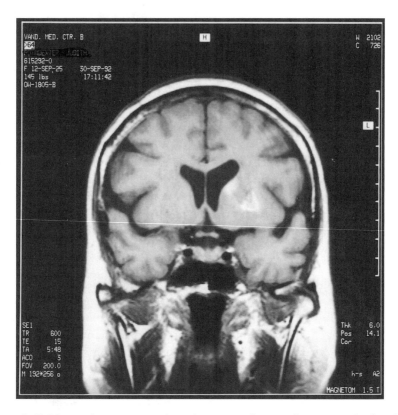

Figure 9–5 Magnetic resonance imaging scan shows a lesion in the head of the caudate, anterior putamen, and anterior limb of the internal capsule, resulting in a mild subcortical aphasia characterized by hesitant speech and anomia. The patient showed good recovery after a period of speech therapy.   Source: Courtesy of Howard S. Kirshner, M.D. (Department of Neurology, Vanderbilt University School of Medicine, Nashville, Tennessee.)

Alexander and Naeser (1988) have suggested that four distinct syndromes exist. Each is associated with a different subcortical anatomic site or combination of sites. These sites include (1) striatal lesions (basal ganglia alone), (2) internal capsule lesions, (3) striatal and internal capsular lesions, and (4) insular and capsule lesions. Figure 9–6 lists the signs and symptoms of each of the subcortical speech or language disorders that Alexander and Naeser identified. Other findings have been described in the literature as well. For example, disproportionate impairment of writing has been reported with subcortical lesion (Tanridag & Kirshner, 1985).

There is a question as to whether lesions of subcortical structures give rise to transient or persistent aphasia. It has been suggested that

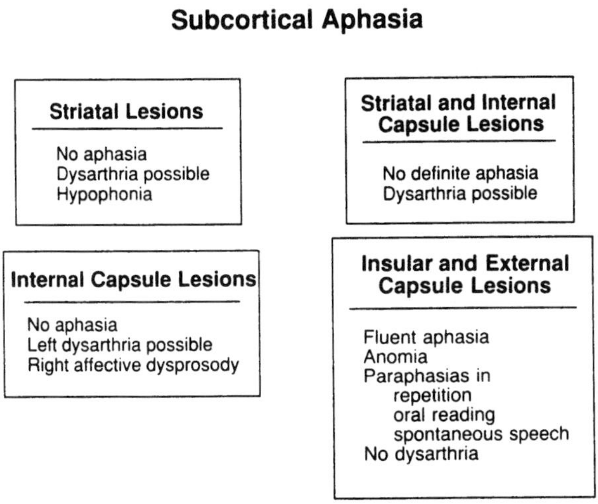

Subcortical Aphasia

Striatal Lesions	Striatal and Internal Capsule Lesions
No aphasia Dysarthria possible Hypophonia	No definite aphasia Dysarthria possible

Internal Capsule Lesions	Insular and External Capsule Lesions

No aphasia
Left dysarthria possible
Right affective dysprosody
	Fluent aphasia
	Anomia
	Paraphasias in
	  repetition
	  oral reading
	    spontaneous speech
	No dysarthria

Figure 9–6 The signs and symptoms of language and speech disorders associated with subcortical lesions. Source: Adapted with permission from M. Alexander and M. Naeser, "Cortical-Subcortical Differences in Aphasia." In F. Plum (Ed.), *Language, Communication and the Brain* (New York: Raven Press, 1988).

subcortical aphasia is transient, but as yet there are very few data to support this assertion.

The correlation of behavioral state and lesion localization is an evolving study to which information is being added daily. A simplified localization scheme based on current knowledge for all major aphasia syndromes is found in Table 9–2.

Testing for Aphasia

Aphasia testing has had a long history in neurology and speech-language pathology. Broca reportedly tested his patients with conversational questions in addition to testing tongue movements, writing, and arithmetic. He also described their gestures. In 1926 the British neurologist Henry Head (1861–1940) published the first systematic aphasia examination in English. The test was not standardized and contained some items that were even difficult for healthy people to perform. Since the appearance of the Head tests, several unstandardized scales as well as many psychometrically sound test batteries have been developed to assess language disturbance in brain injury.

Aphasia tests have been constructed to serve many purposes and have been based on a variety of theoretical biases concerning the nature of the impairment in aphasia. The recent standardized tests generally measure

Table 9–2 Localization of the
Aphasias in the Central Language
Mechanism

Aphasias of the perisylvian zone
Broca's aphasia
Wernicke's aphasia
Global aphasia
Conduction aphasia
Transcortical aphasias of the border zone
Transcortical motor aphasia
Transcortical sensory aphasia
Mixed transcortical aphasia
Aphasias of the subcortical areas
Thalamic aphasia
Striatal disorders
Internal capsule disorders
Striatal or capsular disorders
Insular or capsular disorders

primary language ability while deemphasizing intelligence and educational achievement. These tests are capable of separating language performance that is normal from performance that is abnormal, and most allow the experienced speech-language pathologist to determine whether the language disturbance is truly aphasic in nature and not a nonaphasic language disorder. This determination is accomplished by comparing the pattern of language performance on the test to the language performance of known aphasic patients.

Most standardized aphasia tests assess a wide variety of language functions over a broad range of severity. Some tests yield an overall score of severity, but all tests provide a profile of deficits in the major language modalities. Most tests once provided a system of classifying the aphasic performance by clinical type, but the majority of tests in use today have not been constructed with the classical neurologic model of Wernicke as their theoretical foundation. Speech pathologists and psychologists have been more concerned about developing aphasia tests that precisely measure language behavior under standardized conditions than about providing tests that predict and confirm possible lesions or verify the validity of classical models of neurologic language mechanisms.

Two aphasia tests use a classification based on the classic aphasia syndromes predicted by the Wernicke model. These are the *Boston Diagnostic Aphasia Examination* and the *Western Aphasia Battery*. The *Boston* examination became commercially available in 1972 and was then revised in a second edition (Goodglass & Kaplan, 1983). It yields a diagnosis of the presence of and clinical type of aphasia, plus it offers suggestions of the possible location of brain damage. The *Boston* examination is a comprehensive battery of 27 subtests, and it may take more than one test session to complete. Statistically derived profiles are available for Broca's, Wernicke's, and anomic aphasia. Case histories are provided to aid in classification of conduction and transcortical sensory aphasia. Statistical data can be used to identify global aphasia utilizing deviations from *z*-score measures. Information from the Cookie-Theft Picture responses and other data from the *Boston* examination allow diagnosis of language impairment in Alzheimer's disease. Supplementary nonverbal tests from the *Boston* examination can be used to assess some of the hemispheric disconnection syndromes.

The *Western Aphasia Battery* (Kertesz, 1983) is a shorter version of the *Boston* examination. Its administration time is approximately 1 hour, and it yields a single overall score, the aphasia quotient (AQ), which separates normal language performance from abnormal language performance. The AQ is derived from auditory and speech tests and may also be used as an index of recovery. A performance quotient is derived from tests for reading, writing, and nonverbal functions. The score derived from subtests is the cortical quotient (CQ). Means, standard deviations, and graphic profiles are provided for eight aphasic syndromes: global, Broca's, isolation, transcortical motor, Wernicke's, transcortical sensory, conduction, and anomic. Correlations between computerized tomography scan data for the *Boston* examination and the *Western Aphasia Battery* suggest that, in most cases, these two tests generally predict classical lesion sites and tend to verify major elements of the Wernicke central language model.

Speech-language pathologists should be aware of other major aphasia tests in use today, which are not based on a classic neurologic model. The description of these tests, not as closely based on a specific neurologic theory as the *Boston* examination and the *Western Aphasia Battery*, is beyond the purpose of this book. These aphasia tests include the comprehensive batteries such as Schuell's *Minnesota Test for the Differential Diagnosis of Aphasia* (1965), *the Porch Index of Communicative Ability* (Porch, 1969, 1971), Wepman and Jones' *Language Modalities Test for Aphasia* (Wepman & Jones, 1961), and the *Neurosensory Center Comprehensive Examination for Aphasia* (Spreen & Benton, 1969). Shorter screening tests and scales of aphasia include Eisenson's *Examining for Aphasia* (Eisenson, 1954), the *Halstead-Wepman-Reitan Aphasia Screening Test* (DeMyer,

1980), Schuell's *Short Examination* (Schuell, 1966), and Keenan and Brassell's *Aphasia Language Performance Scales* (Keenan & Brassell, 1975).

Clinical neurologists usually assess language and aphasia disturbances as part of the mental-status examination of higher cerebral functions, which is part of the traditional neurologic examination. The mental-status examination assesses major functions of the total nervous system and lateralizes and localizes dysfunction when it is present.

Testing for aphasia in the mental-status examination at bedside is one of the oldest parts of the traditional clinical neurologic examination. The techniques are not standardized but vary from one neurologic examiner to another. Generally, the goals of examination are to determine the presence or absence of aphasia, assess its extent in various areas of language function, determine the severity and clinical type of aphasia, and suggest the type and site of the lesion. The neurologist will select language test items that will best achieve these various goals. Commonly employed areas of language that are assessed include the quantity and quality of conversational speech, allowing the identification of possible dysarthria; repetition of spoken speech; evaluation of the comprehension of spoken speech; and identification of deficits in word finding or naming, reading, and writing. The language functions tested by the neurologist are found in Table 9–3. An example of a bedside examination of speech and language designed for the clinical neurologist is found in Appendix C.

Associated Central Disturbances

Agnosia

The term *agnosia* was introduced into neurology by Sigmund Freud (1856–1939) in 1891. Agnosia is a disorder of recognition due to cerebral injury. Table 9–4 defines the agnosia syndromes. Classic theory places the lesion responsible for the disorder in the sensory association areas of the cerebral cortex, leaving the primary sensory receptor areas intact. To diagnose the classic disorder correctly, certain precautions must be observed. First, one must be certain that the lesion is at the level of the cortical association area rather than at the level of sensory receptor, the sensory pathway, or the primary sensory receptor area in the cortex. Second, one must rule out unfamiliarity with the test item as a reason for failure to recognize the sensory stimuli. To establish basic knowledge of an item, it often is a good procedure to have the patient match items. If an item can be matched or recognized in other modalities, unfamiliarity can be ruled out as a possible cause for the lack of

Table 9–3   Language Functions of Major Classic Aphasias

	Spontaneous Speech	Compre-hension	Repetition	Reading	Writing
Broca's	Nonfluent	+	−	±	−
Wernicke's	Fluent	−	−	−	Paragraphic
Conduction	Fluent	+	−	+	−
Global	Mute	−	−	−	−
Anomic	Disorder of word recall	+	+	+	+
Transcortical motor	Nonfluent	+	+	+	−
Transcortical sensory	Fluent	−	+	+	−
Mixed transcortical (isolation of speech area)	Nonfluent	−	+	−	Paragraphic

Symbols: +, relatively intact; −, impaired.

Source: Developed by Howard S. Kirshner, M.D., Department of Neurology, Vanderbilt University School of Medicine, Nashville, Tennessee.

Table 9–4   The Agnosias

Agnosia	A disorder of recognition due to damage to cortical sensory association areas or pathways
Visual agnosia	Inability to recognize objects, colors, and pictures
Auditory agnosia	Inability to comprehend speech and/or nonspeech sounds (pure forms = *auditory nonverbal agnosia* and *pure word deafness*)
Tactile syndrome	Inability to recognize objects by touch; characterized by bilateral parietal lobe lesions
Gerstmann syndrome	Includes finger agnosia, right-left disorientation, acalculia, and agraphia; usually characterized by left parietal lobe lesions

recognition. The concept of agnosia has been highly criticized in contemporary neurology.

Geschwind has argued that most of the agnosias can be best understood in the light of newer disconnection theory. Many of the classical agnosias, he maintains, are really isolated disturbances of the naming function resulting from lesions that isolate the language areas in the left hemisphere from the perceptual recognition areas of the right or both hemispheres (Geschwind, 1965).

Visual Agnosia

Analyzed in disconnection terms, classical visual agnosia is produced when visual associations are lost because there is a disconnection of the visual areas from the language area. Also known as *associative visual agnosia,* it results in difficulty in recognizing pictures and objects with surprisingly good ability to describe, copy and match visual stimuli. Patients correctly name the stimulus after tactile or auditory presentation of it. Bilateral occipital lobe lesions with extension on one side or the other into the medial temporal lobe involving the hippocampus have been found on autopsy. With such lesions both the naming and the memory of objects presented visually would be affected.

Visual agnosia may also result from unilateral lesions. With destruction of the left visual cortex in addition to a lesion of the splenium of the corpus callosum or extensive involvement of the white matter of the association cortex of the left occipital and parietal lobes, a unilateral left visual agnosia may result.

Benson (1979) observes that in the few cases of visual agnosia reported, associated findings are common. These may include hemianopsia and prosopagnosia, a visual agnosia for faces. In addition, other associated disorders include constructional impairment, alexia without agraphia, amnesia, and some degree of anomia. A color-naming defect may also be present; this inability to match seen colors to their spoken names is called *color agnosia* by Benson (1979) and a *color anomia* by Geschwind. Lesions in the calcarine fissure and splenium are usually present. These lesions, according to Geschwind, disconnect the right visual cortex from the left language areas.

Auditory Agnosia

The term *auditory agnosia* usually refers to the inability to identify auditory nonlinguistic stimuli though many will use the term when referring to inability to recognize nonlinguistic as well as verbal stimuli. Most appropriate is the label *auditory nonverbal agnosia* for a pure deficit in which identification of nonlinguistic stimuli is impaired and the term *pure word deafness* if referring to the disorder in which nonverbal stimuli can be identified but speech cannot be understood. All auditory agnosias occur in the face of normal hearing acuity. The site of lesion for auditory nonverbal agnosia is in dispute but is assumed to be in the auditory association areas of both hemispheres.

Pure word deafness is an uncommon syndrome in which the patient cannot comprehend verbal language, but usually reads, speaks, and writes functionally. Paraphasic errors in speech are often noted and there may be a mild aphasia. Both unilateral and bilateral temporal lobe lesions have been described. Unilateral lesions are those deep in the temporal lobe in the fibers projecting to Heschl's gyrus. Bilateral lesions have usually been described as occurring in the midportion of the superior temporal gyri of both hemispheres. Geschwind (1965) notes that in pure word deafness with a unilateral lesion, the lesion must be located subcortically in the left temporal lobe so that the auditory radiations as well as the callosal fibers from the opposite auditory region will be interrupted, preventing Wernicke's area from receiving auditory stimulation.

In bilateral pure word deafness, the lesions in the temporal lobe spare Heschl's gyrus. It is assumed that the lesions on the left cut off connections between the primary auditory receptor cortex and Wernicke's area. A lesion on the right would cut off the origin of the callosal fibers from the right auditory cortex. It may be that auditory nonverbal agnosia, in addition to pure word deafness, is the basis of the syndrome known as *cortical deafness*, which is probably associated with bilateral temporal lobe lesions.

Tactile Agnosia

Geschwind (1965) has argued that many instances of classical tactile agnosia should more correctly be called *tactile aphasia*. Tactile aphasia is characterized by the inability to name objects by touching them; the ability to name on the basis of auditory or visual stimulation is preserved, as is intact spontaneous speech. The basis of this disorder is demonstrated by the ability to respond to somesthetic stimulation when the response is demanded from the same hemisphere, but an inability to do so if the response is demanded from the opposite hemisphere. A lesion in the somesthetic association area of the left parietal lobe destroys the connection between the left somesthetic cortex and the left language area and produces a tactile naming disorder in association with the right hand. This disconnection syndrome is better called a *unilateral tactile aphasia* than a *tactile agnosia*. A lesion in the right somesthetic association area or in the corpus callosum is more likely to produce a true tactile agnosia in the right hand.

Beauvois et al. (1978) have reported a syndrome, which they have named *bilateral tactile aphasia*, in a bilaterally damaged patient. This aphasia is analogous to the auditory and visual agnosia disorders. The patient was unable to name objects on touching them, but could give the name upon hearing the sound an object made. The lesion is presumed to be in both parietal lobes.

Gerstmann Syndrome

This well-known syndrome includes an agnosia for the fingers as well as right-left disorientation, acalculia, and agraphia. It has been assumed since Joseph Gerstmann's original description in 1931 that when the four symptoms of the syndrome are present, there is a left parietal lesion. Critics of the syndrome have pointed out that it is rare and that frequently the syndrome is assumed to be present without all four symptoms being identified. Benson has also suggested that the classic Gerstmann syndrome is part of a larger left angular gyrus syndrome including alexia, mild fluent aphasia, and mild constructional impairment.

The clinical procedure for testing for finger agnosia and right-left disorientation is simple. The patient is provided with a method of finger identification by numbering the fingers on each hand from one to five, usually beginning with the thumb. The patient then is asked to close his or her eyes, and the examiner randomly touches a finger on either the right or the left hand. The patient is asked to identify the finger touched by the examiner and to indicate whether the finger in question is on the right or the left hand. Each of the ten digits is systematically assessed. If the patient shows confusion in identifying fingers on the right or left hand, further assessment should be done by having the patient point to objects to his or her right and left. A quick test to assess the integrity of directional orientation is to ask the patient to touch the right hand to the left ear. The remainder of the symptoms may be tested by having the patient write and print words and sentences from dictation to identify agraphia. Simple arithmetic problems that can be calculated both mentally and on paper are useful in identifying acalculia.

Although finger agnosia and right-left disorientation are associated most commonly with left parietal lesions, they also have been seen with right-hemisphere damage in the parietal lobe. A similar syndrome has been identified in children beyond the age of 5 or 6 years and has been called *developmental Gerstmann syndrome* (Benson & Geschwind, 1970).

Apraxias

Apraxia is a disorder of learned movement that is not caused by paralysis, weakness, or incoordination and cannot be accounted for by sensory loss, comprehension deficits, or inattention to commands, according to Geschwind (1975). It has also been defined as a disorder of motor planning. Apraxia is a high-level motor disturbance of the integration of the motor components necessary to carry out a complex motor act.

Apraxias are important to the speech-language pathologist because certain types of apraxia may affect the motor programs of the speech muscles directly. Other forms of apraxia often accompany the aphasias and other cerebral language deficits in the cortical motor association areas and the association pathways of the brain. The major apraxias are defined in Table 9–5.

Hugo Liepmann (1863–1925) is credited with elucidating the concept of apraxia around the turn of the century, although John Hughlings Jackson described an apraxic disturbance of the tongue as early as 1866. Liepmann used early disconnection theory to explain apraxia and demonstrated lesion sites to support the variety of apraxias he described (Liepmann, 1900).

Ideomotor Apraxia

Ideomotor apraxia is the most common type of apraxia. In this condition the patient fails to carry out a motor act to the examiner's verbal command. Impairments are found in the oral muscles, the upper and lower limbs, and the trunk muscles. Generally, simple motor gestures

Table 9–5   The Apraxias

Apraxia	A disorder in performing voluntary learned motor acts, due to a lesion in motor association areas and association pathways, in which similar automatic gestures are intact
Ideomotor apraxia	A disorder in which motor plans are intact, but individual motor gestures are disturbed
Ideational apraxia	A disorder in performing the steps of complex motor plans
Constructional disturbance	A disorder in which constructing in space is disturbed
Apraxia of speech	A disorder of motor programming of speech
Oral apraxia (buccofacial apraxia)	A disorder of nonspeech movements of the oral muscles
Developmental apraxia of speech	A disorder in which motor speech programming is disturbed in childhood

are disturbed when attempts are made to elicit them by verbal command, but the level of ideation for the plan of the motor gesture is retained.

Ideomotor apraxia can be demonstrated on examination. For example, a patient may be unable to lick his lips with his tongue on command but may show appropriate licking movements during eating. This deficit in tongue movements involves an apraxia of oral muscles. Difficulties, for instance, in saluting or waving the hand or in kicking a ball on command are called *limb apraxias*. Difficulties in bending at the waist in a bow or swinging an imaginary baseball bat are called *trunk apraxias*.

Evaluation of ideomotor praxis is best done in a series of hierarchical steps. The most difficult level requires the patient to carry out a spontaneous motor act alone to a verbal command. The examiner must not provide nonverbal cues for the motor gesture. Assume the examiner says, "Show me how to use a screwdriver." Correct performance involves gesturing to place the tool into a screwhead and twisting the wrist. If the patient fails at the spontaneous level, the examiner asks the patient to imitate him or her. Imitation of a motor act for a patient with ideomotor apraxia is usually easier, but often the improvement in motor performance is only partial. If the patient fails at the imitative level, an actual object is provided and the verbal command is given again. Use of the actual object is the easiest mode in which to perform the required motor act. Many patients who fail at the levels of spontaneous performance and imitation will execute movements markedly better with an actual object. Generally, failure at the spontaneous level, coupled with improvement in motor performance during imitation or in object use, allows a positive diagnosis of ideomotor apraxia.

Since ideomotor apraxia may coexist with aphasia, it is necessary for the examiner to make certain the patient understands the verbal commands given when praxis is tested. This approach avoids potential misdiagnoses on two counts. First, a diagnosis of apraxia is avoided when there is actually a verbal comprehension deficit caused by aphasia. Second, a misdiagnosis of a verbal comprehension deficit is not made when the actual failure in performance is due to an apraxic disturbance.

The ability to perform learned movements on verbal command is associated with the integrity of the language areas in the dominant left hemisphere. Since adequate verbal comprehension is a prerequisite for testing praxis, Wernicke's area in the left hemisphere must be intact. After the verbal command is recognized and comprehended through the linguistic processing of Wernicke's area, neural impulses are probably transmitted to the left supramarginal gyrus for matching to kinesthetic memories of required motor acts. This information is then transmitted forward by neural impulse along the arcuate fasciculus to the premotor area where a motor plan for the required gesture is evoked. This motor plan is relayed to the motor area of the precentral gyrus. At the precentral gyrus the pyramidal tract is activated to carry out the motor gesture. Presumably, according to disconnection theory, a lesion at any point in this complex pathway will produce an apraxic disturbance on the right side, since motor activities on the right are controlled by motor areas and pathways in the left hemisphere.

A verbal command to the right motor cortex for a learned movement on the left side of the body must be transferred from the left premotor cortex to the right premotor cortex by the anterior fibers of the corpus callosum. Any interruption of the anterior callosal fibers will produce an apraxia of the left side, particularly left-handed apraxia. This has been called a *sympathetic apraxia* in individuals who have a Broca's aphasia and a right hemiplegia. It has been also called a *callosal apraxia*. This disorder was described by Liepmann in 1900 and elaborated on by Geschwind in 1975.

The posterior callosal fibers could theoretically transmit motor information to the right premotor area, but as Geschwind (1975) points out, lesions in the posterior callosal area rarely result in a left apraxic hand. Apparently the posterior callosal pathway is rarely used to transmit interhemispheric motor impulses that are affected in such a way that apraxia results.

Another motor disorder, called *limb-kinetic apraxia*, was originally described by Liepmann. Currently, the disorder is not considered a true apraxia. Often seen in Broca's aphasia, this motor disorder is a mild disturbance in the limb and hand opposite the cerebral lesion. The disturbance is thought to result from a mild pyramidal tract disorder, and it is often characterized by clumsiness of the hand and involuntary grasp reflexes.

Oral Apraxia

Speech-language pathologists recognize a nonspeech ideomotor disorder of the oral muscles called *oral apraxia*, the inability to perform nonspeech movements with the muscles of the larynx, pharynx, tongue, and cheeks although automatic and sometimes imitative movements of the same muscles may be preserved. This disorder is not the result of paralysis, weakness, or incoordination of the oral musculature, and it may be isolated or coexist with an apraxia of speech (discussed later). Oral apraxia is usually called *buccofacial apraxia* by neurologists.

Oral praxic disturbance must be differentiated from disorders of the motor pathways involved in upper motor neuron and lower motor neuron systems. A careful cranial nerve examination will usually indicate whether the disturbance is on the higher level of motor planning of praxis as opposed to being a lower level motor deficit associated with either supranuclear lesions or cranial nerve lesions. Generally, motor involvement affects both voluntary and reflexive oral acts in lower level motor deficits of the central and peripheral nervous systems. Voluntary oral motor acts will be limited by paralysis, weakness, and incoordination, and the more reflexive acts of mastication and deglutition will be affected as well. Supranuclear lesions are associated with typical tongue deviation, hypertonic oral muscles, palatal paresis, hyperactive gag reflex, and lower facial paresis. Lower motor neuron lesions are associated with tongue deviation and atrophy, hypotonic oral muscles, palatal paresis, and a hyporeflexive gag reflex. Facial paresis is hypotonic. Extrapyramidal lesions produce involuntary movements of oral muscles, and ataxic movements of oral muscles are found in cerebellar disorders.

Oral apraxia testing is completed on a spontaneous level to verbal command and on an imitative level. Commands requiring oral-facial movements such as "lick your lips" or "clear your throat" may be used. Failure to perform appropriately on a number of similar commands suggests a diagnosis of oral apraxia in brain-injured adults. Love and Webb (1977) used a 20-item informal test for assessing oral apraxia. Published tests of apraxia of speech usually include tasks for assessing nonverbal oral apraxia.

Apraxia of Speech

Apraxia of speech is an impaired ability to execute voluntarily the appropriate movements for articulation of speech in the absence of paralysis, weakness, or incoordination of the speech musculature. In 1900 Liepmann discussed a form of ideomotor apraxia that could be localized to the speech muscles; some 40 years earlier, Broca described elements of this disorder as part of *aphemia*. Aphemia, the defect in speech and language that Broca believed to result from damage to the third left frontal convolution of the brain, has become known as *Broca's aphasia*. The disorder is marked by effortful groping for articulatory movements produced in an apparently trial-and-error manner. There is inconsistent articulation on repeated utterances. The speech is dysprosodic, with great difficulty in initiating utterance.

Oral apraxia and speech apraxia may appear independently or may coexist with each other. Oral apraxia may be the basis of a speech apraxia. Speech apraxia may appear in a pure form or may be accompanied by a language disorder, as seen in a classic Broca's aphasia. Some neurologists and speech-language pathologists deny that what is called *apraxia of speech* is a pure disorder of praxis. They view the apraxic elements in Broca's aphasia as more of a linguistic problem than a motor problem. Evidence is not yet available to resolve the issue.

Pure apraxia of speech has been traditionally associated with the left frontal lobe, and it is presumed that the lesion is localized specifically to Broca's area or deep to it. Apraxia of speech as an element of a classic Broca's aphasia with linguistic disorder implies a lesion extending beyond Broca's area into regions other than the frontal lobe. The issue of lesion site is not yet settled, since sites beyond Broca's area have also been suggested as contributing to speech apraxic symptoms (Dronkers, 1993).

If the speech-language pathologist is presented with a case that appears to be a pure speech apraxia, it is necessary to differentiate it from dysarthria. In speech apraxia, articulation is impaired by inconsistent initiation, selection, and sequencing of articulatory movements; in dysarthria, articulatory movements are more consistent, with distortion errors predominating. Speech apraxias do not display consistent disturbances of phonation, respiration, and resonance, whereas dysarthrics almost always display consistent phonatory, resonance, and respiratory disorders. Dysarthrics show impairment of nonspeech musculature, including paralysis, weakness, involuntary movement, and/or ataxia. Speech apraxics do not have these neurologic impairments of the oral musculature.

Developmental Apraxia of Speech (Developmental Verbal Dyspraxia)

Developmental apraxia of speech is a childhood condition reportedly similar to apraxia of speech seen in the adult. The disordered movements of the articulators very frequently appear to contribute to a serious phonologic problem in the school-age child. If an apraxic disorder of the oral muscles is present in the preschool years, it may well delay the development of speech and language, and the language developmental milestones of one-word utterances, two-word combinations, and three-word sentences may be disrupted. A clear-cut syndrome has not yet emerged, despite considerable clinical research on the topic. It appears that the prime sign of the disorder is awkward movement of the speech muscles that cannot be attributed to developmental dysarthria. This single sign appears to be the only clearly reliable and consistent feature for diagnosis of the disorder. There is some question whether the articulation errors of children diagnosed as having speech apraxias can reliably and validly be separated from the articulation errors of children with severe functional developmental phonologic disorders.

It is also difficult to accept the disorder in a true apraxic context. Apraxia of adulthood has been unequivocally associated with verified brain lesions; in children, however, this has not been the case. In some instances no brain lesion has been demonstrated at all; in other instances inconsistent *soft signs* have been found (see Chapter 11), and there has been doubt in these cases about the actuality of cerebral dysfunction because there has been no demonstrable structural lesion or evidence of dysfunction. Issues concerning the validity of this syndrome are discussed in greater length in Love and Fitzgerald (1984). The diagnosis of developmental apraxia of speech remains controversial from the standpoint of both speech pathology and neurology.

Ideational Apraxia

Ideational apraxia, also described by Liepmann (1900), is a higher order disturbance of complex motor planning than is found in ideomotor apraxia. Ideational apraxia is an inability, as the result of cerebral injury, to carry out a hierarchical complex motor plan. It is the converse of ideomotor apraxia, where individual movements are not available to the patient voluntarily. In ideational apraxia, individual movements can be called up, but a complex motor plan involving all elements of a motor act cannot successfully be executed. For instance, in the simple act of striking a match against a matchbox, the patient with ideational apraxia may strike the match on the wrong side of the box, use the wrong end of the match to strike the matchbox, or even strike another object such as a candle on the matchbox. The patient appears to have lost the overall concept of how to proceed to complete the motor task; he or she can carry out individual motor acts in a series but cannot complete a hierarchical sequence.

Ideational apraxia is a complex disability that is most often seen with bilateral lesions in brain disease. It is frequently associated with the dementias, but any diffuse cerebral disease, particularly one involving the parietal lobes, may show elements of ideational apraxia. It is likely that failure to carry out a series of motor tasks in diffuse brain disease is due to some element of ideational apraxia, but often other cognitive deficits play a role in the failure. Certainly memory is frequently impaired, and verbal comprehension deficits may be present in persons with this apraxic disorder. Patients with ideational apraxia seem to have particular difficulty in recognizing the use of objects. For instance, the patient who strikes a candle on a matchbox demonstrates this recognition deficit. In addition, the individual is unable to structure a logical series of steps of action.

The cognitive losses and confusion seen with ideational apraxia have serious consequences. The patient cannot manipulate the environment for survival. He or she cannot cook a meal, make a bed, or carry out to completion the normal activities of daily living. Generally, the presence of ideational apraxia serves as a sign of serious generalized intellectual deterioration.

Constructional Disturbances

In 1922 Karl Kleist (1879–1960) described a high-level nonverbal constructional disability that he called *construction apraxia*. He defined it as a cortical deficit in which patients were unable to form a construction in space. For instance, the inability to copy simple geometric designs (such as a circle, square, or cross) or to reproduce drawings of more complex items (such as a wheel, a wagon, or a bicycle) has been described as a disorder of constructional apraxia. Construction disability is commonly tested by having the patient reproduce drawings, draw to command, construct block designs, or match stick designs. The advantage of testing for constructional disturbances to the speech-language pathologist and neurologist is that the task provides an excellent method for detecting organic brain disease.

Constructional ability is the capacity to draw or construct two- or three-dimensional figures or designs from one- and two-dimensional models. This high-level nonverbal cognitive function is said to involve integration of much of the brain. Occipital, parietal, and frontal lobe functions are employed. With the extensive cerebral functions involved in constructional performance, it is a highly sensitive objective task with which to suggest brain disorder in patients with few other signs of neurologic impairment. Assessment of constructional ability involves much more than testing the capacity to perform high-level learned movements.

The term *constructional disturbance* to describe constructional deficits is preferable to the old term *construction apraxia* since the latter is more limited than the former. The parietal lobes serve as the primary cerebral areas for visual motor integration involved in constructional tasks. Visual receptor areas of the occipital lobe and motor areas of the frontal lobe are used in construction tasks, but the parietal lobes are responsible for the integration of activity in construction tasks. Both right and left parietal lobes contribute to construction performance. Lesions in either parietal lobe will produce a construction deficit. Right-hemisphere lesions tend to produce more deficits than do left-hemisphere lesions. Generally, specific lesions of the right parietal lobe result in more severe constructional deficits than do left parietal lesions. For the speech pathologist, constructional disturbance serves as a good general indicator of adult parietal lobe damage. It may be necessary, however, to have a neuropsychologist or an experienced neurologist interpret constructional errors to determine the possible hemispheric lateralization of the lesion. On occasion, anterior lesions in the frontal lobe may even produce a constructional deficit, so parietal lobe localization is not always reliable.

Certain clinical groups with construction disturbances are of particular interest to the speech-language pathologist. The patient with a right-hemisphere constructional disability may have difficulty in verbal attempts to describe and explain his or her visual-spatial motor performance. Patients with bilateral cerebral lesions, as in dementia, show dramatic constructional disturbances. In fact, the constructional disorder is often seen as an early sign of impending dementia. Language is usually disturbed in these patients as a result of the deficit.

Speech-language pathologists frequently use or become familiar with common tests of constructional abilities. The *Boston Diagnostic Aphasia Examination* (Goodglass & Kaplan, 1983) contains a series of supplementary nonlanguage tests including drawing to command, stick construction, and construction of three-dimensional block designs. The widely used *Bender Gestalt Tests* for adults and children (Koppitz, 1964; Pascal & Suttel, 1951) ask subjects to reproduce drawings. The tests are very sensitive to parietal lobe involvement. Since many adults and children with speech and language disorders that are not of obvious neurologic origin are suspected to have brain dysfunction, these tests have been routinely employed in some speech and language clinics.

Standardized developmental drawing tests and other constructional tests also have been used to assess the maturational level of perceptual motor development in children. Children with delayed language development sometimes show delays in constructional abilities as well, so these tests may be part of the assessment battery of the speech-language pathologist. The *Developmental Test of Visual Motor Integration* (Berry & Butenica, 1989) is an example of a developmental constructional test.

Alexia

Alexia is an inability to comprehend the written or printed word as the result of a cerebral lesion. Terms relating to alexia and agraphia are found in Table 9–6. In current usage, *alexia* is an acquired reading disorder, in contrast to *dyslexia*, an innate or constitutional inability to learn to read. The childhood disorder is often called *developmental dyslexia*. Although this distinction in terms is not universal, it is becoming popular. The classic term *word-blindness* is rarely used in neurology or speech pathology. When employed, it implies difficulty in reading words while letter recognition is more intact. The term *literal alexia* means inability to recognize letters; *verbal alexia* indicates that letters are recognized but words are not. *Pure alexia* is a reading disorder without a writing disorder

Table 9–6   The Alexias and Agraphias

Alexia	A disorder of reading due to cerebral injury
Agraphia	A disorder of writing due to cerebral injury
	Types of alexia
Alexia with agraphia	The lesion is usually in the dominant parietal lobe in the angular gyrus area
Alexia without agraphia	The lesion site is controversial; there are often two lesions, one in the dominant occipital lobe, the other in the splenium of the corpus callosum, according to Dejerine
Frontal alexia	The lesion is in the dominant frontal lobe in Broca's area and adjacent deep structures; it is associated with a nonfluent aphasia
Aphasic alexia	The lesions are the same as in the major aphasias
	Agraphias
All agraphias	The lesions are in the left frontal or parietal lobe or in the complex pathways necessary for writing

(*agraphia*). A variety of terms and types of alexia have been reported, but a limited number of alexic syndromes are widely accepted. The modern understanding of alexia is attributed to Joseph Dejerine (1849–1917), who in 1891 and 1892 described two classic syndromes, alexia without agraphia and alexia with agraphia.

Alexia Without Agraphia

This alexia is also known as *posterior alexia* or *occipital alexia*. The cardinal feature of this uncommon syndrome is loss of the ability to read printed material, with retained ability to write both to dictation and spontaneously. Generally, other language functions are intact. The alexia occurs suddenly as the result of a left posterior cerebral artery occlusion in a right-handed person. A striking clinical feature is the patient's ability to write lengthy meaningful messages, with a contrasting inability to read his or her own writing. The patients generally are able to understand words spelled aloud. Initially pure alexics may show difficulty with letters and words, but letters are easier. With some recovery, the patient is able to read in a letter-by-letter fashion, combining them into syllables and words after saying them. Patients are usually able to regain some reading ability, but reading usually remains quite an effort. The writing seen in the syndrome is not entirely normal, but retained writing capacity is impressive when compared with the minimal reading ability. Often the patient writes better to dictation or spontaneously than when copying. There is usually a right homonymous hemianopsia.

Dejerine found a cerebral infarct in the left occipital lobe and involvement in the splenium of the corpus callosum in a patient with alexia without agraphia. Since the left visual cortex was damaged, all visual information entered the right hemisphere. The right visual cortex perceived the written material but could not transfer it to the left hemisphere because of the callosal lesion. The inferior parietal lobe in the dominant hemisphere, known as the angular gyrus, combined the visual and auditory information necessary in both reading and writing; however, the inferior parietal lobule was disconnected from all visual input. Since the lobule and its connections with the language area were intact, the patient was able to write normally.

Other deficits may be associated with an alexia without agraphia. Patients may be found to have short-term memory problems, a mild anomia, and/or a visual agnosia. A common accompaniment to pure alexia is a *deficit in color naming*. The patient presents this deficit despite good object naming. Not all cases of pure alexia show defective color identification. Disconnection theory explains this disorder as a loss of pure verbal association similar to that in the reading disorder. The patient recognizes the color but is unable to call up its name because of a disconnection between visual recognition areas and language areas.

Alexia With Agraphia

Also known as *central alexia* or *parietal alexia*, this syndrome was classically described as an almost total reading disorder, with limited writing ability, only minimal aphasia, and acalculia. In clinical practice the language symptoms vary more widely than in alexia without agraphia. Some authors separate alexia with agraphia into two different types, one being the classical syndrome just described and the other being the reading and writing disorder that we discuss as *aphasic alexia* below. In most accounts of the syndrome there is some aphasia and it is always a fluent aphasia. The Gerstmann syndrome is sometimes present. A right homonymous visual field defect is frequently reported but not consistently present.

Deficits in reading letters, words, and musical notes are usually seen. Number reading is disordered, and defects of calculation are frequently observed. Writing disturbance is variable in severity but not severe enough to preclude writing of letters. Patients often cannot copy letters, unlike patients with alexia without agraphia, who copy laboriously and slowly. Also unlike pure alexics, these patients do not comprehend words spelled aloud.

Dejerine localized the neuropathology in alexia with agraphia to the angular gyrus of the dominant parietal lobe, and this localization has been universally confirmed since 1891. Dejerine surmised that the angular gyrus in the inferior parietal lobule was essential for the recall of written letters and that its destruction results in disturbances in reading and writing in adults.

Frontal Alexia

In 1977 Benson described a third alexia, which he indicated could be clearly separated from the classic syndromes documented by Dejerine and just described. The alexia is associated with the frontal lobe pathology that produces a Broca's aphasia. Frontal alexia, also known as *anterior alexia*, differs from the two classic alexias of Dejerine in that the patient understands content lexical items better than syntactical and relational lexical items. In fact, there is an inability to comprehend syntax and difficulty in maintaining verbal sequence in reading. Some patients cannot read letters or nonsense syllables, but do recognize words. This is a literal alexia sign.

Frontal alexia usually has an accompanying right hemiparesis and a transitory gaze paresis. The lesion is in the anterior part of the brain in the dominant frontal lobe, usually implicating Broca's area and adjacent deep structures.

Aphasic Alexia

The most common type of alexia is the reading disturbance that accompanies the major clinical types of aphasia. In most instances significant aphasic symptoms produce so much disturbance of language that reading is secondarily involved. It is generally realized in aphasiology that alexic symptoms in aphasia belong properly in a classification of aphasia, not in an outline of alexia. Reading disturbances in each of the major aphasic syndromes were described earlier in this chapter.

Psycholinguistic Classifications of Dyslexia

In the 1970s, British psychologists became very interested in reading disorders; literature began to include references to new classifications of reading disorders. The British refer to these disorders as *dyslexias*, even though they are acquired not developmental disorders (Marshall & Newcombe, 1973; Coltheart, Patterson, & Marshall, 1980). Three types of reading disorder classifications have resulted from psycholinguistic models of patient performance on tasks requiring primarily reading aloud of single words. These disorders are known as *deep dyslexia, surface dyslexia,* and *phonological alexia.* These classifications have become fairly well accepted and the symptoms often identified in patients.

Deep dyslexia is identified by the presence of semantic errors in reading aloud. Reading errors, such as saying "child" for "girl" or "quiet" for "listen" are common. Derivational errors such as reading "invitation" for "inviting" are present as are visual confusions. Deep dyslexia implies that the dyslexia reader goes directly to the semantic value of a word from its printed form without appreciating the sound of the word. Deep dyslexia has also been called phonemic, syntactic, or semantic dyslexia.

Surface dyslexia is distinguished by poor ability to use grapheme-to-phoneme conversion rules, although the reader relies heavily on these rules. The errors are phonologically similar to the target and there is great sensitivity to spelling regularity. Therefore, though many nonsense words can be pronounced, irregularly spelled words (like "yacht") are impossible for the patient to pronounce correctly. There is little sensitivity to meaning; the patient may not recognize that the word does not fit with the context.

Phonological alexia (Beauvois and Derousne, 1979) is characterized by an inability to read nonsense words with some difficulty noted with low-frequency words. Errors are often visual errors. It is assumed that these patients are impaired in the ability to use letter-to-sound conversion rules of the language.

Agraphia

Writing is a complex learned motor act that involves a conversion of oral language symbols into written symbols. It is assumed that the language symbols to be written originate in the posterior language areas in the dominant hemisphere of the brain. These oral symbols are translated into visual symbols in the inferior parietal lobe. The linguistic message is then sent forward to the frontal lobe for motor processing. Lesions in any of these language areas or pathways may produce the writing disorder called *agraphia*. The most common type of agraphia is secondary to aphasia and known as *aphasic agraphia*. Agraphia also may be seen in the absence of aphasia.

A rare agraphia has been described in which there is a writing disturbance in the left hand only. Patients with lesions of the anterior corpus callosum display this syndrome. The lesion disconnects the right motor cortex in the frontal area from the posterior language areas of the left hemisphere. Writing with the right hand is normal because of intact connections between left motor cortex and the left language areas. The callosal lesion disrupts language messages going to the right motor area, which controls the left hand.

Dementia

Cummings and Benson adopted the following operational definition of *dementia*: "an acquired persistent impairment of intellectual function with compromise in at least three of the following spheres of mental activity: language, memory, visuospatial skills, emotion or personality, and cognition (abstraction, judgment, executive function, and so forth)" (Cummings & Benson, 1992, pp. 1–2). The definition serves well to emphasize that dementia is acquired, is persistent, and does not affect all aspects of intelligence equally. It is important for the neurologist and the speech-language pathologist specializing in neurogenic communication disorders to recognize the early features of this syndrome so that the patient and family, if they so desire, can be proactive to prevent the serious social, economic, and vocational consequences of unrecognized intellectual deterioration.

The incidence and prevalence of dementia are difficult to determine as studies differ vastly depending on how dementia is defined and what particular population is studied. It is agreed by all that the incidence of dementia is rapidly increasing, with an increasing percentage of the population being affected. This is especially true because most dementias are found in persons over age 65 and the number of elderly people in the population is increasing rapidly. It has been estimated that the cost of caring for demented patients in the United States is approximately $30 billion annually.

The etiologies of dementia are many, and determination of the cause is critical since some dementias can be reversed. The most familiar, dementia of the Alzheimer's type (DAT), is not curable—although research is promising. Beyond DAT, other etiologies of dementia include Pick's disease, ischemic episodes resulting in multiple infarctions, extrapyramidal syndromes (including Huntington's and Parkinson's diseases), depression, hydrocephalus, metabolic disorders, toxic disorders, trauma, neoplasms, central nervous system infections, and demyelinating diseases.

Cummings and Benson (1992) classify the dementias into two basic patterns of neuropsychological impairment with identified neuroanatomical correlates: *cortical* and *subcortical* dementias. A third category of *mixed* is also noted. Cortical dementias, found in Alzheimer's disease and Pick's disease, have clinical characteristics that resemble focal lesions in cortical areas. These may include visuospatial and constructional problems, memory disturbance for new learning and for remote memory, cognitive deficits (including problems with calculation, judgment, and abstract thinking), and language disturbances affecting naming, reading, writing, and auditory comprehension. There may be disinhibition or a lack of concern and interest, but premorbid personality may be otherwise relatively preserved. In most cases, it is not until the later stages of the disease that gait, posture, tone, and speech are compromised.

Subcortical dementias may accompany extrapyramidal syndromes, depression, some white matter diseases (such as multiple sclerosis and AIDS-related encephalopathy), and some vascular diseases causing lacunar states. With subcortical dementias there is a slowing and progressive deterioration of cognition. Forgetfulness and alterations of affect are noted. Retrieval in memory is often aided by cues and by structure. In mood, the person may appear very depressed or apathetic with decreased motivation. The cognitive impairment has been described as one of *dilapidation*. Patients seem to be unable to synthesize and manipulate information to produce sequential steps to solve a complex problem though they may correctly perform individual steps accurately. The neurological examination of these patients will be abnormal with motor, posture, tone, and speech problems noted.

The mixed cortical-subcortical dementias result from such entities as multiple infarcts, toxic and metabolic encephalopathies, trauma, neoplasms, and anoxia. The mixture of characteristics will depend on the parts of the brain affected by the disease, trauma, or dementing process.

Alzheimer's disease afflicts a high percentage of the patients with cortical dementia. It is projected that there will be 14 million individuals with Alzheimer's disease in the United States in 10 years (*Scientific American*, 1995). The neuropathology of Alzheimer's disease shows the presence of neurofibrillary tangles in the cytoplasm of nerve cells. These tangles are pronounced in certain granular layers of the inferior temporal lobe, which has connections with the hippocampus (Davis, 1993). Tangles also tend to accumulate in posterior association regions of the cortex. In an individual there may be differences between the two hemispheres in the density of the tangles. Microscopic examination of the brain tissue of persons with DAT also shows neuritic plaques, which are remains of degenerated nerve fibers.

One of the most frustrating aspects of DAT for both physicians and patients is that definitive diagnosis is difficult in the early stages. Postmortem brain tissue examination is the only way at present to confirm the diagnosis. Thus, the National Institutes of Health diagnostic criteria refer to the disease as *probable dementia of the Alzheimer's type*. New techniques using magnetic resonance imaging have shown promise in identifying brain changes in patients with probable Alzheimer's. An even simpler test using a very dilute solution of tropicamide (used to dilate the pupil in eye examinations) has been studied at Harvard. Patients with probable Alzheimer's disease showed pronounced dilation even with a solution 1/100th as strong as that ordinarily used in eye tests (*Scientific American*, 1995).

Cummings and Benson (1992) report that the clinical course of DAT can be divided into three stages, the characteristics of which are fairly agreed on by most experts. These stages and their characteristics are summarized in Table 9–7.

Assessment and Treatment of Communication Disorders in Dementia

The speech-language pathologist is usually called on to help identify subtle language disorders that may signal intellectual deterioration since language is highly sensitive to even mild changes in brain function. In more advanced cases, the clinician may be asked to assess the effect of the intellectual deterioration on functional communication and suggest ways that family and other caregivers might improve communication with the patient.

Table 9–7   Clinical Features of the Different Stages of Dementia of the Alzheimer's Type

Stage	*Characteristics*
Stage I: mild	Memory for new learning is defective, and remote recall is mildly impaired. Language shows word retrieval problems and some difficulty understanding humor, analogies, and complex implications. The patient may be vague and may not initiate conversation when appropriate. The patient may also show indifference, anxiety, and irritability.
Stage II: middle	Memory for recent and remote events is more severely affected, and language shows vocabulary diminishment. The patient repeats ideas, forgets topics, has difficulty thinking of words in a category, loses sensitivity to conversational partners, and rarely corrects mistakes. Comprehension is reduced, and language may rely on jargon and paraphasias. The patient becomes increasingly indifferent, irritable, and restless.
Stage III: late	Memory is severely impaired, as are all intellectual functions. Language is rarely used meaningfully, and some patients are mute or echolalic. Motor function is compromised with limb rigidity and flexion posture.

Speech-language pathologists often use a simple measure of mental status to screen the patient if adequate information is not available about the possible presence of dementia. The *Mini-Mental Status Exam* (Folstein et al., 1975) and the *Global Deterioration Scale* (Reisberg et al., 1982) are two frequently used tools. Some patients may be seen after having extensive neurological workups and neuropsychological testing.

The purpose of the assessment by the speech-language pathologist may be assisting in making the differential diagnosis by trying to determine whether there is a true aphasia, apraxia, or an amnesia without language involvement. In these cases, aphasia testing and other traditional test batteries may be quite useful. As Bayles (1994) points out, however, the pragmatic and semantic language domains seem to be the most disordered in dementia patients, and many aphasia batteries do not adequately assess these domains with tasks that are active, generative, and dependent on logical reasoning. Bayles and Tomoeda (1991) developed the *Arizona Battery for Communication Disorders of Dementia* and standardized it on patients with Alzheimer's disease. Tasks such as the word fluency measure (Borkowski et al., 1967) and the similarities subtest of the *Wechsler Adult Intelligence Scale* (Wechsler, 1981) are also sensitive to the communication disorders caused by a dementing illness.

Dysphagia is another area of assessment for patients with dementia in which the speech-language pathologist will have primary involvement. Horner and colleagues (1994) did a cross-sectional study of 63 patients with Alzheimer's disease. They looked at correlates of aspiration and found that the significant variable was severity of dementia. There was a trend toward significance for oral praxis, eating dependency, swallow response delay, and impaired physical status. In a longitudinal study of 24 patients with Alzheimer's disease, Horner et al. found that the incidence of aspiration increased from 13 to 21 percent over a period of 1 year. This increase seemed to be associated with worsening dementia, increased eating dependence, declining physical status, and worsening oral apraxia.

Management of the communication and swallowing disorders accompanying irreversible dementia usually does not primarily involve direct treatment. Management includes education of the family and other caregivers as to how to maximize the communicative effectiveness of the mildly impaired patient. For patients with more advanced disease, caregivers must be taught specific strategies to help them communicate more effectively with the person. Specific strategies for feeding may also be suggested, including type of food, environment, adaptations, and the effect of medication. The speech-language pathologist also provides important information to the physician and caregiver by periodic reassessment of the communicative status of the patient since the correlation between performance on language tests and severity of dementia is strong. More proactive planning may be necessary if increased communication difficulty is predicted.

Acute Confusional States

Several etiologies produce confusion, which is characterized by rapid onset over a period of hours or days. The causes of confusion include metabolic imbalance, adverse drug reactions, and alcohol and drug withdrawal reactions. Patients generally are inattentive, incoherent, and irrelevant; they demonstrate fluctuating levels of consciousness. Agitation and hallucinations, usually visual, are often present. Acute confusional states generally respond to primary medical treatment. Confusional states are not usually the result of focal brain lesions; there is generally widespread cortical and subcortical neuronal dysfunction. Confusional symptoms are also seen during the period of posttraumatic amnesia in traumatic head injury.

Symptomatic language impairment is seen in the confusional states. The language disturbance may be viewed as a secondary symptom of the confusional state. Halpern, Darley, and Brown (1973) reported on the language symptoms of patients with confused language in contrast to other language impairments of cerebral involvement. Lesions in these patients were either bilateral or multifocal. Generally, vocabulary and syntax were normal. The most striking feature of the language of these confused patients was its irrelevancy and confabulatory nature. Other investigators have also found irrelevant language response and confabulation in dementia, so it is not a pathognomic feature of confused states.

Confabulation is the verbal or written expression of fictitious experiences, generally filling a gap in memory. It is less marked in the presence of aphasia, since it is a response in which the language areas must be relatively intact. Confabulation is more often associated with generalized cerebral deficit or dysfunction rather than with focal lesions. Some instances in which focal lesions are associated with confabulation are in the Wernicke-Korsakoff's amnestic syndrome and in ruptured aneurysms of the anterior communicating artery.

Traumatic Brain Injury

Traumatic brain injury (TBI) or closed head injury occurs approximately once every 16 seconds in the United States, with approximately 400,000 new head injuries each year (Friedman, 1988). Knowledge about the resulting deficits has greatly increased over the past 10 years, as have the number of rehabilitation programs and treatment method-ologies devoted to TBI. Patients usually display the language of confusion but often present a more serious and pervasive language deficit now termed a *cognitive communication disorder* or a *cognitive-linguistic disorder.*

The predominant type of injury is an acceleration-deceleration injury, where the head is accelerated and then suddenly stopped, as in a motor vehicle accident. Discrete focal lesions may result from direct impact forces. Contusions may be found at the point of direct impact, and contre-coup damage may be present at the site opposite the point of direct impact. The frontal (frontopolar and orbitofrontal) and temporal (anterior temporal, but not necessarily medial temporal) lobes are the most likely sites of focal cortical contusions (Adamovich & Henderson, 1990).

Very frequently in TBI, there is no evidence of focal lesions, but there is diffuse brain injury resulting from molecular commotion. The molecu-lar structure of the brain is disrupted after impact as the impact force causes acceleration, rotation, compression, and expansion of the brain within the skull. Brain tissues are compressed and torn apart and sheared on the bony prominences of the skull, causing diffuse axonal injury (DAI) and permanent microscopic alterations of both white and gray matter.

Diffuse axonal injury, even severe DAI, may occur without skull fracture or cortical contusion. It has been demonstrated in nonhuman primate models that DAI can be produced on rapid acceleration of the head with no impact and in cases of mild brain injury in which the nonhuman primate has only transitory alterations in the level of consciousness.

The DAI and focal lesions are primary mechanisms of injury in traumatic brain insult. Secondary mechanisms that occur as a result of the initial direct forces also cause further brain damage. These secondary mechanisms of injury include ischemia, hypoxia, edema, hemorrhage, brain shift, and raised intracranial pressure, and they all produce further deleterious effects on brain function.

The neurobehavioral sequelae of traumatic brain injury are usually divided into two classes: focal deficits and diffuse deficits. *Focal deficits* may be manifested as a specific language deficit or as a paralysis of specific muscles or muscle groups. Disorders such as mutism, dysarthria, palilalia, stuttering, voice disorder, hearing loss, and visual or auditory perceptual dysfunction may be considered focal deficits.

Diffuse deficits are more common and are most often manifested as cognitive disorganization. Ylvisaker and Szekeres (1994) note that the cognitive processes of attention, perception, memory, learning, organiza-tion, reasoning, problem-solving, and judgment are affected. These aspects of cognition and the possible effect of their disruption on behavior and language are outlined in Table 9–8.

Table 9-8 Cognitive Impairment Following Traumatic Brain Injury: Effect on Behavior and Language

Aspect of Cognition	Effect on Behavior	Effect on Language
	Attention	
Holding objects, events, words, or thoughts in consciousness	Short attention span; distractable; weak concentration	Decreased auditory comprehension; confused or inappropriate language; poor reading comprehension; poor topic maintenance
	Perception	
Recognizing features and relationships among features	Weak perception of relevant features; possible specific deficits (including field neglect); poor judgement based on visual or auditory cues; stimulus-bound (i.e., focus on part of the whole); spatial disorganization	Difficulty in reading and writing; poor comprehension of facial and intonation cues
	Memory and learning	
Encoding: recognizing, interpreting, and formulating information, including language, into an internal code (knowledge base, personal interests, and goals affect what is coded). *Storage*: Retaining information over time. *Retrieval*: Transferring information from long-term memory to consciousness.	Memory problems; inability or inefficiency in learning new material	Difficulty following multistep directions; word-finding problems; difficulty with reading comprehension and spelling; poor integration of new and old information. Language may be fragmented, lacking logic, order, specificity, and precision; difficulty with math is also seen.

Table 9-8 *(continued)*

Aspect of Cognition	Effect on Behavior	Effect on Language
Organizing Processes		
Analyzing, classifying, integrating, sequencing, and identifying relevant features of objects and events, comparing for similarities or differences; integrating into organized descriptions, higher-level categories, and sequenced events	Poor organization of tasks and time; difficulty setting and maintaining goals; poor problem-solving, self-direction, self-confidence, and social judgment	Disorganized language (verbal and written); difficulty discerning main ideas and integrating them into broader themes; poor conversational skills (may get lost in details); difficulty outlining material for study; difficulty with math
Reasoning		
Considering evidence and drawing inferences or conclusions; involves flexible exploration of possibilities (divergent thinking) and use of past experience	Concrete, impulsive, and reactionary; may be easily swayed; vulnerable to propaganda; difficulty discerning cause-and-effect and consequences of behavior; poor social judgment	Difficulty understanding and expressing abstract concepts; socially inappropriate; lack of tact; difficulty using language to persuade, understanding humor, learning academic subjects, and following complex conversation
Problem-solving and judgment		
Problem-solving: Ideally it involves identifying goals, considering relevant information, exploring possible solutions, and selecting the best solutions. *Judgment:* Deciding to act, or not to act, based on consideration of relevant factors, including prediction of consequences.	Impulsive; uses trial-and-error approach; difficulty predicting consequences of behavior; shallow reasoning; poor safety and social judgment; inflexible thinking; poor self-direction and poor use of compensatory strategies	Difficulty understanding and expressing steps in problem-solving to get a particular outcome; difficulty in math and higher academic tasks; socially inappropriate behavior; lack of tact; difficulty in understanding explanations for behavior

Source: Adapted from S. F. Szekeres, M. Ylvisaker, & A. L. Holland, "Cognitive Rehabilitation Therapy: A Framework for Intervention." In M. Ylvisaker (Ed.), *Head Injury Rehabilitation: Children and Adolescents.* (San Diego: College-Hill Press, 1985).

Testing and Treating the Language Impairment in Traumatic Brain Injury

Although standard aphasia batteries are used in assessing the language impairment in TBI, testing must extend beyond these batteries in most cases. As examination of Table 9–8 reveals, the cognitive and communicative deficits of TBI can be quite different from the aphasia of a patient with a vascular lesion. The speech-language pathologist must attempt to determine which cognitive processes underlying language performance are disrupted, and to what degree, and must also determine if there is a true aphasic component to the language impairment.

The speech-language pathologist working with TBI patients is usually part of a rehabilitation team, at least in the initial stages of recovery and rehabilitation. Informal or formal testing and observation using such assessment scales as the *Rancho Los Amigos Levels of Cognitive Recovery* (Hagen & Malkmus, 1979) will help the team members identify the patient's best level of cognitive functioning throughout the course of rehabilitation. Specific treatment approaches for each level of cognitive functioning have been developed by Hagen (1986). Ylvisaker and Szekeres (1994) have outlined treatment methods for the middle and later stages of recovery, and Solberg and Mateer (1989) have developed the *process-specific approach* to cognitive rehabilitation which is also used by many speech-language pathologists providing services to the TBI patient.

Right-Hemisphere Lesions

The neurology of right-hemisphere lesions is of special interest to speech-language pathologists despite the fact that only a small percentage of the population has right-hemispheric or bilateral representation of language functions. The person who is right-hemispheric dominant for language is usually left-handed or ambidextrous, but not all left-handers or ambidexters have right or bilateral representation for language. Milner (1974), reporting on the results of the *Wada Test* in the left-handed, suggests that 70 percent of left-handers have language represented in the left cerebral hemisphere, 15 percent show bilateral representation, and 15 percent have language represented in the right hemisphere. It appears that in the left-hander there are gradients of hemispheric specialization for language that vary from absolute dominance of one hemisphere to an equal contribution of both hemispheres. For the population as a whole, the left hemisphere is dominant for language regardless of handedness.

If a left-hander becomes aphasic, the language disturbance is usually milder than it is in the right-hander who is left-language dominant.

Generally, left-handers with presumed lesions in the right hemisphere recover more quickly and thoroughly than do right-handers who are left-dominant.

The role of the right hemisphere in recovery of language functions after damage to the left, language-dominant, hemisphere is not completely understood. Neurologists, from the era of Wernicke and his contemporaries, however, have attributed language recovery to the action of the right hemisphere. In 1922 the Scandinavian neurologist Salomon E. Henschen (1847–1930) formulated this principle into a statement that has become known as *Henschen's axiom* in neurology. Henschen's axiom asserts that restitution of speech is often due to the activity of the opposite hemisphere.

Evidence from hemispherectomies and callosal sections suggests that the right hemisphere can assume some language function, although the extent of recovery may be limited. In adult hemispherectomies with no cortical tissue remaining, language behavior is similar to that of a global aphasic with extensive infarction of the perisylvian area. What language remains appears to be completely the product of the right hemisphere. The mechanisms of right-hemisphere recovery are speculative. Some experts believe that language is relearned by the right hemisphere; others believe that right-hemisphere substitution is the release of already-learned language functions of the right hemisphere. Further, there may be considerable individual variation in hemisphere substitution, and some patients may make more use of commissural connections and right-hemisphere mechanisms than do others. Although the precise mechanism of right-hemisphere language in left-hemisphere aphasia is unknown, it is probable that the right hemisphere does play some role in language recovery after cerebral insult to the left hemisphere.

In right-hemisphere lesions of the nondominant hemisphere, a broad spectrum of deficits is seen. The most dramatic deficits are neglect, inattention, denial, visual and spatial perceptual disorders, and constructional disturbances. Language disorders from right-hemisphere lesions, for the most part, are milder than those resulting from left-hemisphere lesions. Some common right-hemisphere lesion syndromes are discussed below.

Neglect, Inattention, and Denial

Neglect is a syndrome in which a patient fails to recognize one side of the body and the environmental space surrounding that side. Patients may use only one half of their bodies, even using only one sleeve in their shirts, even though the neglected side of the body is free of paralysis. Neglect of half of the environmental space is not the result of a visual field defect.

The exact neurologic locus of the neglect syndrome with right-hemisphere lesions is not exactly known. Chronic parietal lobe damage shows a high correlation with the syndrome. *Unilateral inattention* may be considered a subtle form of the neglect syndrome. Neurologists test for unilateral inattention through a procedure called *double simultaneous stimulation*, in which all sensory modalities are tested. In tactile testing, corresponding points on the body are touched at the same time with equal intensity. Visual testing involves having the patient fixate on a point on the neurologic examiner's face. The examiner moves his or her fingers into both the right and left peripheral visual fields, and the patient reports where the fingers are seen. Auditory testing is performed by having the examiner stand behind the patient and provide a stimulus of equal intensity to both ears.

Extinction is present when the patient suppresses stimuli from one side. Extinction may occur in all modalities or in a single modality. When extinction is elicited, the degree of inattention can be assessed by increasing the strength of the stimulus on the inattentive side.

Anatomically, *global attention* is related to the ascending reticular activating system in the pons, the midbrain, and an extension of tegmentum into the diencephalon. The ascending reticular activating system is a nonspecific neuronal system that is coupled with the cerebral cortex to control levels of consciousness and attention. The limbic system also contributes to focusing attention by adding emotional significance to the object of attention. Unilateral inattention probably results from damage to the brainstem reticular formation or to the cortex. Midbrain lesions of the ascending reticular activating system are rare, but general inattention is commonly seen in bilateral diffuse brain dysfunction caused by metabolic disturbance, drug intoxication, cerebral infection, or postsurgical states of the brain. Extensive bilateral cortical damage also produces inattention. Unilateral inattention to double simultaneous stimulation appears to result from a contralateral lesion to the parietal lobe. Right parietal lobe lesions produce more unilateral inattention than do left-hemisphere lesions. The reason for this asymmetry in unilateral attention defects is unknown.

Many patients develop a dramatic *denial* of their neurologic illness; the denial may range from mild to severe. An example of severe denial is the patient's lack of recognition of a hemiplegia. The condition was documented by the Russian neurologist Joseph Babinski (1857–1932), who had a patient with a left-sided hemiplegia and left-sided sensory loss who appeared completely unaware of his neurologic deficit. If the patient's hemiplegic arm was placed on the bed along his left side and the neurologist placed his own arm across the patient's waist, the patient would lift the physician's arm aloft. If he were asked to grasp his left arm with his nonparalyzed right arm, he would grasp the physician's arm. Asked to move his paralyzed arm even though his arm was completely hemiplegic, the patient would emphatically say that he could move his arm. Babinski used the term *anosognosia* to describe this unawareness. Anosognosia is sometimes used to describe symptoms of denial other than the ones described here, but it probably is best to limit it to the specific denial impairment Babinski described. This example of denial is highly common in right-hemispheric lesions and much less common in left-hemispheric lesions. Anosognosia does not appear to be based on a psychological mechanism but, rather, a more fundamental neurological mechanism of gnostic loss.

Prosopagnosia

Prosopagnosia refers to the inability to recognize familiar faces and their expressions. The patient recognizes individuals by voice rather than visual perception. The disorder may be a memory disturbance for the category of faces plus a disorder of fine visual discrimination. Bilateral lesions are usually found in the occipital-temporal areas in this disorder. The lesion in the right hemisphere is usually specifically in the right temporal-occipital region. A specific type of color agnosia often accompanies prosopagnosia. The lesions that cause the facial recognition deficit also cause the color agnosia.

Agraphagnosia

Agraphagnosia is the inability to recognize letters and numbers traced on the skin or fingertips when the eyes are closed. If there is a lack of number, letter, or character recognition on the left hand, a right parietal lobe lesion may be suspected.

Visual-Perceptual and Reading Deficits

Right-hemisphere lesions are associated with deficits in meaningful interpretation and recall of complex visual structures. Deficits in the perception and recall of letters, words, and numbers may produce problems in reading.

Spatial Organizational Deficits

As noted earlier in this chapter, constructional disturbances are present when there are either right or left parietal lobe lesions. In most instances, right-hemisphere lesions tend to cause more frequent and severe constructional deficits, but constructional deficits can also indicate a left-hemisphere lesion.

Language Disorders of Visual-Spatial Perception

Rivers and Love (1980) reported on the language performance of patients with right-hemisphere lesions when the patients were asked to respond to a series of visual spatial processing tasks. The language was judged poorer than that of normal controls, but not as poor as that of the majority of aphasic controls with left-hemisphere lesions. The patients with right-hemisphere lesions showed dysnomia in oral storytelling based on a series of visual stimuli but ability to name pictured objects did not differ from normal subjects. Other investigators have reported mild agrammatism and telegraphic speech plus anomia in a variety of right-hemispheric conditions.

Paralinguistic and Prosodic Deficits

Although patients with damage to the right hemisphere rarely display symptoms of a serious aphasia, they do show a variety of language disturbances beyond those mentioned in the preceding paragraphs. Patients have impairments in comprehending the meaning of single words, with difficulty in understanding connotative meanings but not denotative meanings (Brownell et al., 1984). They also have problems in making judgments of semantic relatedness involving picture-word matching.

Patients are often quite literal. They may show superficially intact understanding of single sentences but miss the point of the whole conversation, as well as of jokes and stories. They also have difficulty with the interpretation of complex themes of linguistic information. When compared with control patients and patients with left-hemisphere damage, patients with right-hemisphere damage have greater difficulty if the themes in stories are placed at the end of a paragraph (Hough & Pierce, 1993).

A common defect in the right-hemisphere syndrome is known as *aprosodia*. Prosody, among other things, conveys appropriate emotional affect. Prosody also carries pragmatic information, allowing a listener to discriminate between questions, statements, and explanations. When normal stress or emphasis is disturbed in a sentence, it is often difficult to convey new information.

The neurologist G. H. Monrad-Krohn (1963) was among the first to distinguish various types of prosodic disturbances. He cited a dramatic case of aprosody which has become a classic in the neurological literature. A Norwegian patient who suffered right frontal brain damage during World War II developed *hyperprosody*, an increase in "intonation variation," to such a degree that it was thought she had the accent of a person from Germany.

Elliot Ross (1981) has reported widely on patients with deficits of both prosodic production and comprehension. Patients often show the inability to provide variations in their voices so that they have a "flat" emotional tone. Comprehension defects are called *affective aprosodia* and may include several distinct components. However, they report being able to feel emotions and hear emotion in the voices of others. Ross has developed a set of eight aprosodias and proposed that *motor aprosodia* is associated with right frontal damage. He has also suggested that *sensory aprosodia* is associated with right posterior damage. A motor aprosody on the right is analogous to a motor aphasia in Broca's area, and a sensory aprosodia on the right is analogous to a Wernicke's aphasia on the left.

Many other neurologists have confirmed the presence of prosodic defects in both comprehension and expression, but lesion localization for these and other symptoms in Ross' scheme have not been found consistently in the literature. Various lesion sites of left- and right-hemisphere aprosodias have been associated with lesions in the basal ganglia of the right or left hemispheres and in the anterior temporal lobe. Ross initially believed that right-hemisphere aprosodia was associated with corpus callosal lesions.

Dysarthria

A dysarthria involving primarily the articulatory aspects of speech has frequently been reported in patients with right-hemisphere lesions. This dysarthria has sometimes been called a pathognomonic sign of nondominant-hemisphere damage. Since dysarthria occurs in lesions of either or both hemispheres, it cannot be viewed as an unequivocal sign for the diagnosis of right-hemisphere lesions; however, it may be used as a corroborating sign of the syndrome of right-hemisphere lesions.

In sum, the speech and language disturbances of the right hemisphere are not as striking as those of the left hemisphere; however, without an intact right hemisphere, communication in its broadest sense cannot be fully realized. At present, speech-language pathologists do not have at their disposal an assessment battery to identify all the behavioral linguistic and extralinguistic deficits associated with right-hemisphere lesions syndromes. Meyers (1994) suggests using selected subtests of published tests along with informal measures and observations.

Pharmacology in Aphasia

The use of medication by the neurologist to aid the language-impaired patient has been attempted for many years. In general, results have not been particularly encouraging and even when they were, the results lacked methodological strength: sample sizes were small, and double-blind studies in which some subjects received a placebo while matched subjects did not were rarely employed.

In recent years, however, intensive study of the actions of neurotransmitter systems has increased the use of drugs in aphasia rehabilitation. It has been found that selected linguistic functions such as verbal fluency and verbal memory can be influenced by specific neurotransmitter systems. Of the more than 20 neurotransmitters identified to date, only a few appear to be cognitive enhancers, and that those drugs, at best, often have only secondary, nonspecific benefits on the speech and language systems.

Dopaminergic networks appear specifically to mediate verbal fluency. Strong clinical evidence indicates that dopamine exerts control of fluency in Parkinson patients. Speech volume, timing, phrase structure, and syntactic constructions have been improved with L-dopa. Paraphasias have also been reduced. Aphasics who reportedly benefited from dopamine agonists had nonfluent aphasia but not all nonfluent aphasias improved with drug administration.

Patients with transcortical motor aphasia have been more responsive to dopaminergic agents, since damage to dopamine networks underlying lesion sites produces transcortical motor aphasia in the supplementary motor area. The supplementary motor area, together with the anterior cingulate, forms a link with midbrain dopaminergic centers.

Of the dopaminergic agonists, the drug bromocriptine has been most widely used because it does not require preservation of presynaptic function as does L-dopa. However, sufficient studies have not yet been carried out to point to a clear preference in drug usage (Minura, Albert, & McNamara, 1995).

Pharmacologic therapy for fluent aphasia may also be feasible. Cholinergic networks, utilizing acetylcholine, are known to influence verbal memory. Anticholinergic drugs such as scopolamine impair verbal memory and produce verbal intrusions and preservations in normal subjects. Deficits produced by lack of cholinergic agents have been thought to produce memory deficits in elderly persons and patients with Alzheimer's disease. It has been hypothesized that cholinergic therapy may be effective in fluent aphasia. Cholinergic networks are specifically found in the left posterior brain areas. The internationally known Russian neurologist Alexander Luria was one of the first to utilize a powerful anticholinesterase agent, *galanthamine* to improve speech and gnostic and praxic functions in brain-injured individuals (Luria et al., 1969). Different cholinergic drugs appear to be effective with fluent aphasia.

In brief, it appears that biochemical intervention may be a powerful adjunct to the more traditional methods of behavioral therapy used with aphasics. Drug therapy certainly will not supersede traditional methods of therapy, but the future appears brighter for more effective drug therapies combined with other approaches for the rehabilitation of aphasia.

Summary

The exact neurophysiology of the central language mechanism is not completely known, but a model developed by Carl Wernicke over a century ago, in 1874, has proved to be the most valid and reliable construct for the explanation of the wide array of aphasic symptoms seen clinically. The model has gained wide acceptance among neuroscientists, linguists, and speech-language pathologists. There is growing support for the model from neurosurgical data, brain and computerized tomography scans, and other neurodiagnostic procedures.

The Wernicke model assumes a large perisylvian speech area on the left cerebral cortex that includes all the major anterior and posterior language areas (Broca's, Wernicke's, angular gyrus, and supramarginal gyrus) and the intra- and interhemispheric connective pathways—namely, the arcuate fasciculus and the corpus callosum. Recently, subcortical language mechanisms important in memory and naming have been confirmed at the thalamic level. Thalamic aphasia, without cortical involvement, has also become an accepted aphasic syndrome. Other subcortical aphasic syndromes have recently been reported.

Although aphasic classification systems are abundant, the Wernicke model is the source of the most widely used current classifications. Aphasias of the perisylvian zone include Broca's aphasia, Wernicke's aphasia, conduction aphasia, and global aphasia. Aphasia syndromes outside the perisylvian speech area are called *transcortical aphasias* and include transcortical motor aphasia, transcortical sensory aphasia, mixed transcortical aphasia, and the isolated speech area syndrome. Anomic aphasia is usually associated with bilateral lesions or mild involvement of the perisylvian speech area. Other anomic patients show no demonstrable lesions.

Aphasia syndromes have often been dichotomized into fluent or nonfluent disorders in terms of spontaneous speech performance. Nonfluent aphasia is usually associated with anterior lesions and fluent aphasia with posterior lesions.

There are many associated central disturbances seen alone or with aphasia. Agnosias (recognition syndromes) are uncommon. Bilateral visual agnosia, auditory agnosia, and its two subtypes—pure word deafness and agnosia for nonspeech sounds—are currently accepted as clinical syndromes. Isolated cases of bilateral tactile agnosia have been described but are uncommon.

The Gerstmann syndrome is controversial. It is said to include finger agnosia, left-right disorientation, acalculia, and agraphia as the result of left parietal lobe lesions; it may be seen independently or with aphasia. A developmental form of the syndrome has also been described.

Apraxia is a disorder of motor programming due to brain injury. The terminology of apraxia is confusing. The historical classification of Hugo Liepmann, including ideational and ideomotor aphasia, is accepted by many clinical neurologists. Limb apraxia, construction disturbance, and buccofacial apraxia (oral apraxia) are frequently reported in the neurologic and neuropsychologic literature. Apraxia of speech is well-accepted by speech-language pathologists. Developmental apraxia of speech remains controversial to both neurologists and speech-language pathologists.

Alexia is a reading disturbance that may exist with aphasia or may be seen independently. Alexia with agraphia, alexia without agraphia, and frontal alexia are reasonably well-accepted. Aphasia alexia is the most common disorder of reading in adults. Agraphia is a writing disturbance due to brain injury. Dementia, primarily an impairment of intellectual functioning, may present a serious language disturbance. In this chapter, the language of acute confusional states is described, the right-hemisphere lesion syndrome is outlined, and traumatic brain injury is discussed. Drug therapy in aphasia is outlined, but effective results must be considered preliminary.

References and Further Readings

Model of the Central Language Mechanism

Alexander, M. P., Naeser, M. A., & Palumbo, C. L. (1987). Correlations of subcortical CT lesion sites and aphasia profiles. *Brain, 110,* 961–991.

Benson, D. F. (1977). The third alexia. *Archives of Neurology, 34,* 327–331.

Brownell, H., Gardner, H., Prather, P. & Martino, G. (1995). Language, communication and the right hemisphere. In H. Kirshner (Ed.), *Handbook of neurologic speech and language disorders.* New York: Marcel Dekker.

Buckingham, H. W., Jr. (1982). Neuropsychological models of language. In N. Lass, L. McReynolds, J. Northern, & D. Yoder (Eds.), *Speech, language, and hearing* (Vol. 1). Philadelphia: W. B. Saunders.

Caplan, D. (1992). *Language: Structure processing, and disorders.* Cambridge, MA: MIT Press.

Churchland, P. M. (1995). *The engine of reason, the seat of the soul: A philosophical journey into the brain.* Cambridge, MA: MIT Press.

Crosson, B. (1984). Role of the dominant thalamus in language: A review. *Psychological Bulletin, 96,* 491–517.

Crosson, B. (1992). *Subcortical functions in language and memory.* New York: Guilford Press.

Dejerine, J. (1891). Sur un cas de cécité verbal avec agraphie, suivi d'autopsie. *Mem Soc Biol, 3,* 197–201.

Dejerine, J. (1892). Contributions à l'étude anatomo-pathologique et clinique des différentes variétés de cécité. *Mem Soc Biol, 4,* 61–90.

Eggert, G. (1977). *Wernicke's works on aphasia.* The Hague, Netherlands: Mouton.

Ellman, J. L. (1992). Grammatic structure and distributed representations. In S. Davis (Ed.), *Connectionism: Theory and practice. Vol. 3. Vancouver studies in cognitive science.* Oxford: Oxford University Press.

Geschwind, N. (1967). Wernicke's contribution to the study of aphasia. *Cortex, 3,* 449–463.

Geschwind, N. (1969). Problems in the anatomical understanding of aphasia. In A. L. Benton (Ed.), *Contributions to clinical neuropsychology.* Chicago: Aldine.

Geschwind N. (1975). The apraxias: Neural mechanisms of disorders of learned movements. *American Scientist, 63,* 188–195.

Gopnik, M. (1990). Genetic basis of grammar defect. *Nature, 34,* 26.

Hough, M. S., & Pierce, R. S. (1993). Contextual and thematic influences on narrative comprehension of left and right hemisphere brain-damaged adults. In H. H. Browness & Y. Joanette (Eds.), *Narrative discourse in neurologically impaired and normal aging adults.* San Diego: Singular Publishing Group.

Luria, A. R., Naydin, V. L., Tsvetkova, L. S., & Vinarskaya, E. N. (1969). Restoration of higher cortical functions following local brain damage. In P. J. Vinken & G. W. Bruyn (Eds.), *Handbook of clinical neurology. Vol. 3. Disorders of higher nervous activity.* Amsterdam: North Holland Publishing.

Marshall, J. C. (1985). On some relationships between acquired and developmental dyslexias. In F. H. Duffy & N. Geschwind (Eds.), *Dyslexia: A neuroscientific approach to clinical evaluation.* Boston: Little, Brown.

Metter, E. J., Riege, W. H., Hanson, W. R., Jackson, C. A., Kempler, D., & van Lancker, D. (1988). Subcortical structures in aphasia: An analysis based on (F-18)-fluorodeoxyglucose, positron emission tomography, and computed tomography. *Archives of Neurology, 45,* 1229–1234.

Metter, E. J., Riege, W. H., Hanson, W. R., Kuhl, D. E., Phelps, M. E., Squire, L. R., Wasterlain, C. G., & Benson, D. F. (1983). Comparison of metabolic rates, language, and memory in subcortical aphasias. *Brain and Language, 19,* 33–47.

Mimura, M., Albert, M. L., & McNamara (1995). Toward a pharmacology for aphasia. In H. Kirshner (Ed.), *Handbook of neurological speech and language disorders*. New York: Marcel Dekker.

Mohr, J. P., Watters, W. C., & Duncan, G. W. (1975). Thalamic hemorrhage and aphasia. *Brain and Language*, 2, 3–17.

Monrad-Krohn, G. H. (1963). The third element of speech: prosody and its disorders. In L. Halpern (Ed.), *Problems of dynamic neurology*. Jerusalem: Hebrew University.

Naeser, M. A., Alexander, M. P., Helm-Estabrooks, N., Levine, H. L., Laughlin, S., & Geschwind, N. (1982). Aphasia with predominantly subcortical lesion sites. *Archives of Neurology*, 39, 2–14.

Penfield, W. G., & Roberts, L. (1959). *Speech and brain mechanisms*. Princeton, NJ: Princeton University Press.

Robin, D. A., & Schienberg, S. (1990). Subcortical lesions and aphasia. *Journal of Speech and Hearing Disorders*, 55, 90–100.

Roeltgen, D. P., & Heilman, K. M. (1985). Review of agraphia and a proposal for an anatomically-based neuropsychological model of writing. *Applied Psycholinguistics*, 6, 205–230.

Springer, S. P., & Deutsch, G. (1989). *Left brain, right brain* (3rd ed.). San Francisco: W. H. Freeman.

Wallesch, C. W., & Papagno, C. (1988). Subcortical aphasia. In Rose, F. C., Whurr, R., & Wyke, M. A. (Eds.), *Aphasia*. London: Whurr Publishers.

Wernicke, K. (1874). *Der Aphasische Symptomkomplex*. Breslau: Kohn and Neigert.

Whitaker, H. A. (1971). *On the representation of language in the human brain*. Edmonton: Linguistic Research.

Aphasia Classification and Testing

Benson, D. F. (1979). *Aphasia, alexia, and agraphia*. New York: Churchill Livingstone.

DeMyer, W. (1980). *The technique of the neurologic examination* (3rd ed.). New York: McGraw-Hill.

Eisenson, J. (1954). *Examining for aphasia*. New York: The Psychological Corporation.

Goodglass, H., & Kaplan, E. (1983). *The assessment of aphasia and related disorders* (2nd ed.). Philadelphia: Lea & Febiger.

Head, H. (1926). *Aphasia and kindred disorders of speech*. Cambridge: Cambridge University Press.

Keenan, J. S., & Brassell, E. G. (1975). *Aphasia language performance scales*. Murfreesboro, TN: Pinnacle Press.

Kertesz, A. (1983). *The Western Aphasia Battery.* New York: Grune & Stratton.

Kirshner, H. S. (Ed.) (1995). *Handbook of neurological speech and language disorders.* New York: Marcel Dekker.

Porch, B. E. (1967). *Porch Index of Communicative Ability. Vol. 1. Theory and development.* Palo Alto, CA: Consulting Psychologists Press.

Porch, B. E. (1971). *Porch Index of Communicative Ability. Vol. II. Administration, scoring and interpretation* (rev. ed.). Palo Alto, CA: Consulting Psychologists Press.

Schuell, H. M. (1965). *Minnesota Test for Differential Diagnosis of Aphasia.* Minneapolis: University of Minnesota.

Schuell, H. M. (1966). A reevaluation of the short examination for aphasia. *Journal of Speech and Hearing Disorders,* 31, 137–147.

Spreen, O., & Benton, A. L. (1969). *Neurosensory Center Comprehensive Examination of Aphasia,* Victoria, BC, Canada: Neuropsychology Laboratory, University of Victoria.

Tanridag, O., & Kirshner, H. S. (1985). Aphasia and agraphia in lesions of the posterior internal capsule and putamen. *Neurology,* 35, 1797–1801.

Weisenburg, T. H., & McBride, K. E. (1935). *Aphasia.* New York: Commonwealth Fund.

Wepman, J. M., & Jones, L. V. (1961). *Studies in aphasia: An approach to testing.* Chicago: Education Industry Service.

Associated Central Disturbances

Adamovich, B. L. B., & Henderson, J. A. (1990). Traumatic brain injury. In L. L. LaPointe (Ed.), *Aphasia and related neurogenic language disorders.* New York: Thieme.

Adams, R., & Sidman, R. L. (1968). *Introduction to neuropathology.* New York: McGraw-Hill.

Alexander, M. P., & Naeser, M. A. (1988). Cortical-subcortical differences in aphasia. In F. Plum (Ed.), *Language, communication and the brain.* New York: Raven Press.

Bayles, K. A. (1994). Management of neurogenic communication disorders associated with dementia. In Chapey, R. (Ed.), *Language intervention strategies in adult aphasia* (3rd ed.). Baltimore: Williams & Wilkins.

Bayles, K. A., & Tomoeda, C. K. (1991). *Arizona Battery for Communication Disorders of Dementia.* Tucson, AZ: Canyonlands Publishing.

Beauvois, M. F. & Derousne, J. (1979). Phonological alexia: Three dissociations. *Journal of Neurology, Neurosurgery and Psychiatry,* 42, 1115–1124.

Beauvois, M. F., Sailliant, B., Meininger, V., & Lhermitte, F. (1978). Bilateral tactile aphasia: A tacto-verbal dysfunction. *Brain*, 101, 381–402.

Benson, D. F. (1979). *Aphasia, alexia and agraphia*. New York: Churchill Livingstone.

Benson, D. F., & Geschwind, N. (1970). Developmental Gerstmann syndrome. *Neurology*, 20, 293–298.

Berry, K. E. (1989). *Developmental Test of Visual Motor Integration* (3rd rev. ed.) Chicago: Follet.

Borkowski, J. G., Benton, A. L., & Spreen, O. (1967). Word fluency and brain damage. *Neuropsychologica*, 5, 135–140.

Brownwell, H. H., Potter, H. H., Michelson, D., Gardner, H. Sensitivity to lexical denotation and connotation in brain damaged patients: A double dissociation. *Brain and Language* 22: 253–265.

Code, C. (Ed.) (1990). *The characteristics of aphasia*. New York: Taylor and Francis.

Coltheart, M. (1987). Functional architecture of the language processing system. In M. Coltheart, G. Samtori, & R. Fob (Eds.), *The cognitive neuropsychology of language*. London: Lawrence Erlbaum and Associates.

Coltheart, M., Patterson, K., & Marshall, J. C. (Eds.) (1980). *Deep dyslexia*. London: Routledge and Kegan Paul.

Cummings, J. L., & Benson, D. F. (1992). *Dementia: A clinical approach* (2nd ed.). Boston: Butterworth-Heinemann.

Davis, G. A. (1993). *A survey of adult aphasia and related disorders* (2nd ed.). Englewood Cliffs, NJ: Prentice-Hall.

Dronkers, N. (1993). Cerebral localization of production disorders in aphasia. Telerounds #9, 3/31/93. Tempe, AZ: National Center for Neurogenic Communication Disorders, Arizona Board of Regents.

Folstein, M. F., Folstein, S. E., and McHugh, P. R. (1975). "Mini-Mental State": A practical method for grading the mental state of patients for the clinician. *Journal of Psychiatric Research*, 12, 189–198.

Friedman, S. G. (Ed.) (1988). National head injury foundation information pamphlet. Southborough, MA: National Head Injury Foundation.

Gennarelli, T. A., Adams, J. H., & Thibault, L. B. (1982). Diffuse axonal injury and traumatic coma in the primate. *Annals of Neurology*, 12, 564–574.

Gerstmann, J. (1931). Zur symptomatologie der Hirnlasionem im Obergangs-gebiet der unteren Parietal und mittern Oppitalwindung. *Nervenarzt*, 3, 691–695.

Geschwind, N. (1965). Disconnection syndromes in animals and man. *Brain*, 88, 237–294, 585–664.

Geschwind, N. (1975). The apraxias: Neural mechanism of disorders of learned movements. *American Scientist*, 63, 188–195.

Hagen, C. (1986). Language disorders in head trauma. In J. M. Costello & A. L. Holland (Eds.), *Handbook of speech and language disorders*. San Diego: College Hill Press.

Hagen, C., & Malkmus, D. (1979). Intervention strategies for language disorders secondary to head trauma. American Speech-Language-Hearing Association Convention, Atlanta, GA.

Halpern, H., Darley, F. L., & Brown, J. R. (1973). Differential language and neurologic characteristics in cerebral involvement. *Journal of Speech and Hearing Disorders*, 32, 162–173.

Henschen, S. E. (1920–1922). *Klinische und Anatomische Beitige zur Pathologie der Gehirns* (Vols. 5–7). Stockholm: Nordiska Bokhandeln.

Horner, J., Alberts, M. J., & Dawson, D. V. (1994). Swallowing in Alzheimer's Disease. *Alzheimer's Disease and Associated Disorders*, 8, 177–189.

Jennett, B. (1986). Head trauma. In A. K. Asbury, G. M. McKhann, & W. J. McDonald (Eds.), *Diseases of the nervous system*. Philadelphia: W. B. Saunders.

Kirshner, H. S., Webb, W. G., Kelly, M. P., & Wells, C. E. (1984). Language disturbance: An initial symptom of cortical degenerations and dementia. *Archives of Neurology*, 41, 491–496.

Kliest, K. (1922). In O. Schjemings (Ed.), *Handbuch der argblichen Erfahrugen*. Leipzig: Banth.

Koppitz, E. M. (1964). *The Bender gestalt for young children*. New York: Grune & Stratton.

Liepmann, H. (1900). Daskrankheitshild der Apraxia (motorischen) Asymbolie. *Mtschr Psychiat*, 8, 15, 44, 102–132, 182–197.

Love, R., & Fitzgerald, M. (1984). Is the diagnosis of developmental apraxia of speech valid? *Australian Journal of Human Communication Disorders*, 12, 71–89.

Love, R. J., & Webb, W. G. (1977). The efficacy of cueing techniques in Broca's aphasia. *Journal of Speech and Hearing Disorders*, 42, 170–178.

Marin, O. S. M. (1982). Brain and language: The rules of the game. In M. A. Arbib, D. Caplan, & J. C. Marshall (Eds.), *Neural models of language processes*. London: Academic Press.

Marshall, J., & Newcombe, F. (1973). Patterns of paralexia: A psycholinguistic approach. *Journal of Psycholinguistic Research*, 2, 175–199

Mesulam, M. M. (1987). Primary progressive aphasia—Differentiation from Alzheimer's disease. *Archives of Neurology*, 22, 533–534.

Meyers, P. S. (1994). Communication disorders associated with right-hemisphere brain damage. In Chapey, R. (Ed.), Language intervention strategies in adult aphasia (3rd ed.) . Baltimore: Williams and Wikins.

Milner, B. (1974). Hemispheric specializations: Scope and limits. In F. 0. Schmidt & F. G. Worden (Eds.), *The neurosciences: The third study program.* Cambridge, MA: MIT Press.

Pascal, G., & Suttel, B. (1951). *The Bender Gestalt Test.* New York: Grune & Stratton.

Reisberg, B., Ferris, S. H., DeLeon, M. J., and Crook, T. (1982). The Global Deterioration Scale (GDS): An instrument for the assessment of primary degenerative dementia (PDD). *American Journal of Psychiatry, 139,* 1136–1139.

Rivers, D. L., & Love, R. J. (1980). Language performance on visual processing tasks in right hemisphere cases. *Brain and Language, 10,* 348–366.

Ross, E. (1981). Aprosodia: Functional-anatomic organization of the affective components of language in the right hemisphere. *Archives of Neurology, 38,* 561–569.

Rothi, L. G., & Moss, S. E. (1985). Alexia/agraphia in brain-damaged adults. Paper presented at the American Speech-Language-Hearing Association Convention, Washington, DC.

Sapin, L. R., Anderson, F. H., & Pulaski, P. D. (1989). Progressive aphasia without dementia: Further documentation. *Annals of Neurology, 25,* 411–413.

Scientific American. (1995). Putting Alzheimer's to the tests: Several new techniques may detect the disease. *Scientific American, 272,* 2, 12–13.

Solberg, M. M., & Mateer, C. A. (1989). *Introduction to rehabilitation: Theory and practice.* New York: Guilford Press.

Wechsler, D. (1981). *Wechsler Adult Intelligence Scale—Revised Manual.* New York: Psychological Corporation.

Whitehouse, P. I., Jr. (1986). The concept of subcortical and cortical dementia: Another look. *Annals of Neurology, 19,* 1–6.

Ylvisaker, M., & Szekeres, S. F. (1994). Communication disorders associated with closed head injury. In R. Chapey (Ed.), *Language intervention and strategies in adult aphasia* (3rd ed.). Baltimore: Williams & Wilkins.

10

□ □ □
□ □ □
□ □ □

Language Mechanisms in the Developing Brain

"In a child, speech is a new acquisition, and as with most recently evolved faculties it is sensitive. Like an orchard blighted by a late frost, a child loses its speech easily, and he may show a taciturnity or even mutism for a variety of reasons. In such cases there may be no focal lesion of the brain, but only a presumed thinly spread minor cerebral affection. . . . Though vulnerable, speech in the child is also a highly resilient faculty. Hence a considerable restitution of function is always possible and speech may return to normal with little delay."

—Macdonald Critchley, *Aphasiology*, 1970

Brain Growth

Acquisition of speech and language is clearly tied to physical development and maturation in the infant and child, yet the exact nature of the interaction of growth and development with emerging speech is unknown. It is known, however, that the course of speech and language development is a correlate of cerebral maturation and specialization. Having noted that, a critical question still remains to be answered: What indices of cerebral maturation are of significance to language acquisition? It is clear that there are critical periods in the maturation of the brain as well as growth gradients in different brain structures. Can these critical periods be applied equally to the stages of language acquisition?

Brain Weight

One obvious index of neurologic development is the change in gross brain weight with age. The most rapid period of brain growth is during the first 2 years of life. The brain more than triples its weight in the first 24 months. At birth, the brain is about 25 percent of its adult weight, and at 26 months it has reached 50 percent of its full weight. At 1 year, the average age at which the first word appears, the brain is 60 percent of its adult weight. Thus, the brain makes its most rapid growth in the first year of life. By 2.5 years, the brain has reached about 75 percent of its full growth, and at 5 years it is within 90 percent of its complete maturation. Table 10–1 illustrates this increase in brain weight. It is not until 10 years of age that the brain achieves approximately 95 percent of its ultimate weight. By about 12 years, or puberty, full brain weight is reached.

In brief, the brain grows very rapidly during the first 2 years after birth. It moves at a slower, but still accelerated, pace between 2 and 5 years and finally completes its growth at the physical landmark of puberty. The late neurolinguist Eric Lenneberg (1921–1975) argued that the accelerated curve of brain growth in the first years of life matched the course of rapid early acquisition of language of the child. He further claimed that primary linguistic skills were achieved by the age of 4 or 5 years and that the ability to acquire language diminished sharply after puberty, when accelerating brain growth reached a plateau.

Differential Brain Growth

Just as the total brain grows at different rates at different ages, so do its different parts—and various brain structures reach their peak growth rates at different times. For instance, brainstem divisions, such as the midbrain, pons, and medulla, grow rapidly prenatally and less rapidly postnatally. The cerebellum develops rapidly from before birth to the age of 1 year. The cerebral hemispheres, important in language development, grow rapidly early, contributing about 85 percent to total brain volume by the sixth fetal month.

Table 10–1 Language and Brain Growth from Birth to 2 Years

Age	Language Milestones	Brain Weight in Grams
Birth	Crying	335
3 months	Cooing and crying	516
6 months	Babbling	660
9 months	Voicing intonated jargon	750
12 months	Approximating first word	925
18 months	Early naming	1,024
24 months	Making two-word combinations	1,064

The differential growth of the cortex of the cerebral hemispheres is of vital importance for speech and language function because the majority of neural structures for communication are integrated there. Most cortical neurons are in place at birth, but brain growth may be measured through the development of synaptic connections and myelination. One method of establishing a schedule of cortical growth gradients in cerebral maturity is to determine what cortical areas are most developed in myelination at birth. The motor area of the precentral gyrus of the frontal lobe is the first cortical area developed at birth. It is soon followed by the somatosensory area of the postcentral gyrus of the parietal lobe. Next, very soon after birth, the primary visual receptor area of the occipital cortex matures. The primary auditory area, Heschl's gyrus in the temporal lobe, matures last. The medial surface of the hemispheres shows the final development of the brain.

The cortical association areas lag behind the development of the cortical receptor areas that are present and active at birth. In fact, the major association areas devoted to speech and language mature well into the preschool years and even beyond. The progressive development of Broca's area, the frontal motor area for the face area on the motor strip, and the development of Wernicke's area, the posterior auditory association area, are related to progressive stabilization of the phonological system. As the phonemic motor planning system matures, the auditory association system increases its ability to process longer and more complex sequences of connected phonemes. The arcuate fasciculus connecting Broca's and Wernicke's areas apparently begins myelination in the first year and continues for some time afterward.

At 1 year the normal child has a vocabulary of one or more word approximations, usually names for objects that have been seen and sometimes touched. This stage of language development requires the ability to mix neural information from the auditory, somesthetic, and visual association areas. The association area of the inferior parietal lobe is where information from the temporal auditory association areas, the occipital visual association area, and the parietal association area combine to provide the neural bases for the feat of naming that the 1-year-old child displays. The rapid growth of vocabulary in the second and third years of life, therefore, may well be a correlate of the maturation of this significant posterior association area in the parietal lobe, which combines information from surrounding association areas. It no doubt is a master association area, rightly named by Geschwind as the "association area of association areas."

The left hemisphere is destined to serve as the primary neurologic site for speech and language mechanisms in most infants, children, and adults. The left hemisphere shows early structural differences that will support later language dominance. The sylvian fissure is longer on the left in fetal brains, and the planum temporale on the left is larger in the majority of fetal and newborn brains. Although the temporal lobe appears well-differentiated from early life, Broca's area is not differentiated until 18 months, and the corpus callosum is not completely myelinated until age 10. The inferior parietal lobe, the master association area, is not fully myelinated until adulthood, often well into the fourth decade.

Myelination for Language

Myelination has been considered one of the more significant indices of brain maturation and is often a prime correlate of speech and language. Myelination allows more rapid transmission of neural information along neural fibers and is particularly critical in a cerebral nervous system that is dependent on several long axon connections between hemispheres, lobes, and cortical and subcortical structures. Lack of maturation of myelin in language association fibers and language centers has frequently been suggested as a cause for developmental delays in language. Immaturity of myelogenesis has not been definitely proved as a demonstrable cause in speech-language delay, but the available data suggest it as a likely factor.

Myelogenesis is a cyclic process in which certain neural regions and systems appear to begin the process early and others much later. In some instances the myelogenetic cycle is short, in other cases much longer. Clear differences in rate of myelogenesis exist between different pathways. Myelination of the cortical end of the auditory projections extends beyond the first year, whereas myelination of the cortical end of the visual projections is complete soon after birth. There is a similar discrepancy between myelination of the auditory geniculotemporal radiations and visual geniculolocalcarine radiations. These myelogenetic cycles appear to underlie the early visual maturity and slowly developing auditory maturity of the infant. Myelination cycles can be roughly correlated with the milestones of speech and language development, but since there is no behavioral way of assessing myelogenetic maturation in the living brain of the child with language delay, the concepts have little or no clinical utility for the speech-language pathologist.

Cerebral Plasticity

Children who have begun to develop language normally and then sustain cerebral injury, particularly to the left hemisphere, show a language disturbance of an aphasic nature. The younger the child, however, the more quickly the language disturbance appears to resolve itself and the child appears to become grossly normal or near normal in language function. This fact is in relatively sharp contrast to the adult who sustains left cerebral injury. In adult brains, resolution of aphasic difficulty following focal injury to the left hemisphere rarely reaches the level of normality of functioning that is apparent in the child.

One explanation given for this phenomenon is that the child's brain demonstrates considerable plasticity of function, so that undamaged areas are capable of assuming language function. In terms of language function, *cerebral plasticity* is defined as a state or stage in which specific cortical areas are not well-established because of the brain's immaturity. The brain is more plastic during the most rapid periods of brain growth, and damage to the left hemisphere before the end of the first year of life is often associated with a shift of language function to the right hemisphere. By contrast, injury to the left hemisphere after this critical period is less likely to be associated with a functional reorganization of the brain. Studies from various neurosurgical centers show that approximately one third of the cases with left-hemisphere damage before 1 year continue to have speech mediated exclusively by the left hemisphere. In those cases where left-hemisphere dominance for speech continues even in the face of damage, it is dependent primarily on the integrity of the frontal and temporal-parietal language areas. This explanation of cerebral plasticity of speech and language mechanisms rests on the concept of a transfer of functional areas from the left hemisphere to uncommitted areas in the right hemisphere. However, it has been argued that in certain cases recovery of language is so rapid that transfer and learning by the right hemisphere is unlikely. Another explanation for the rapid recovery of language in children assumes that both hemispheres contain mechanisms for language and that language need not be relearned on the right. If there is a genetic predisposition to develop the mechanisms of the left hemisphere for language, in most normal infants the mechanisms of the right will be inhibited as the left side develops complex language mechanisms. With damage to the left hemisphere, however, there is assumed to be a release of the mechanisms of the right brain. This explanation also implies that damage to the right hemisphere in the child may be associated with aphasia more frequently than it is in the adult.

Development of Language Dominance

An overriding fact of brain functioning is that the cerebral hemispheres demonstrate asymmetry and that language is dominant in one of them. Cerebral dominance appears to be a developing function because, although there are anatomic differences favoring the temporal lobe in the left hemisphere, there is strong evidence suggesting that language is less fixed in the immature brain. Lenneberg advanced the theory that the course of language lateralization follows the course of cerebral maturation. He argued that lateralization is completed by puberty, based on the assumption that at birth the two hemispheres have equal potential for the development of language mechanisms and that there is gradual lateralization associated with the period of major growth.

This theory has been criticized on several grounds. First, current anatomic evidence suggests that the hemispheres may not have equal potentiality for language and that the left hemisphere is organized differently from the right, with speech mechanisms for language in the left. The planum temporale is larger in adults, in newborns, and in fetuses (Figure 10–1). Second, a reexamination of basic data of language recovery following right and left hemiplegia indicates that lateralization may be basically complete at 5 years, rather than at 10 to 12 years as Lenneberg suggested. Other interpretations of these data have even suggested that lateralization is present at birth and does not follow a developmental course. It is quite clear that the age at which cerebral dominance for language is established is controversial, and a definitive

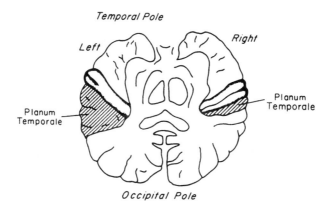

Figure 10–1 Cerebral asymmetry in the planum temporale. Geschwind and Levitsky (1968) demonstrated a larger left planum temporale in 65 adult subjects, a larger right planum temporale in 11 subjects, and equal plana temporale in 24 subjects. The drawing shows an exposed upper surface of the temporal lobe with a cut made at the plane of the sylvian fissure. Note a large left planum lying behind the transverse gyrus of Heschl. On the right there are two transverse gyri and a small planum. Source: Adapted from N. Geschwind, in C. Ludlow and M. Doran-Quine (Eds.), *The Neurologic Bases of Language Disorders in Children: Methods and Directions for Research*, NIH Publication 79–440, August, 1979; N. Geschwind and W. Levitsky, "Left-Right Asymmetries in Temporal Speech Region." *Science*, 1968, 161, 186–187.

statement cannot be made from the available evidence; however, recovery of language after damage is usually excellent before the age of 5.

Cerebral dominance for language has been long associated with laterality of other functions. As long ago as 1865, Jean Bouillaud (1796–1881) suggested that language dominance and handedness were related in some way. For many years it was believed that the preferred hand was contralateral to the cerebral hemisphere dominant for language. This meant that the left cerebral hemisphere was dominant for language in right-handers and the right hemisphere in left-handers. Primarily through the cortical-stimulation studies of Penfield and Roberts, we now believe that the left hemisphere is almost always language-dominant in right-handers, with approximately 95 percent of this group left-brained for language. In left-handers, about 50 to 70 percent also show language dominance in the left hemisphere.

Hand preference is a relevant but not totally reliable index in predicting language dominance. Right-handedness is a relatively universal trait and is usually associated with other preferences in laterality. Human beings also tend consistently to prefer one foot, eye, and ear. There are varying degrees of laterality. Some people are more strongly right-handed than others, but true ambidexters—those who use either hand equally well—are quite rare.

Inconsistency in lateral preferences also is seen often. A person may write with the right hand, throw a ball with the left, and kick a ball with the right foot. This is *mixed laterality* or *mixed dominance*. On occasion mixed laterality has been found to be associated with language retardation or developmental dyslexia in children, but the relationship between mixed laterality and a disorder of cerebral dominance for language is uncertain.

Most right-handed people demonstrate ear preference, which is considered consistent with a contralateral hemisphere laterality for language in the brain. This preference can be demonstrated through dichotic listening tasks in which simultaneous auditory stimuli are presented to both ears at once. Listeners generally show a consistent lateral preference in recognition of stimuli in one ear over the other ear. This is called an *ear advantage*. Only 80 percent of right-handers show a distinct right-ear advantage, so the relationship to cerebral dominance for language is not always clear.

Childhood Language Disorders

Acquired Childhood Aphasia

Acquired aphasia of childhood is usually defined as present in a child who has begun to develop language normally and then sustains a language disturbance as the result of cerebral insult. It is usually distinguished from a primary delay or failure to develop language in childhood. A delay or failure to develop language, as opposed to acquired childhood aphasia, usually goes by many names. Neurologists use the name *developmental dysphasia* and speech pathologists usually use *developmental language disability*. Acquired childhood aphasia is the least common of childhood language problems, but for those experts interested in the mechanisms of language development and the brain, it has assumed a pivotal theoretical role.

Onset of acquired childhood aphasia usually is considered to date from infancy through preadolescence, although there is debate as to its boundaries. The clinical characteristics of the disorder for the most part depend on the same variables of etiology and localization of lesion that are important in adult aphasia, but the age of onset significantly changes the clinical picture for each child. As in the adult, thrombosis, embolism, hemorrhage, and tumor are common causes. Thrombotic stroke appears to be a much more frequent cause than formerly believed (Wood, 1995).

Earlier literature reported that nonfluent aphasia was overwhelmingly common in acquired aphasia in children, but recently more reports of posterior lesions have been documented in children who exhibit nonfluent expressive speech. The lack of receptive abilities in children with posterior lesions may lead to a gradual loss of expressive speech and may account for the fact that nonfluency was noted in most children as a first sign if they were diagnosed with acquired aphasia.

Although the prognosis in early childhood aphasia due to unilateral lesions is very good, complete recovery cannot always be expected. A receptive component usually prolongs recovery. In addition, although language function may appear adequate, it may exceed reading, writing, and numerical skills; writing in particular may show very obvious deficiencies. Of course the earlier the onset of the lesion, the better the prognosis; however, this may be complicated by seizures, which slow the recovery. Generally, it is assumed that the greatest improvement occurs in children in whom there is a complete takeover of language functions by the uninjured hemisphere. As children get older there appears to be less chance of a complete takeover by the uninjured hemisphere, most likely because brain plasticity decreases with increasing age. Rarely is recovered language, even early in life, equal to that of a normal child of the same age (Wood, 1995).

Childhood Aphasia With Abnormal Electroencephalogram Findings: The Landau-Kleffner Syndrome

An important but small subgroup of patients with acquired aphasia is composed of children whose language disturbance is associated with convulsive seizures and electroencephalographic (EEG) abnormalities or Landau-Kleffner syndrome. The clinical picture in this group is extremely varied. The age of onset of the disorder is generally between 18 months and 13 years. The onset of the language disturbance lasts from a few hours or days to over 6 months. The defining sign of the disorder is seizure behavior and/or abnormal EEG discharges from one or both of the temporal lobes. Seizures may occur before or after the aphasic incident. The child may give the impression of being deaf, because the language disturbance usually includes a comprehension disorder. Both expressive and receptive deficits are present, and total mutism may even occur. The underlying etiology producing the seizure behavior that affects language is often unknown. The long-term course is unclear, with recovery seen in a minority of cases; many patients have chronic auditory receptive disorders. Anticonvulsant drugs are usually prescribed.

Developmental Language Disability

By far the most prevalent childhood language abnormalities are the developmental language disorders rather than the acquired ones. Children with a developmental language disability never develop language normally. Technically it is inappropriate to call these children *aphasic*, since their language has not developed normally and then become lost or impaired. Terms such as *congenital aphasia, developmental aphasia,* and *dysphasia* are not often used by speech-language pathologists, who are typically careful not to label children who are not definitely diagnosed as neurologically or genetically impaired. However, children who do show neurologic signs or possible genetic abnormalities are labeled as having *specific language impairment.*

Specific Language Impairment

In recent years in speech-language pathology there has been an increased use of the term *specific language impairment* (SLI). The term has been applied to a subset of children with developmental language disorders, with the implication that many of these children have a consistent history of developmental speech and language delay *and* have evidence of possible organic involvement.

Professionals who employ the term SLI have been particularly concerned with its definition. One critical defining feature of SLI is that the language disorder must not be secondary to a more generalized condition such as peripheral hearing loss, cognitive retardation, a psychiatric disorder (such as autism or childhood schizophrenia), or an acquired neurologic anomaly of the speech mechanism.

Generally SLI is defined as a significant expressive and/or a receptive language disorder with normal performance in other skills, particularly nonverbal cognition. Of importance is the fact that children with SLI are essentially free of frank neurologic symptoms, in contrast to children with acquired childhood aphasia who exhibit obvious hemiplegia.

A striking feature of SLI is that it is highly heterogenous in type and severity as defined by speech-language pathologists. Montgomery, Windsor, and Stark (1991) suggest that there are many possible causal factors, including impaired symbolic representational abilities, auditory perceptive processing disabilities at both the speech sound and sentence level, auditory memory problems, problem-solving difficulties (including impaired hypothesis testing and inferential thinking), impaired cognitive styles in linguistic and nonlinguistic thinking, and deficiencies in metalinguistic tasks.

One must question whether there is a neurologic basis for these behaviors in the child with SLI. Lou, Henderson, and Bruhn (1984) found reduced regional cerebral blood flow in 13 children, 6.5 to 15 years of age, diagnosed with SLI and/or attention deficit disorder. Both cortical and subcortical regions of hypoperfusion were found. Children with dyspraxia of speech showed deficits in the anterior perisylvian area. Children with generalized expressive and receptive disorders showed deficits in both the anterior and posterior perisylvian areas. A single child with a diagnosis of verbal agnosia showed bilateral posterior blood flow problems in both cortical and subcortical areas. Attention-deficit—disordered children showed medial frontal hypoperfusion. Six out of 11 of these children were language-impaired.

Weinberg, Harper, and Blumback (1995) recently have indicated that information on known lesion sites in adults can be used with children to predict lesion sites from a simple neuropsychological test given in the office of the pediatric neurologist. Recently, emphasis has also been placed on genetic evidence of loss of certain grammatic features in children with SLI (Gopnik & Crago, 1990; Pinker, 1994).

Attention Deficit—Hyperactivity Disorder

The lack of evidence of obvious neurologic disturbances in many language-disordered children has led speech-language pathologists over the past 40 years to employ the concepts of *minimal cerebral dysfunction* and, later, *attention deficit—hyperactivity disorder* or *AD-HD* (American Psychiatric Association, 1987) as possible explanatory etiologies in children with developmental language disabilities. It has been long recognized that some children with language impairment also display behavioral disorders, perceptual and attention deficits, and minor neurological deficits, all of which are suggestive of cerebral disorder. Often, however, the neurological deficits are so mild and subtle that they may be overlooked in the routine pediatric neurologic examination.

The minor neurologic signs most frequently reported are impairments of fine coordination of hands, clumsiness, and mild choreiform or athetoid movements. These have been called *soft signs* of possible neurologic damage because they are inconsistent and isolated indications of neurologic disturbance, rarely clustering together to present a classic neurologic syndrome allowing reliable lesion lateralization and location (Tupper, 1987). The diagnosis, therefore, is often made on the basis of behavioral characteristics rather than neurologic signs. For characteristics implying a diagnosis of AD-HD, see Table 10–2. Like children with SLI, not all children with AD-HD show soft signs or are suspected of having a neurological disorder.

Differential Diagnoses of Language Disorders

Hearing Loss

Hearing impairment of any etiology disturbs or delays language in children and may be one of the most important causes of language delay in children referred to a speech-language pathologist or pediatric neurologist. It is not uncommon to see a significant hearing loss associated with brain injury. Many disorders that affect hearing also produce cerebral disorder. Intrauterine infection, hyperbilirubinemia with kernicterus, neonatal anoxia, complications of prematurity, and purulent meningitis are among the well-known causes of hearing loss that also severely affect the nervous system.

Table 10–2   Signs of Attention Deficit—Hyperactivity Disorder

Hyperactivity (hyperkinesis)

Attention disorder

Perseveration

Clumsiness

Emotional lability

Perceptual and cognitive deficits

Memory deficits

Spelling and arithmetic disorders

Speech, language, and hearing disorders

Minor neurologic signs

Nonspecific EEG abnormalities

Hypoxia and kernicterus are accompanied by a typical high-frequency sensorineural loss with a precipitous drop in the primary speech frequencies (500 to 8,000 Hz). If severe, these losses have a significant effect on speech. A profound articulation disorder is present, and in some cases articulatory skills are almost absent.

Generalized Cognitive Deficit: Mental Retardation

Cognitive deficits limit language development, and the linguistic skills of the mentally retarded person are generally poorer than those of the nonretarded child of equivalent chronologic age. Language development in the majority of retarded children proceeds on a slower but normal course until early adolescence, when development reaches a plateau. It has been argued that, as in other children, language development in retarded people is paced by cerebral maturation. The lack of development of adequate speech and language in mental retardation often serves as one of the earliest and most sensitive signs of a degenerative disease of the nervous system for the pediatric neurologist and speech-language pathologist.

Childhood Autism

Autism is a relatively uncommon syndrome in which disturbed communication and delayed language development are key signs. Verbal behavior is often severely involved, and the child may be mute or echolalic. Other disturbances in the syndrome include difficulties in social relationships, abnormal responses to objects, and difficulties in sensory modulation and motility.

The etiology of autism is controversial and basically unknown. Some experts believe that the autistic syndrome is related to early affective or sensory deprivation. Other experts believe that some type of neurologic dysfunction plays a major role in the syndrome. Early brain injury and abnormalities of the cerebral ventricles, brainstem, or cerebellum have been found and cited as possible etiologies. Recent computerized tomography scan studies have not revealed cortical lesions in cases of autism (Dawson, 1989).

Table 10–3 provides a classification of the major childhood language disorders.

Developmental Dyslexia

Reading disorders of childhood are frequently associated with inadequate or inappropriate instruction or emotional disorders. One form of reading disorder, called *developmental dyslexia*, can best be understood in a neurologic context. Known also as *congenital word blindness* or *specific reading disability*, developmental dyslexia is the most common disorder of

Table 10-3   Classification of Neurologic Language Disorders of Childhood

Acquired childhood aphasia

  Landau-Kleffner syndrome (childhood aphasia with convulsions)

Developmental language disability

  Specific language impairment

Developmental language disability secondary to

  Peripheral hearing loss

  Generalized cognitive delay

  Autism

Attention deficit—hyperactivity disorder

Developmental dyslexia

communication found in schoolchildren. It is estimated to occur in 5 to 10 percent of all schoolchildren and is found at all levels of intelligence, from superior to subnormal. The child with dyslexia has great difficulty in attaching sound and meaning to written words. Oral reading is usually very difficult. Words with a similar appearance are often confused, and letters that look alike are reversed. Phonemes may be mispronounced in oral reading, and certain phonemes may be omitted or inserted. Reading comprehension is impaired. Disorders of writing are often present, with reversals, poorly formed letters, rotations, repetition, and omission of letters. Written syntax is poor.

The etiology of developmental dyslexia is not established. Frequently, however, left-handedness or ambidexterity, along with mild generalized abnormal EEG patterns, are seen. Often there is a positive family history, with other members of the family having similar problems. Dyslexia occurs more often in males. Some studies show an autosomal dominant mode of inheritance. Suggestions of focal lesions in the parietal lobe have not been widely supported by neurodiagnostic tests, but it is widely believed that immature development of the parietal lobe may play a role. If there are developmental anomalies of the brain, they are doubtless microscopic and may not be visible on current neurodiagnostic tests. Perceptual impairments, particularly in making visual and auditory associations, have also been found. Usually the problem responds to remedial procedures.

Summary

Development and maturation of the brain paces the emergence of speech and language milestones. Two indices of brain growth—changes in brain weight with advancing age and the differential myelination of cerebral structures—appear to be valid correlates of speech and language development. Neuroanatomic differences, such as larger left plana temporale and longer sylvian fissures on the left (found in the majority of fetuses and infants), provide some support for an early lateralization of language mechanisms. But infants who sustain damage to the left hemisphere before 1 year of age demonstrate a degree of early cerebral plasticity for language mechanisms.

Language lateralization and handedness are often associated, but preference is not a totally reliable index of cerebral dominance for language in the developing brain. Language disability in children has not always been unequivocally related to signs of cerebral damage in children. A recognized but relatively uncommon language disorder syndrome related to clear-cut cerebral injury is acquired traumatic aphasia. Recovery depends on the age of onset, with earlier onset offering a better prognosis for almost full language recovery. Aphasia associated with seizures is also an established syndrome of acquired language disorder. Abnormal EEG activity and transient aphasia are the prime signs in this disorder, which is also known as Landau-Kleffner syndrome.

Developmental language disability without evidence of focal brain lesions has long been associated with the primary etiologies of deafness, mental retardation, and autism. Many children with language delay and disabilities present unknown etiologies but are suspected of cerebral dysfunction. Genetic causation is also suspected, especially in these children who have specific language impairment. Children with hyperactivity and attention deficits often are suspected of having neurologic language impairment.

References and Further Readings

Brain Growth

Jabbour, I., Duenas, D., Gilmartin, R., & Gottlieb, M. (1976). *Pediatric neurology handbook* (2nd ed.). New York: Medical Examination Publishing Company.

Lecours, A. R. (1975). Myelogenetic correlates of development of speech and language. In E. Lenneberg & E. Lenneberg (Eds.), *Foundations of language development* (Vol. 1). New York: Academic Press.

Lenneberg, E. (1967). *Biological foundations of language.* New York: Wiley.

Cerebral Plasticity and Cerebral Dominance

Geschwind, N. (1979). Anatomical foundations of language and dominance. In C. L. Ludlow & M. E. Doran-Quine (Eds.), *The neurologic bases of language in children: Methods and directions for research.* Bethesda, MD: National Institutes of Health (publication no. 79–440, pp. 145–157).

Geschwind, N., & Galaburda, A. M. (Eds.) (1984). *Cerebral lateralization: Biological mechanisms, associations and pathology.* Cambridge, MA: Harvard University Press.

Rasmussen, T., & Milner, B. (1977). The role of early left-brain injury in determining lateralization of cerebral speech functions. *Annals of the New York Academy of Sciences, 299,* 355–369.

Wada, J. A., Clark, R., & Hamm, A. (1975). Cerebral hemispheric asymmetry in humans. *Archives of Neurology (Chicago), 32,* 239–246.

Witleson, S. F. (1977). Early hemispheric specialization and interhemispheric plasticity: An empirical and theoretical review. In S. J. Segalwitz & F. A. Gruber (Eds.), *Language development and neurological theory.* New York: Academic Press.

Neurologic Language Disability in Children

American Psychiatric Association (1987). *Diagnostic and statistical manual of mental disorders* (3rd ed.). Washington, DC: Author.

Bishop, D. V. M. (1985). Age of onset and outcome in "acquired aphasia with convulsive disorder" (Landau-Kleffner syndrome). *Developmental Medicine and Child Neurology, 27,* 705–712.

Chase, R. A. (1972). Neurologic aspects of language disorders in children. In J. V. Irwin & M. Marge (Eds.), *Principles of childhood language disabilities.* New York: Appleton-Century-Crofts.

Cohen, M., Campbell, R. E., & Yaghmi, F. (1989). Neuropathological abnormalities in developmental dysphasia. *Annals of Neurology, 25,* 567–570.

Cranberg, L. D., Filley, C. M., Hart, E. J., & Alexander, M. P. (1987). Acquired aphasia in children: Clinical and CT investigations. *Neurology, 37,* 1165–1172.

Dawson, G. (Ed.) (1989). *Autism: Nature, diagnosis, and treatment.* New York: Guilford Publications.

Dreifuss, F. (1975). The pathology of central communicative disorders in children. In D. B. Tower (Ed.), *The nervous system. Vol. 3. Human communication and its disorders.* New York: Raven Press.

Fenichel, G. M. (1988). *Clinical pediatric neurology.* Philadelphia: W. B. Saunders.

Galaburda, A. M., & Kemper, T. L. (1979). Cytoarchitectonic abnormalities in developmental dyslexia: A case study. *Annals of Neurology, 6,* 94–100.

Galaburda, A. M., Rosen, G. D., & Sherman, G. F. (1989). The origin of developmental dyslexia: Implications for medicine, neurology and cognition. In A. M. Galaburda (Ed.), *From reading to neurons.* Cambridge, MA: MIT Press.

Gopnik, M., & Crago, M. (1990). Familial aggregation of a developmental language disorder. *Cognition, 39,* 1–50.

Hecaen, H. (1983). Acquired aphasia in children: Revisited. *Neuropsychologia, 21,* 581–587.

Lou, H. C., Henderson, L., & Bruhn, P. (1984). Focal cerebral hypoperfusion in children with dysphasia and attention deficit disorder. *Archives of Neurology, 41,* 825–829.

Ludlow, C. L. (1980). Children's language disorders: Recent research advances. *Annals of Neurology, 7,* 497–507.

Miller, J. F., Campbell, T. E., Chapman, R. S., & Weismer, S. (1984). Language behavior in acquired childhood aphasia. In A. Holland (Ed.), *Language disorders in children: Recent advances.* San Diego: College Hill Press.

Montgomery, J. W., Windsor, J., & Stark, R. E. (1991). Specific speech and language disorders. In J. E. Ober & G. W. Hynds (Eds.) *Neuropsychological foundations of learning disorders.* New York: Academic Press.

Murdoch, B. E. (Ed.) (1990). *Acquired neurological speech-language disorders in childhood.* London: Taylor and Francis.

Pinker, S. (1994). *The language instinct.* New York: Morrow.

Rie, H. E., & Rie, E. (Eds.) (1980). *Handbook of minimal brain dysfunctions: A critical view.* New York: Wiley.

Tupper, D. (Ed.) (1987). *Soft neurological signs.* Orlando, FL: Grune & Stratton.

Weinberg, W. A., Harper, C. R., & Blumback, R. A. (1995). Neuroanatomic substrate of developmental specific learning disabilities and select behavioral syndromes. *Journal of Child Neurology, 10* (suppl), 578– 580.

Wood, B. T. (1995). Acquired childhood aphasia. In H. Kirshner (Ed.), *Handbook of neurological speech and language disorders.* New York: Marcel Dekker.

11 ⬜⬜⬜
⬜⬜⬜
⬜⬜⬜

Clinical Speech Syndromes and the Developing Brain

"An examination of infant behavior is an examination of the central nervous system."

—Arnold Gesell and Catherine S. Amatruda,
Developmental Diagnosis, 1947

Developmental Motor Speech Disorders

Early cerebral injury to speech mechanisms of the developing brain will result in conditions that may be classified as developmental motor speech disorders. Included in a classification of the motor speech disorders are the *developmental dysarthrias, developmental anarthrias,* and *developmental apraxias of speech.* Developmental dysarthria is a speech disorder resulting from damage to the immature nervous system; it is characterized by weakness, paralysis, and/or incoordination of the speech musculature. Developmental anarthria refers to a complete lack of speech due to profound paralysis, weakness, and/or incoordination of the speech musculature. Usually the diagnosis implies that useful speech will not develop because of the severity of the oral motor involvement. Developmental apraxia of speech is an impaired ability to execute voluntarily the appropriate movements of speech in the absence of paralysis, weakness, and incoordination of the speech muscles. The syndrome of apraxia of speech, in both adults and children, is described in Chapter 9.

Certain types of developmental dysarthria have been well-studied; other types have received less attention in the speech pathology literature. The developmental dysarthrias of the cerebral palsies, for instance, have been studied extensively for many years, whereas research on the dysarthrias of childhood muscular dystrophy is much less common. The speech signs commonly observed in the developmental dysarthrias are seen in Table 11–1.

Table 11–1   Major Developmental Motor Speech Disorders

Disorder	Speech Signs
	Developmental apraxia of speech
	Disorder in selection and sequencing of articulatory movements, with oral apraxia sometimes present; comprehension intact; expression poor; occasional nonfocal neurologic signs
	Developmental dysarthrias of cerebral palsy
Spastic dysarthria	Bilateral corticobulbar involvement, dysphagia, articulation disorder, hypernasality, slowed rate, and loudness, pitch, and vocal quality disturbances
Dyskinetic dysarthria	Athetosis (usually), dysphagia, hypernasality, articulation disorders, prevocalizations, and loudness, pitch, and vocal quality disturbances
Ataxic dysarthria	Articulation and prosodic disorders; unequal stress, loudness, and pitch; speech has an explosive, scanning quality

Cerebral Palsy

Developmental dysarthria is most commonly seen in children diagnosed as having cerebral palsy. Cerebral palsy is a neurological condition caused by injury to the immature brain; it is characterized by a nonprogressive disturbance of the motor system. Many associated problems are often seen, such as mental retardation, hearing and/or visual impairments, and perceptual problems produced by the infantile cerebral injury. Cerebral palsy is considered a major developmental disability.

The cerebral palsies have been variously classified, but most experts currently accept three major clinical categories of clinical motor disorders: *spasticity*, *dyskinesia*, and *ataxia*. By far the most common type of dyskinesia is athetosis (see Chapter 6).

Table 11–2 presents a classification of the cerebral palsies. As in adult disorders, spasticity implies a lesion in the pyramidal system; dyskinesia, a lesion in the extrapyramidal system; and ataxia, a lesion in the cerebellar system. However, syndromes are often not as clear-cut in the child as they are in the adult. Many children with cerebral palsy show a mixed picture. For instance, a child whose clinical picture is primarily athetoid, with typical slow, writhing movements of the limbs, grimaces of the face, and involuntary movements of the tongue and muscles of respiration, may also display hypertonic muscles and the up-turning toes of the classic

Table 11–2   Classification of the Cerebral Palsies

Lesions	Clinical Signs	Limb Involvement
Pyramidal tracts	Spastic paralysis	Paraplegia (legs only); diplegia (legs more than arms); quadriplegia; hemiparesis (half of body); monoplegia (usually one leg)
Extrapyramidal tracts or basal ganglia	Athetosis, choreoathetosis, dystonia, tremor, rigidity	Arms, leg, neck, and trunk
Cerebellum	Ataxia, sometimes with diplegia	Arms, leg, trunk

Babinski sign. The structural closeness of the pathways of the pyramidal and extrapyramidal tracts in the relatively small infant brain no doubt produces such mixed clinical pictures.

Children with cerebral palsy may also be classified according to topological involvement. Common topological pictures are *hemiplegia, diplegia,* and *quadriplegia.* Occasionally, a *monoplegia, triplegia,* or *paraplegia* will be seen. Children may also be classified by etiology. Common causes are prematurity, anoxia, kernicterus, birth trauma, and infection. Approximately 1 to 2 of every 1,000 schoolchildren has some form of cerebral palsy. Of the three major types, spasticity is the most prevalent, athetosis is next, and ataxia is the least common.

Developmental dysarthria is a major problem in the cerebral palsied population, with 75 to 85 percent of the children showing obvious speech problems. Dysarthria may be complicated by mental retardation, hearing loss, and perceptual disorders in some children. Despite complicating factors, the two major dysarthrias—spastic dysarthria and dyskinetic dysarthria of athetosis—in cerebral palsy can be differentiated. Spasticity and athetosis cannot be identified by articulatory errors alone; however, when vocal and prosodic features are incorporated into perceptual judgments of speech, the two clinical types become distinct, just as spastic and hyperkinetic types are distinct among adult dysarthrias (Meyer, 1982; Workinger & Kent, 1991).

Childhood Suprabulbar Paresis

An isolated paresis or weakness of the oral musculature is sometimes seen in children without major motor signs in the trunk or extremities. This condition results in a form of developmental dysarthria and associated problems. Described by the neurologist Worster-Drought (1974), this condition usually affects the corticobulbar fibers that innervate cranial nerves X (vagus) and XII (hypoglossus). The etiology has been attributed to agenesis or hypogenesis of the corticobulbar fibers, but this theory has not been verified. The muscles of the lips, pharynx, palate, and tongue are involved to varying degrees. The jaw reflex is usually exaggerated. The dysarthria that is present is marked by misarticulations and hypernasality. There may be a history of dysphagia, and occasionally there is laryngeal involvement and drooling.

This condition is called *congenital childhood suprabulbar palsy* because involvement is generally confined to the muscles innervated by the corticobulbar fibers. Paresis of the trunk and limbs is not present as in the child who is obviously cerebral palsied. The condition is brought to the attention of the speech-language pathologist or neurologist because of an isolated dysphagia or dysarthria. Muscles of the oral mechanism are involved, but no other obvious neurologic signs are present in the motor system. Table 11–3 displays neurologic signs seen in the dysarthric syndromes of congenital and acquired suprabulbar paresis of childhood.

Muscular Dystrophy

Next to cerebral palsy, muscular dystrophy is the childhood neurologic disorder most likely to present a developmental dysarthria. The most common type of muscular dystrophy is the *pseudohypertrophic* type, also called *Duchenne dystrophy*. Duchenne dystrophy is associated with a sex-linked recessive gene, occurs primarily in males, and usually is manifest by the third year of life. The disorder is marked by a characteristic progression of muscle weakness starting in the pelvis and

Table 11–3   Dysarthria in Suprabulbar Paresis Syndrome of Childhood

Congenital Signs	Acquired Signs
Articulation disorder	Articulation disorder
Hypernasality	Hypernasality
Lip, tongue, palate, and pharynx paresis	Lip, tongue, palate, and pharynx paresis
Isolated paresis (in some cases)	Some facial rigidity
Possible agenesis of corticobulbar fibers	Encephalitis
Drooling	Traumatic head injury

trunk and eventually involving all of the striated muscles, including those of the speech mechanism. The visceral muscles are usually spared. Enlargement of the calf muscles and occasionally of other muscle groups accounts for the term *pseudohypertrophic* in the name of the disorder. Infiltration of fat and connective tissue produces the pseudohypertrophic effect.

In the later stages of the disease a flaccid dysarthria may appear, marked by articulation disorder and voice quality disturbances. Often the articulation disorder is mild, with only one or two phonemes in error. Dystrophic subjects show reduced oral breath pressure and vocal intensity. They do not sustain phonation as well as healthy children do, and they show serious involvement of the muscles of speech. Rate of tongue movement and strength of the tongue are poor. Retracting and pursing the lips as well as pointing and narrowing the tongue are noticeably disordered, and phonemes requiring tongue and lip elevation are often in error. A broadening and flattening of the tongue is sometimes seen in advanced cases. Respiratory and laryngeal muscles are also weakened, affecting respiratory and phonatory performance. Despite weakness, labial phonemes are generally produced more accurately than are tongue-tip consonants. Table 11–4 presents the speech and physical signs in the developmental dysarthria of pseudohypertrophic muscular dystrophy. Several uncommon

Table 11–4 Developmental Dysarthria in Pseudohypertrophic Muscular Dystrophy

Speech signs (flaccid dysarthria)
Articulation disorder
Reduced vocal intensity
Respiratory weakness
Articulator weakness
Broad flattened tongue
Physical signs
Onset: 3 to 4 years
Proximal weakness
Pseudohypertrophic calf muscles
Proximal atrophy
Hyporeflexia except ankles
Mental retardation (one third of cases)

childhood dysarthrias associated with lower motor neuron disorders are surveyed in Love (1992).

Diagnosis of Neurologic Disorder With Primitive Reflexes

The neurological examination of the newborn child and infant suspected of cerebral damage has relied heavily on the concept of a primitive reflex profile in recent years. Primitive and postural reflexes follow an orderly sequence of appearance and disappearance, beginning in the fetal period and extending through the first years of life. The reflexes are mediated at a subcortical level. First described by Rudolph Magnus (1873–1927), who received a Nobel prize for his efforts, these reflexes can help determine degrees of prematurity or suggest neurologic dysfunction. If a normal reflex pattern does not appear on schedule, or if a reflex pattern persists beyond the age at which it normally disappears, the newborn or infant is considered at risk for cerebral injury or other neurologic involvement. Some pediatric neurologists assert that neurological abnormalities at birth predict a diagnosis of minimal cerebral dysfunction at later ages, but other workers have found a limited association between neonatal abnormalities and neurologic signs, particularly at 1 year and beyond.

Despite questions about the reliability of prediction for a diagnosis of minimal neurologic abnormality, the careful evaluation of early primitive reflexes and later evolving postural reflexes provides a basis for diagnosis and therapy of disturbed motor function. Examination can usually provide a locomotor prognosis, indicating when and how a child with cerebral palsy will walk. Table 11–5 presents a summary of the primitive and postural reflexes of the first year. Although the speech-language pathologist may be more interested in the neurologic status of oral and pharyngeal reflexes, an understanding of the primitive and postural reflexes is essential to assessment of the neurologic maturity of a child suspected of cerebral injury.

There is a notable lack of consensus on the definition of the stimulus and response in the widely tested primitive reflexes. There is also no agreement on how the responses change with time and growth. Seven reflexes are reviewed here. They are commonly assessed by neurologists and pediatricians and they are typical of the first year of life, with the peak development at about 6 months. Carrying out testing during this peak time period avoids assessing the transitory neurologic signs of the newborn but is sufficiently early to allow a neurologic diagnosis before 1 year of age. These seven reflexes also appear to be predictive of later motor function in the child. Of the many infantile reflexes described by neurologists in neurologic literature, these are the most studied.

Table 11–5   Primitive and Postural Infantile Reflexes of the First Year

Reflex	*Response*
Asymmetric tonic neck reflex	Infant extends limbs on chin side and flexes on occiput side when turning head
Symmetric tonic neck reflex	Infant extends arms and flexes legs with head extension
Positive support reflex	Infant bears weight when balls of feet are stimulated
Tonic labyrinthine reflex	Infant may retract shoulder and extend neck and trunk with neck flexion; tongue thrust reflex may occur
Segmental rolling reflex	Infant may roll trunk and pelvis segmentally with rotation of head or legs
Galant reflex	Infant arches body when skin of back is stimulated near vertebral column
Moro reflex	Infant may adduce arm and move it upward, followed by arm flexion and leg extension and flexion

Asymmetrical Tonic Neck Reflex

The asymmetrical tonic neck reflex (ATNR) is probably the most widely known of the early body reflexes. The reflex was shown to be universally present in the healthy infant by the outstanding child developmentalist Arnold Gesell (1880–1961). When the healthy child is supine, he or she may lie with the head turned to one side. There will be an extension of the extremities on that side (the chin side), with a corresponding flexion of the contralateral extremities on the opposite (occiput) side. This position is described as the fencer's position.

To test for the presence of the reflex, the child is placed in a supine position. Observations are made of active head turning and subsequent movement of the extremities. The head is then passively turned through an arc of 180° alternately to each side for 5 seconds. This maneuver is repeated five times on each side. Consistent changes in muscle tone in the extremities generally define the presence of the reflex. A clearly positive response is visible extension of extremities on the chin side and flexion on the occiput side when the head is passively turned. If extension of the extremities on the chin side and flexion on the occiput side lasts more than 30 seconds, the response may be called *obligatory*.

If the response is found beyond the eighth or ninth month, it is indicative of possible cerebral damage and poor motor development and suggests that the cortical control of upper motor neurons is not on schedule and that motor behavior is still controlled at subcortical levels. Obligatory tonic neck reflexes persisting into the second year and beyond are usually incompatible with independent standing and walking; they may disappear later, however, and the child may learn to walk alone. The ATNR may be seen in various types of cerebral palsy, predicting brain injury, but it is not useful for distinguishing between spastic and dyskinetic types. The ATNR is suggestive of brain injury only, and it is in no way completely diagnostic for cerebral palsy or its subtypes. The ATNR can reemerge after a catastrophe such as cardiac arrest and also may be present in progressive disease. It has little or no effect on the development of speech and shows very little relationship to the oral and pharyngeal reflexes. Elicitation procedures for the ATNR are illustrated in Figure 11–1.

Symmetrical Tonic Neck Reflex

The symmetrical tonic neck reflex (STNR) is analogous to the ATNR, but the head is manipulated in flexion and extension in midline rather than turned laterally. The resulting responses are differences between upper and lower extremities, rather than right-left differences in extremities. The normal reflex is an extension of the arms and flexion of the legs if the head is extended in midline. Flexion of the head will have the opposite effect: the arms will flex and the legs will extend.

The technique of eliciting the reflex is first to ask the child to flex and extend his neck. The neck is then passively extended and flexed. This is repeated five times each for extension and flexion. If the reflex sign is absent at 5 to 6 months or persists into the second year, it is a symptom of motor abnormality. The STNR does not appear to elicit any associated oral or pharyngeal reflexes (Figure 11–2).

Positive Support Reflex

Magnus saw the positive support reflex (PSR) as necessary for support of erect posture. When the balls of the foot are stimulated, there is contraction of opposing muscle groups to fix the joints of the lower extremities so that they bear weight. To test the reflex, the infant is suspended around the trunk below the armpits with the head in midline and flexed slightly. The child is bounced on the balls of the feet five times. The feet are then placed in contact with the floor, and the degree to which the infant can support his or her weight is assessed. The PSR is seen in fetal life and is considered abnormal if it persists beyond 4 months. A persistent strong response has been associated with spastic

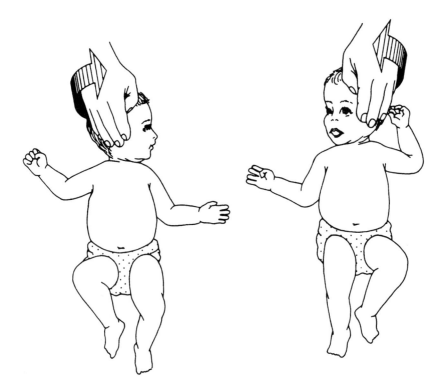

Figure 11–1 The asymmetrical tonic neck reflex is elicited by turning the head to each side for 5 seconds. This movement should be repeated five times to each side. The reflex is pathologic if there is obligatory extension and flexion of limbs for more than 60 seconds. Source: Adapted from A. Capute et al., *Primitive Reflex Profile* (Baltimore: University Park Press, 1978).

quadriparesis. The PSR does not appear to elicit associated oral or pharyngeal reflexes (Figure 11–3).

Tonic Labyrinthine Reflex

The tonic labyrinthine reflex (TLR) is associated with the changes in tone associated with different postures. The position of the extremities changes with respect to the position of the head in space, due to the orientation of the labyrinths of the inner ear. The TLR is tested in both a supine and a prone position.

To test in the prone position, the child is held in prone suspension. The head is extended about 45° below the horizontal plane. Changes of posture and tone in the extremities are evaluated, with special attention to the shoulder area. When the head is flexed, a normal response involves

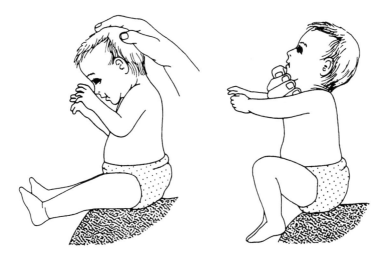

Figure 11–2 The symmetrical tonic neck reflex is elicited by passively extending and flexing the neck five times. The reflex is pathologic if there is obligatory arm extension or leg flexion with neck extension for more than 60 seconds. Source: Adapted from A. Capute et al., *Primitive Reflex Profile* (Baltimore: University Park Press, 1978).

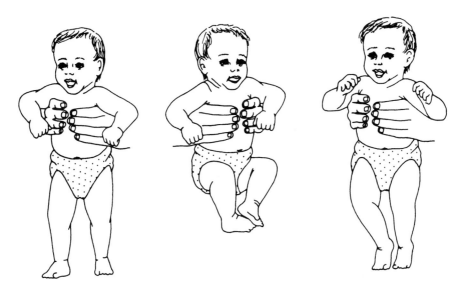

Figure 11–3 The positive support reflex is elicited by suspending the child so that the balls of the feet may be bounced on a flat surface. The reflex is pathologic if the child remains on his or her toes and cannot move out of the position for 60 seconds or more. Source: Adapted from A. Capute et al., *Primitive Reflex Profile* (Baltimore: University Park Press, 1978).

protraction of the shoulders or flexion of the lower extremities. Consistent tone changes should be present in at least one upper and lower extremity for the reflex to be considered present (Figure 11–4).

In testing the TLR in the supine position, support is placed between the shoulders so that the head is extended at 45°. Position and tone of the shoulders are assessed. Active neck flexion and grasp in midline are elicited. If the flexion and grasp responses are not noted, the head is flexed with the back supported and the midline grasp is sought again (Figure 11–4).

The normal response is shoulder retraction if the head is in extension. Trunk and leg extension accompanies shoulder retraction. Neck flexion results in shoulder protraction in 5 seconds and the disappearance of an extension posture.

An abnormal TLR may be accompanied by extensor hypertonia, and a persistent abnormal response may prevent the infant from rolling over normally. A pathologic response may make the legs so rigid that when the child is pulled to a sitting position, he or she will stand instead. The TLR is not always present in healthy children, but it is more common in children with pathologic conditions. Of the reflexes reviewed, it is the only one that may be routinely associated with oral reflexes. With the head extended 45°, a tongue reflex or tongue thrust may occur in the cerebral palsied child.

Segmental Rolling Reflex

The normal newborn baby will show a log-rolling response in turning that is a reflex associated with the activity of turning over. It is primarily a neck-righting reflex action. This early rolling response develops into a segmental rolling (SR) response, in which turning of the head produces a reaction in which the infant attempts to undo the applied rotation by twisting the body at the waist, allowing one segment of the body to turn at a time. This corkscrew reaction allows the infant to roll over with a minimum of effort because only one segment of the body moves at a time. Abnormal responses are indicated by perseveration of a simple log-rolling response in which head rotation produces the simultaneous turning of the upper and lower extremities with no segmental control. The response is seen in motor-handicapped children with cerebral palsy.

To test the SR response, the child is placed in a supine position. The response is tested in two maneuvers: first, the child is rotated from the head; second, the child is rotated from the legs. For head rotation, the child's head is first flexed to approximately 45° and then slowly rotated so that the shoulders are turned. The rotation is observed. The child's head is usually rotated with one hand on the side of the face near the chin and the other hand on the occiput of the head. When the child is rolled

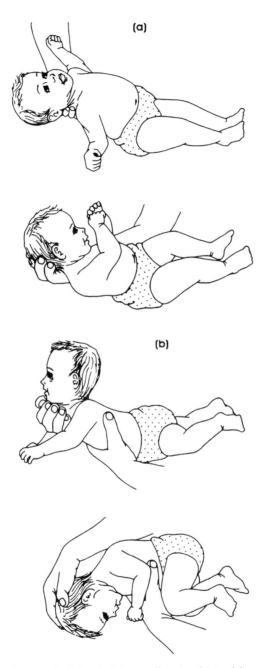

Figure 11–4 (a) The tonic labyrinthine reflex is elicited by putting support between the shoulders to extend the head 45°. The head is flexed 45°. The reflex is pathologic if there is severe extensor trust or opisthotonos. (b) Extension and flexion. Source: Adapted from A. Capute et al., *Primitive Reflex Profile* (Baltimore: University Park Press, 1978).

to the right, the examiner's left hand is the face hand and the right is the occiput hand. When the child is rolled to the left, the position of the examiner's hands is reversed (Figure 11–5).

To test the leg response, one leg of the child is flexed at the hip and knee. The examiner holds the flexed leg below the knee, and the child is rotated to turn the pelvis toward midline. Rotation patterns are then observed (Figure 11–6). Rotation responses have not been associated with oral and pharyngeal reflexes.

The Galant Reflex

The Galant reflex is an arching of the infant's body when the skin of the back near the vertebral column is stroked. The arching is usually forward, toward the stimulation. Arching in the other direction indicates the child is attempting to evade the stimulus. The responses

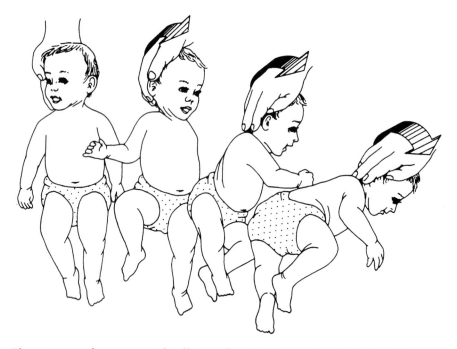

Figure 11–5 The segmental rolling reflex (with rotation of the head) is elicited by rotating the head to turn the shoulders and by rotating the legs (Figure 11–6) to turn the pelvis. The reflex is pathological if the child is obliged to roll in a log-rolling manner and cannot inhibit the reflex.
Source: Adapted from A. Capute et al., *Primitive Reflex Profile* (Baltimore: University Park Press, 1978).

may vary from total absence of response to an exaggerated hip flexion. In the majority of newborns, the response is present bilaterally; unilateral responses have been reported in athetoid cerebral palsy. The response normally disappears by 2 months of age but persists in athetosis beyond that time. The Galant reflex is thought to be associated with delay of trunk stabilization and head control in athetoid cerebral palsy. It is assumed that persistence of the response beyond 6 months may interfere with sitting balance. No association with oral or pharyngeal reflexes has been reported (Figure 11–7).

The Moro Reflex

The Moro reflex, along with the ATNR, is one of the best-known and best-studied reflexes of child neurology, and it is present in almost all newborns except for small premature babies. With sudden head lowering, there is a rapid and symmetrical abduction and upward movement of the arms. The hands open, and there is a gradual adduction and flexion of the arms. The lower limbs also show extension and then flexion.

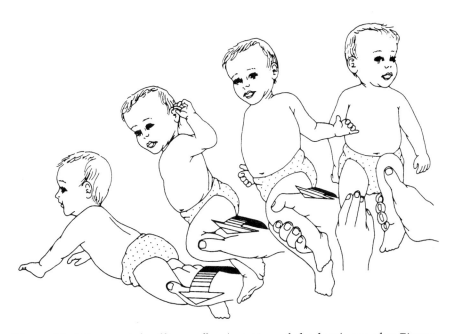

Figure 11–6 Segmental rolling reflex (rotation of the legs); see also Figure 11–5. Source: Adapted from Capute et al., *Primitive Reflex Profile* (Baltimore: University Park Press, 1978).

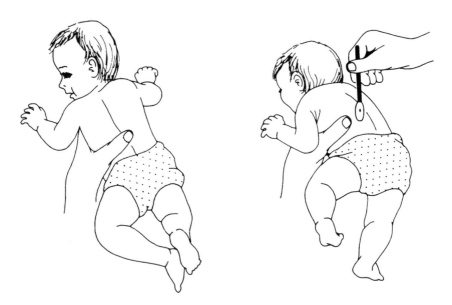

Figure 11–7 The Galant reflex is elicited by stroking the back in the lumbar region with a blunt object. The reflex is pathologic if there is persistent curvature of the back and elevation of the hips. Source: Adapted from A. Capute et al., *Primitive Reflex Profile* (Baltimore: University Park Press, 1978).

There has been some debate about whether the Moro response and the startle response are continuous patterns. Both responses appear in the newborn, so they are thought to be discontinuous. The Moro usually reaches a peak at 2 months and diminishes by 4 months. A persistent reflex has been associated with cerebral palsy and mental retardation.

To test for the Moro reflex, the child is held in the examiner's arms, well-supported at the head, trunk, and legs. The examiner suddenly lowers the child's head and body in a dropping motion (Figure 11–8).

The most significant aspect of the stimulus is the quality of suddenness. It is known that primitive and postural reflexes sometimes reinforce more circumscribed reflexes, but there is no evidence that the primitive Moro reflex tends to reinforce oral and pharyngeal reflexes in children with cerebral palsy. The persisting Moro reflex is much less valuable to the neurologist as a sign of cerebral injury than is the ATNR.

In summary, persisting infantile primitive and postural reflexes have been a classic sign of central nervous system dysfunction. In particular, they have been extremely useful in the early diagnosis of cerebral palsy. Infantile reflex behavior also has been incorporated in motor treatment programs for children with cerebral palsy. An important fact for the speech-language pathologist is that the primitive and postural body reflexes,

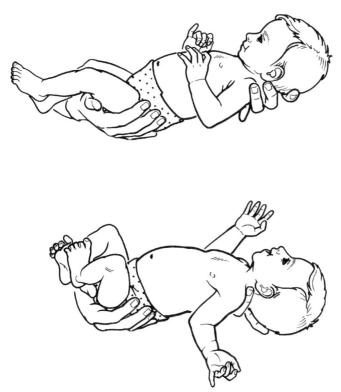

Figure 11–8 The Moro reflex is elicited by dropping the head. The reflex is pathologic if there is a persistent symmetrical abduction and upward movement of the arms with fingers splayed, followed by flexion of the arms in clasp manner. The back arches.

with some exceptions, appear to have limited influence on oral and pharyngeal reflexes. While these neonatal and early reflexes are important in assessing delayed development of motor function before age 12 to 18 months, they are of only limited use in the pediatric neurologic examination for the older child. The more conventional neurologic signs of altered muscle tone and abnormal muscle stretch and superficial reflexes, as well as the results of objective neurodiagnostic tests, are of equal value in making a diagnosis for the examining pediatric neurologists.

Oral and Pharyngeal Reflexes

Over the past half century, study of the normal infant reflexes and their relation to brain disease has prompted speech-language pathologists and others interested in the management of cerebral palsy to consider another set of reflexes—the oral and pharyngeal reflexes. Table 11–6 summarizes the major oral reflexes. Some speech specialists have assumed that abnormal oral and pharyngeal reflexes will play a significant role in the speech development of the child with cerebral palsy who is dysarthric or is likely to develop dysarthria with the onset of speech. Absent or persisting reflexes, they argue, are predictive of dysarthria. Neurologists are more likely to argue that when the oral and pharyngeal reflexes are integrated into a spontaneous feeding pattern, they become more diagnostically and prognostically significant in neurologic disease. Similarly, speech-language pathologists are beginning to question whether the isolated artificially elicited reflexes of the first few months of life have as much diagnostic and prognostic importance in speech performance as do the dysphagic symptoms commonly seen in many children with cerebral palsy.

The type, number, and reliability of abnormal oral and pharyngeal reflexes found in cerebral palsied subjects varies from research study to study. Research (Love, Hagerman, & Tiami, 1980) strongly suggests that there is little or no correlation between the presence and number of abnormal oral and pharyngeal reflexes and the severity of dysarthria in cerebral palsy as defined by a measure of articulation proficiency. In fact, the dysphagic symptoms—disordered biting, sucking, swallowing, and chewing—are slightly better predictors of articulation proficiency than are an elicited set of neonatal oral and pharyngeal automatisms. The correlation, however, between speech impairment and dysphagic symptoms is not particularly strong either. This limited relation between speech and dysphagia strongly implies that motor control for speech and the feeding reflexes may be mediated at different levels in the nervous system. Evidence indicates that the feeding reflexes are mediated at the brainstem level and that voluntary speech is controlled at the cortical, subcortical,

Table 11–6   Infantile Oral Reflexes

Reflex	Stimulus	Age of Appearance	Age of Disappearance
Rooting	Oral area being touched	Birth	3–6 months
Suckling	Nipple in mouth	Birth	6–12 months
Swallowing	Bolus of food in pharynx	Birth	Persists
Tongue	Tongue or lips being touched	Birth	12–18 months
Bite	Pressure on gums	Birth	9–12 months
Gag	Tongue or pharynx being touched	Birth	Persists

and cerebellar levels, with the prime voluntary pathways for speech being the corticobulbar fibers. Brainstem reflex pathways apparently subserve only vegetative and reflex functions and are inactive during the execution of normal speech. Therefore, early motor speech gestures probably are not directly related to the development of motor reactions in feeding during infancy and childhood, even though some of the motor coordinations and refinements in speech acquisition are analogous to some of the biting and chewing gestures in feeding.

Even though early oral motor behavior in feeding may only have a limited resemblance to actual motor patterns for speech, management programs to improve muscle function and coordination in eating have been initiated as a possible prophylactic measure for future dysarthria. The assumption of these programs is that any improvement in motor activity of the oral musculature gained through feeding therapy might conceivably result in improvement in speech performance, since the parallel activities of speech and feeding have muscles in common. At the very least, feeding therapy will probably make eating faster and easier. This, of course, is an important consideration in the total management of the child with cerebral palsy, one that should not be overlooked by speech-language pathologists and neurologists. In fact, dysphagia may be just as disturbing as dysarthria in the young cerebral palsied person. Direct motor training of the muscles during speech, rather than feeding training, appears to be the most effective method for improving the dysarthria, since cortically mediated speech activities drive the muscles at a more rapid and coordinated rate than do brainstem-mediated feeding activities.

The feeding reflexes have sometimes been used diagnostically by speech-language pathologists in planning management programs in cerebral palsied children. Persistent abnormal oral reflexes have also been factors considered in coming to the decision to elect an augmentative communicative system with a nonspeaking motor-handicapped child. One pair of experts have asserted that "of all factors investigated, obligatory persistence of oral reflexes can in isolation lead to a decision to elect an augmentative communication system" (Shane & Bashir, 1980). Their assumption is that retained oral reflexes indicate a very poor prognosis for oral speech development. This claim may have to be reevaluated in the light of the aforementioned findings concerning the poor correlation between articulatory proficiency and the number of retained oral reflexes in a cerebral palsied population (Love et al., 1980).

Despite the controversy about oral reflexes and speech in diagnosis, management, and prognosis, a description of six commonly tested oral pharyngeal reflexes is offered for the speech-language pathologist who may wish to consider this aspect of disturbed oral motor functions in the cerebrally injured infant and child. In the typical infantile oral motor evaluation, it is probably best first to elicit each of these infantile automatisms artificially one by one to determine whether they are absent or abnormally persisting. Next it is appropriate to assess the spontaneous functions of mastication and deglutition in the feeding act to determine how these neonatal reflex behaviors have become integrated into a more complex and voluntary oral-pharyngeal pattern of feeding. Infantile mastication and deglutition utilize the six cranial nerves (V, VII, IX, X, XI, XII) important for future speech, so evaluation of early feeding allows cranial nerve assessment for the child who is too immature to cooperate in standard cranial nerve testing.

Rooting Reflexes

If the perioral face region is touched, two responses in combination make up the rooting reflex. The side-to-side head turning reflex is usually elicited by gently tapping on the corners of the mouth or cheek. The response is the head alternately turning toward and away from the stimulus, ending with the lips brushing the stimulus. Occasionally the response will occur without the stimulus when the infant is hungry.

This activity usually precedes any actual suckling. The side-to-side head-turning response is present in the full-term baby and premature infant. The reflex usually disappears by 1 month of age and is replaced by the direct head-turning response, a simple movement of the head toward the source of stimulation. The source is grasped with the lips and sucked. In the direct head-turning response, if the stimulus is applied to the corners of the mouth, the bottom lip usually lowers and the head and tongue orient toward the stimulus. The direct head-turning response is established at 1 month and disappears by the end of the sixth month of life. Persistence beyond a year may suggest cerebral injury, and asymmetry of response indicates damage to one side of the brain or facial injury. The cranial nerves involved in the reflex are V, VII, XI, and XII. The reflex is mediated by the pons, medulla, and cervical spinal cord (Figure 11–9).

Suckling Reflex

If a finger or nipple is placed in the infant's mouth, bursts of suckling behavior will occur, interspersed with periods of rest. The suckling reflex is integrated at birth, but within 2 or 3 months the action develops more purpose, and jaw activity is incorporated into the pattern. Involuntary suckling may disappear between 6 months and a year. Persistent suckling beyond a year suggests brain injury. The reverse, inability to suckle, may also be an early sign of cerebral injury. The cranial nerves involved in suckling are V, VII, IX, and XII. The reflex is mediated at the pons and medulla (Figure 11–10).

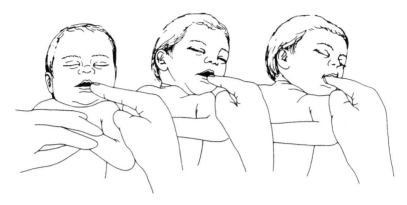

Figure 11–9 The rooting reflex is elicited by stimulating the cheek lateral to the mouth. From birth, the infant normally will turn the head toward the stimulus and then grasp the stimulus in the mouth. The reflex is pathologic if it is absent in infants from any cause or if it persists beyond the fourth month.

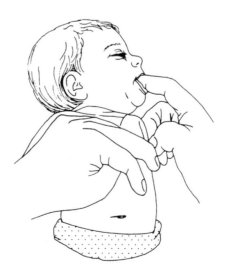

Figure 11–10 The suckling reflex is elicited by putting the index finger 3 to 4 centimeters into the mouth of the infant. From birth, the infant will normally engage in rhythmic sucking of the finger. The reflex is pathologic if it is absent or exaggerated or if it persists beyond the fourth month.

Swallowing Reflex

The swallowing reflex develops after the suckling reflex is integrated into a total feeding pattern. Suckling activities produce saliva, which accumulates in the reflexogenic area of the pharynx. The swallowing reflex is triggered, and swallowing may be observed by visible upward movement of the hyoid bone and thyroid cartilage of the larynx. The upward movement of the thyroid cartilage of the larynx may also be felt through palpation during the swallow. It is sometimes difficult to separate suckle and swallow, since swallow may precede a suck or follow a first or second swallow. The act of deglutition involves muscles of the mouth, tongue, palate, and pharynx and is dependent on a highly coordinated movement pattern. Cranial nerves V, VII, IX, X, and XII are involved in the act of swallowing. An immature swallow with tongue thrusting is sometimes seen until about 18 months. A mature swallow is present afterwards. The reflex is mediated at the level of the brainstem in the medullary reticular formation. Disturbances in swallowing are frequent manifestations of neurologic deficits in the infant and child, and they make up the most important sign of neurologic disorder among the feeding reflexes.

Tongue Reflex

This reflex may be considered part of a suckle-swallow reaction in which the tongue thrusts between the lips. If lips or tongue are touched, cranial nerve XII predominates. Excessive thrusts beyond 18 months are abnormal. The reflex is mediated at the medulla.

Bite Reflex

Moderate pressure on the gums elicits jaw closure and a bite response. This reflex is present at birth; in the normal infant, it disappears by 9 to 12 months, when it is replaced by a more mature chewing pattern. The reflex may be exaggerated in the brain-injured child and may interfere with feeding and dental care. Its persistence inhibits the lateral jaw movements of chewing seen in the spontaneous mastication pattern. A weak response is seen with brainstem lesion, and corticobulbar lesions exaggerate the response. Cranial nerve V innervates the reflex, which is mediated at the low midbrain and pons.

Gag Reflex

A stimulus applied to the posterior half of the infant tongue or on the posterior wall of the pharynx causes rapid velopharyngeal closure. This primary action is accompanied by mouth opening, head extension, and depression of the floor of the mouth with elevation of the larynx and diaphragm. This reflex is present at birth and continues throughout life. The gag serves as a protective mechanism for the esophagus. Brain-damaged children often show a hyperactive gag. In the severely motor-involved child, the gag may be difficult to elicit. In the ataxic child, the gag is sometimes hypoactive. Cranial nerves IX and X innervate the gag, and the reflex is mediated at the level of the pons and medulla (Figure 11–11).

Assessing Mastication and Deglutition

In the infant and child at risk for neurologic injury, the clinical evaluation of neural control of the oral and pharyngeal activities involved in chewing and swallowing allows the speech-language pathologist to estimate the motor potential of those muscles, which will ultimately fall under the control of higher nervous centers devoted to the production of speech. The fact that speech and feeding are mediated at different levels within the nervous system implies that evaluation of chewing and swallowing will predict future muscle activity in speech in only a very limited manner. It is probable that only gross estimates of muscle potential for speech can be derived from any nonspeech examination because of the semiautonomous control of the muscles for the dual function.

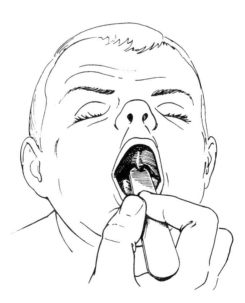

Figure 11–11 The gag reflex is elicited by stimulating the posterior half of the infant's tongue with a tongue blade or stimulating the posterior pharyngeal wall. The reflex is present from birth, and it is pathologic when absent or exaggerated.

In addition to gross estimation of muscle function in mastication and deglutition, the infantile oral motor examination of the cranial nerves for speech permits the speech-language pathologist and neurologist to observe signs of possible neurologic disorder that may not be readily apparent in other motor behaviors. Mastication and deglutition, as relatively complex motor behaviors in the repertoire of infant motor activity, are highly sensitive to neurologic dysfunction. Dysphagia may be an early and even sometimes isolated sign of brain injury.

Modified Feeding

Examination of chewing and swallowing is best accomplished through the technique of modified feeding. In the prespeaking child, this technique can replace the more traditional procedures of the adult speech cranial nerve test, which requires a level of maturity not yet developed in the infant and very young child. By selectively placing small morsels of solid food in different locations in the oral cavity of the child, an examiner can judge the integrity of the bulbar muscles and the brainstem neural pathways innervating these muscles. Healthy children from birth to 36 months respond well to the technique, which may also be used with motor-handicapped children with oral motor involvement well beyond 3 years of age. In the healthy child, spontaneous feeding emerges from the neonatal oral and pharyngeal reflexes and reaches its full maturity at about age 3. Experiences with solid foods provide a gradual refinement and integration of movements of the lips, tongue, palate, and pharynx for chewing and swallowing.

When testing the infant or motor-handicapped child without sitting balance, it is usually best to place the child in a chair in which the body and head can be well-supported (for example, a tumble-form chair) or in the primary caregiver's or clinician's lap in a well-supported position. In the child with some sitting balance, placement in a relaxed sitting position with adequate head support is preferred for the examination.

Cranial Nerve VII

Placing a small food bolus on the lower lip in midline and observing the child's oral reaction to it will provide evidence of the ability to use the muscles of the lip and lower face purposefully. Pursing the lips during rooting and sucking indicates intact facial movement. Lack of a smiling response may be suggestive of severe bilateral facial muscle involvement. The healthy baby smiles to a human face at 2 to 4 months of age. A sober expression and sluggish grin must be carefully evaluated as possible neurologic signs of a bilateral corticobulbar system involvement ultimately affecting the paired nerves of cranial nerve VII. An asymmetrical smile with a unilateral flattening of the nasal fold on one side of the face may be associated with unilateral paresis. This sign is not as obvious in the infant and young child as it is in the adult. Lack of lip tonicity may be present, and lip seal may not be maintained. In the brain-damaged child, drooling may result from the poor lip seal.

Cranial Nerve XII

The child with cerebral injury is often unable to shape, point, and protrude the tongue in retrieving food from the lower lip by licking. The lack of tongue protrusion is common in both spastic and athetoid children. In the brain-injured infant, the tongue often will not cup, even during crying. Neither will the tongue thin, nor will the tip elevate with precision. This inability to produce any fine tongue movements suggests motor involvement of both the intrinsic and the extrinsic tongue musculature.

Unilateral or bilateral atrophy of the tongue may be seen in young children, and this loss of muscle bulk suggests lower motor neuron disease. However, fasciculations are rarely seen in the tongue muscles of infants.

Excessive tongue thrust, sometimes called the *tongue reflex*, is common in children with severe brain damage. It is particularly common in athetosis, and it may be associated with orthodontic problems and excessive drooling. In addition, occasional wave-like involuntary movements are seen in the body of the tongue, mimicking the involuntary movements of limb and trunk in extrapyramidal athetosis.

Cranial Nerve V

When confronted with a small food bolus on the lips or tongue, the young child begins the total act of deglutition by initiating voluntary mastication. The aim of the evaluation at this point is to determine whether the bolus of food can be pulverized and whether the particles of food can be selectively manipulated to be transported to the back of the oral cavity. With a large food bolus, the tongue is usually elevated, so the bolus is placed between the tongue surface and the anterior hard palate and crushed. Smaller boluses of food are crushed between the hard palate and tongue, and the tongue directly begins a wave-like, peristaltic movement, carrying the food to the pharynx. If the food bolus is large, the tongue often acts in a whip-like fashion to propel the food laterally between the molars for grinding and pulverization. Observation of the vigorous tongue actions will confirm the integrity of the neural control of the tongue. Disorders involving neurologic integrity of the tongue and jaw innervation often limit cerebrally damaged children to eating only diced or liquefied food.

Adequate biting and vigorous anterior-posterior movements of the mandible plus lateral grinding action of the jaws assure the speech-language pathologist that cranial nerve V innervation is intact and that muscles innervated from the pons are functional. On the other hand, an exaggerated and too powerful bite may be a manifestation of an abnormal jaw reflex, suggesting an upper motor neuron lesion above the level of the pons. In older children with brain damage, a firm tap on the lower jaw may elicit a clonus, suggesting a hyperactive jaw reflex. If the lower jaw deviates to one side on opening or during mastication, there may be pterygoid muscle weakness on the side of deviation. In athetosis the jaw may become a major articulator, producing the motor power for elevating a poorly controlled tongue in achieving tongue-tip—alveolar ridge contacts and other tongue-elevation gestures.

Integration of Cranial Nerves V, VII, IX, X, and XII

When the food bolus is well-masticated, the final, involuntary stage of deglutition is initiated. The nasopharynx is closed by the action of the muscles of the soft palate and the pharyngeal constrictors. Cranial nerves IX and X produce this closure. Saliva or the food bolus is pushed through the palatal fauces, into the pharynx, and on to the esophagus in a peristaltic wave. Muscles of the soft palate, the pharyngeal constrictors, and muscles of the tongue and larynx work in intricate coordination to propel the food bolus to the esophagus. In one sense, swallowing becomes the ultimate integration of the nervous mechanisms to be used later in motor expression of speech.

Speech, however, requires more intricate coordination of muscles than do chewing and swallowing. This fine coordination is accomplished through increasing cortical and cerebellar control of the pontine and bulbar muscles. Certain other complex motor adjustments are seen in speech that are not seen in chewing or swallowing. As an example, the grooved fricative /s/ requires finer motor control than is seen in mastication. To produce an adequate /s/, a central groove in the tip and blade of the tongue must be formed, with the sides of the tongue firmly anchored between the lateral dentition. This specific tongue configuration, common to speech, is not seen in brainstem-mediated functions. Intricate coordination of intrinsic and extrinsic tongue muscles is needed for the grooved fricatives. These fine motor configurations are not present in feeding. Thus, assessment of mastication and deglutition in a prespeaking child suspected of neurologic impairment is most appropriate, but when speech emerges, the evaluation should be based on the motor control for phonemes, syllables, words, and sentences assessed in the traditional articulation test format and on the results of a standard oral examination that includes assessment of the speech cranial nerves (Chapter 7).

The actions of the cranial nerves for speech and of the corticobulbar system, which activate the cranial nerve nuclei, can be assessed in infancy through observation of chewing and swallowing. All of the nervous action of the bulbar muscles is integrated into the single act of feeding in infancy.

Summary

The developmental motor speech disorders include developmental dysarthria, developmental anarthria, and developmental apraxia of speech. Developmental dysarthria is by far the most common of the motor speech disorders and is most frequently seen in children with cerebral palsy. Cerebral palsy is primarily a movement disorder due to damage to the immature brain. The three major clinical syndromes of cerebral palsy are spasticity, athetosis, and ataxia. Most cerebral palsied children present multiple disabilities in addition to their motor disorder.

Next to cerebral palsy, childhood muscular dystrophy is the most common motor disorder in children. Pseudohypertrophic muscular dystrophy is the largest subgroup of the childhood dystrophies. Flaccid dysarthria may appear in the later stages of this progressive degenerative disease. An uncommon syndrome is isolated motor involvement of the oral muscles. This disorder has been called congenital suprabulbar paresis.

The diagnosis of early neurologic injury depends on a total pediatric neurologic examination that usually includes an assessment of the primitive reflexes of the first year of life. Absent or highly persistent reflexes are usually indicative of abnormality. Among the best-studied reflexes are the asymmetrical tonic neck reflex, symmetrical tonic neck reflex, positive support reflex, tonic labyrinthine reflex, segmental rolling reflex, Galant reflex, and Moro reflex. Only the tonic labyrinthine reflex may activate an oral response of tongue thrusting.

The influence of persistent oral reflexes or dysphagic symptoms on later speech production in developmental dysarthria is controversial, but speech-language pathologists and pediatric neurologists usually recognize the following oral reflexes as often disturbed by early cerebral injury: the rooting reflex, suckling reflex, swallowing reflex, bite reflex, tongue reflex, and gag reflex. These infantile oral reactions are mediated at a brainstem level, whereas speech movements are initiated and carried out through the corticobulbar system and are influenced by other motor systems.

In the infant and older prespeaking child, a gross estimate of the movement potential of the oral muscles can be obtained by observing the muscle action in mastication and deglutition in modified feeding activities. Chewing and swallowing involve integration of the action of the cranial nerves V, VII, IX, X, and XII, those nerves that are critical for normal speech production. In the older child, a standard cranial nerve examination suggests the degree of motor involvement on speech production.

References and Further Readings

Cerebral Palsy

Hardy, J. C. (1983). *Cerebral palsy*. Englewood Cliffs, NJ: Prentice-Hall.

Meyer, L. A. (1982). A study of vocal, prosodic and articulatory parameters of the speech of spastic and athetotic cerebral palsied individuals. Ph.D dissertation, Vanderbilt University.

Neilson, P. D., & O'Dwyer, N. J. (1981). Physiopathology of dysarthria in cerebral palsy. *Journal of Neurology, Neurosurgery and Psychiatry*, 44, 1013–1019.

Scherzer, A. I., & Tscharnuter, I. (1982). *Early diagnosis and therapy in cerebral palsy*. New York: Marcel Dekker

Thompson, G. H., Rubin, I. L., & Bilenker, R. H. (1983). *Comprehensive management of cerebral palsy*. New York: Grune & Stratton.

Workinger, M. S., & Kent, R. D. (1991). Perceptual analysis of the dysarthrias in children with athetoid and spastic cerebral palsy. In C. A. Moore, K. M. Yorkston, & D. R. Beuklman (Eds.), *Dysarthria and apraxia of speech*. Baltimore: Paul H. Brooks.

Childhood Suprabulbar Paresis

Worster-Drought, C. (1974). Suprabulbar paresis. *Developmental Medicine and Child Neurology*, 16 (suppl 30), 1–30.

Muscular Dystrophy

Love, R. J. (1992). *Childhood motor speech disability*. Columbus, OH: Merrill.

Sanders, L. J., & Perlstein, M. A. (1965). Speech mechanism in pseudohypertrophic muscular dystrophy. *American Journal of Diseases of Children*, 109, 538–543.

Walton, J. N. (1981). *Disorders of voluntary muscle* (4th ed.). London: Churchill-Livingstone.

Primitive Reflexes

Capute, A. J., Accardo, P. I., Vining, E. P. G., & Rubenstein, J. E. (1978). *Primitive reflex profile.* Baltimore: University Park Press.

Oral and Pharyngeal Reflexes

Anderson, D. J., & Mathews, B. (1976). *Mastication.* Bristol: Wright.

Dubner, R., Sessle, B. I., & Storey, A. T. (1978). *The neural basis of oral and facial function.* New York: Plenum.

Love, R. J., Hagerman, E. L., & Tiami, E.G. (1980). Speech performance, dysphagia and oral reflexes in cerebral palsy. *Journal of Speech and Hearing Disorders, 45,* 59–75

Shane, H. C., & Bashir, A. S. (1980) Election criteria for adoption of an augmentative communication system: Preliminary considerations. *Journal of Speech and Hearing Disorders, 45,* 408–414.

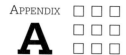
Prevalence of Neurological Disorders

Tables A–1 and A–2 show the approximate point prevalence rates per 10,000 population, all ages, of common and less common neurological disorders, respectively.

Table A–1 Point Prevalence Rates per 100,000 Population, All Ages: Most Common Neurological Disorders

Disorders	Rate
Migraine	2,000
Other severe headaches	1,500
Brain injuries	800
Epilepsy	650
Acute cerebrovascular disease	600
Lumbosacral pain syndrome	500
Alcoholism	500
Sleep disorders	300
Ménière's disease	300
Lumbosacral herniated nucleus pulposus	300
Pulposus	250
Cerebral palsy	250
Dementia	250
Parkinsonism	200
Transient ischemic attacks	150
Febrile fits	100
Persistent postconcussive syndrome	80
Herpes zoster	80

Disorders	Rate
Congenital malformations of the central nervous system	70
Signal seizures	60
Multiple sclerosis	60
Benign brain tumor	60
Cervical pain syndrome	60
Down's syndrome	50
Subarachnoid hemorrhage	50
Cervical herniated nucleus pulposus	50
Transient postconcussive syndrome	50
Spinal cord injury	50

Source: Modified from J. F. Kurtze, "Neuroepidemiology." In W. G. Bradley, R. B. Daroff, G. M. Fenichel, & D. C. Marsden, (Eds.), *Neurology in Clinical Practice* (Vol. 1) (Boston: Butterworth-Heinemann, 1991).

Table A–2 Point Prevalence Rates per 100,000 Population, All Ages: Less Common Neurological Disorders

Disorders	Rate
Tic douloureux	40
Neurological symptoms without defined disease	40
Mononeuropathies	40
Polyneuropathies	30
Dorsolateral sclerosis	30
Peripheral nerve trauma	30
Other head injury	30
Acute transverse myelopathy	15
Metastatic brain tumor	15
Chronic progressive myelopathy	10
Optic neuritis	10
Encephalitides	10
Vascular disease, spinal cord	9
Hereditary ataxias	8
Syringomyelia	7
Motor neuron disease	6
Polymyositis	6
Progressive muscular dystrophy	6

Table A–2 *(continued)*

Disorders	Rate
Malignant primary brain tumor	5
Metastatic cord tumor	5
Meningitides	5
Bell's palsy	5
Huntington's disease	5
Charcot-Marie-Tooth disease	5
Myasthenia gravis	4
Familial spastic paraplegia	3
Intracranial abscess	2
Cranial nerve trauma	2
Myotonic dystrophy	2
Spinal muscular atrophy	2
Guillain-Barré syndrome	1
Wilson's disease	1
Acute disseminated encephalomyelitis	0.6
Dystonic musculorum deformans	0.3

Source: Modified from J. F. Kurtze, "Neuroepidemiology." In W. G. Bradley, R. B. Daroff, G. M. Fenichel, & D. C. Marsden, (Eds.), *Neurology in Clinical Practice* (Vol. 1) (Boston: Butterworth-Heinemann, 1991).

Medical Conditions Related to Communication Disorders

I. Congenital disorders
   A. *Cerebral palsy*: Defect of motor power and coordination related to damage of the immature brain
   B. *Congenital hydrocephalus*: Condition marked by excessive accumulation of fluid, dilating the cerebral ventricles, thinning the brain, and causing a separation of cranial bones; caused by a developmental defect of the brain
   C. *Craniostenosis*: Contraction of the cranial capacity or narrowing of the sutures by bony overgrowth
   D. *Down's syndrome*: Syndrome of mental retardation associated with many and variable abnormalities, caused by representation of at least a critical portion of chromosome 21 three times instead of twice in some or all cells
   E. *Idiopathic mental retardation*: Mental retardation of unknown cause
   F. *Minimal cerebral dysfunction*: Syndrome of neurologic dysfunction in children usually marked by impairment of fine coordination, clumsiness, and choreiform or athetoid movements; learning disorders are often associated with this diagnosis
   G. *Neurofibromatosis*: Condition in which small, discrete, pigmented skin lesions develop in infancy or early childhood, followed by the development of multiple subcutaneous neurofibromas that may slowly increase in number and size over many years

II. Vascular disorders

     A. *Cerebral embolism*: Obstruction or occlusion of a vessel in the cerebrum by a transported clot or vegetation, a mass of bacteria, or other foreign material

     B. *Cerebral hemorrhage*: Bleeding in the brain; a flow of blood, especially if very profuse, into the substance of the cerebrum, usually in the region of the internal capsule; caused by rupture of the lenticulostriate artery

     C. *Cerebral thrombosis*: Obstruction or occlusion of a vessel in the cerebrum by a fixed clot developing on the arterial wall

     D. *Pseudobulbar palsy*: Muscular paralysis from bilateral upper motor neuron lesions of the cranial nerves; often accompanied by signs of dysarthria, dysphagia, and emotional lability with outbursts of uncontrolled crying and laughing

     E. *Recurrent cerebral ischemia or transient ischemic attacks*: Temporary disruptions of the blood supply that produce specific neurological signs; experienced as sudden, transient blurring of vision, weakness, numbness of one side, speech difficulty, vertigo or diplopia, or any combination

     F. *Subdural hemorrhage*: Extravascularization of blood between the dural and arachnoid membranes

III. Infections

     A. *Acute anterior poliomyelitis*: Inflammation of the anterior cornu of the spinal cord due to an acute infectious disease marked by fever, pains, and gastroenteric disturbances; followed by flaccid paralysis of one or more muscular groups and later by atrophy

     B. *Cerebral abscess*: Intracranial abscess or abscess of the brain, specifically of the cerebrum; a collection of pus in a localized area

     C. *Encephalitis*: Inflammation of the brain

     D. *Jacob-Creutzfeldt disease*: Spastic pseudosclerosis with corticostriatospinal degeneration and subacute presenile dementia; characterized by slowly progressive dementia, myoclonic fasciculations, ataxia, and somnolence with gradual onset; usually fatal within a few months to years

     E. *Meningitis*: Inflammation of the membranes of the brain or spinal cord

     F. *Neurosyphilis*: Syphilis, an infectious venereal disease caused by a microorganism, affecting the nervous system

     G. *Sydenham's chorea*: Acute toxic or infective disorder of the nervous system, usually associated with acute rheumatism, occurring in young persons and characterized by involuntary semipurposeful but ineffective movements; movements involve the facial muscles and muscles of the neck and limbs and are intensified by voluntary effort but disappear in sleep

IV. Trauma
   A. *Penetrating head injury*: Open head injury, which causes altered consciousness and can produce fairly definitive and chronic aphasias
   B. *Closed head injury*: Injury to the head in which there is no injury to the skull or in which injury is limited to an undisplaced fracture; also known as *nonpenetrating head injury*; can produce loss of consciousness and often produces diffuse effects

V. Tumors
   A. *Astrocytomas (grades 1 and 2) and oligodendrogliomas*: Less common glial cell tumors, with a better prognosis than glioblastoma multiforme; slow growing; usually treated with surgery and radiation therapy, with an average survival rate of 5 to 6 years after surgery
   B. *Glioblastoma multiforme*: Also known as *malignant glioma* or *astrocytoma* (grades 3 and 4), this is the most common primary brain tumor in adults; most frequent sites are frontal and temporal lobes, although tumors may occur anywhere in the brain; infiltrative and rapidly growing, with an average survival rate of about 1 year
   C. *Meningioma*: Benign tumor arising from the arachnoid cells of the brain; slow growing and usually occurring at the lateral areas and base of the brain; generally does not invade the cerebral cortex; favorable prognosis

VI. Degenerative diseases
   A. *Dementia of the Alzheimer's type*: Progressive mental deterioration with loss of memory, especially for recent events
   B. *Parkinson's disease*: Degenerative disease resulting from damage to the dopamine-producing nerve cells of the striatum and the substantia nigra; characterized by rest tremor, rigidity of muscles, paucity of movement, slowness of movement, limited range, limited force of contraction, and failure of gestural expression

C. *Wilson's disease*: Genetic metabolic disorder caused by inadequate processing of dietary intake of copper and characterized by motor symptoms, with a significant dysarthria

D. *Huntington's chorea*: Chronic progressive hereditary disease characterized by irregular, spasmodic, involuntary movements of the limbs or facial muscles; sometimes accompanied by dementia and dysarthria

E. *Friedreich's ataxia*: Hereditary disease characterized by degeneration principally of the cerebellum and dorsal half of the spinal cord; ataxic dysarthria is often an accompanying sign

F. *Dystonia musculorum deformans*: Hereditary disease occurring especially in children; characterized by muscular contractions producing peculiar distentions of the spine and hip and by bizarre postures

G. *Multiple sclerosis*: Inflammatory disease mainly involving the white matter of the central nervous system and characterized by scattered areas of demyelination causing impairment of transmission of nerve impulses; may cause a variety of symptoms, including paralysis, nystagmus, and dysarthria, depending on the lesion sites

VII. Metabolic and toxic disorders

A. *Reye's syndrome*: Sudden loss of consciousness in children following the initial stage of an infection, usually resulting in death with cerebral edema (swelling) and marked fatty change in the liver and renal system; surviving children often have motor, cognitive, and speech problems

VIII. Neuromuscular disorders

A. Progressive muscular atrophies

1. *True bulbar palsy*: Disorder caused by involvement of nuclei of the last four or five cranial nerves and characterized by twitching and atrophy of the tongue, palate, and larynx, drooling, dysarthria, dysphagia, and finally respiratory paralysis; usually a manifestation of amyotrophic lateral sclerosis

2. *Amyotrophic lateral sclerosis*: Disease of the motor tracts of the lateral columns of the spinal cord causing progressive muscular atrophy, increased reflexes, fibrillary twitching, and spastic irritability of muscles

B. Muscular dystrophy

1. *Pseudohypertrophic (Duchenne) type*: Type of muscular dystrophy characterized by bulky calf and forearm muscles and progressive atrophy and weakness of the thigh, hip, and back muscles and shoulder girdle; occurs in the first 3 years of life, usually in boys and rarely in girls

2. *Facioscapulohumeral type*: Type of muscular dystrophy causing atrophy of the muscles of the face, shoulder, girdle, and upper arms; occurs in either sex, with onset at any age from childhood to late adult life; characterized by prolonged periods of apparent arrest

3. *Ocular myopathy*: Type of muscular dystrophy affecting external ocular muscles, causing ptosis, diplopia, and occasional total external ophthalmoplegia; sometimes associated with upper facial muscle weakness, dysphagia, and atrophy and weakness of neck, trunk, and limb muscles

C. *Myasthenia gravis*: Disorder characterized by marked weakness and fatigue of muscles, especially those muscles innervated by bulbar nuclei

D. Congenital neuromuscular disorders

1. *Möbius syndrome*: Congenital disorder characterized by paresis or paralysis of both lateral rectus muscles and all face muscles; sometimes associated with other musculoskeletal anomalies

IX. Other

A. *Epilepsy*: Chronic disorder characterized by paroxysmal attacks of brain dysfunction (seizures) usually associated with some alteration of consciousness; seizures may remain confined to elementary or complex impairment of behavior or may progress to a generalized convulsion

B. *Wernicke-Korsakoff syndrome*: Cerebral disorder characterized by confusion and severe impairment of memory, especially for recent events; patient compensates for memory loss by confabulation; often seen in chronic alcoholics and associated with severe nutritional deficiency

APPENDIX ☐ ☐ ☐
C   ☐ ☐ ☐
     ☐ ☐ ☐

Bedside Neurological Examination

I. Mental status
   A. Orientation: person, place, time
   B. Memory and information
      1. Three objects at 5 minutes
      2. Presidents back to Kennedy
   C. Language
      1. Spontaneous speech characterization
      2. Confrontation naming
      3. Auditory comprehension (commands, yes/no questions)
      4. Repetition (words, phrases)
      5. Reading (printed commands)
      6. Writing (signature, words, and sentences to dictation)
   D. Calculations
      1. Serial 7s (count by 7s to 100)
      2. Subtract $0.43 from $1.00
   E. Visuospatial ability
      1. Clock drawing
      2. Copying of figures
   F. Insight, judgment

II. Cranial nerves
   A. I: Smell
   B. II: Visual fields, pupillary reactions, optic fundi
   C. III–IV: Extraocular movements
   D. V: Facial sensation
   E. VII: Facial symmetry
   F. VIII: Hearing
   G. IX and X: Articulation, palatal movement, gag reflex
   H. XI: Sternomastoid and trapezius strength
   I. XII: Tongue movement

III. Motor examination
  A. Bulk
  B. Spontaneous movements (fasciculations, tremor, movement disorders)
  C. Strength
    1. Evaluation of strength on right and left
      a) deltoid
      b) biceps
      c) triceps
      d) hip flexion
      e) knee flexion
      f) ankle dorsiflexion
      g) ankle plantar flexion
  D. Reflexes
    1. Evaluation of reflexes on right and left
      a) biceps
      b) triceps
      c) brachioradialis
      d) ankle
      e) plantar
      f) jaw
  E. Stance and Romberg
  F. Gait
    1. Spontaneous gait
    2. Tandem gait
    3. Tiptoe gait
    4. Heel gait
  G. Sensory examination
    1. Pinprick
    2. Touch
    3. Vibration
    4. Position
    5. Stereognosis, graphesthesia ("cortical" sensory modalities)
  H. Cerebellar
    1. Finger–nose–finger
    2. Rapid alternating hand movements
    3. Fine finger movements
    4. Heel–knee–shin

Source: Courtesy of Howard Kirshner, M.D., Department of Neurology, Vanderbilt University School of Medicine, Nashville, Tennessee.

Screening Neurologic Examination for Speech-Language Pathology

I. Mental status

A. *General behavior and appearance*: Is the patient normal, hyperactive, agitated, quiet, immobile? Is he neat, slovenly? Is he dressed in accordance with peers, background, and sex?

B. *Stream of talk*: Does the patient respond to conversation normally? Is her speech rapid, incessant, under great pressure? Is she very slow and difficult to draw into spontaneous talk? Is she discursive, able to reach the conversational goal?

C. *Mood and affective responses*: Is the patient euphoric, agitated, inappropriately cheerful, giggling? Or is he silent, weeping, angry? Does his mood swing in a direction appropriate to the subject matter of the conversation? Is he emotionally labile?

D. *Content of thought*: Does the patient have illusions, hallucinations or delusions, and misinterpretations? Is she preoccupied with bodily complaints, fears of cancer or heart disease, and other phobias? Does she feel that society is maliciously organized to cause her difficulty?

E. *Intellectual capacity*: Is the patient bright, average, dull, obviously demented, mentally retarded?

F. *Sensorium.*

1. *Consciousness*: Note whether the patient is alert, drowsy, or stuporous.

2. *Attention span*: Note response in cerebral function test.

3. *Orientation*: Note whether the patient can answer questions about his person, location, and time.

4. *Memory*: Note recent and remote memory deficits, as disclosed during history taking.
5. *Fund of information*: Note in history taking.
6. *Insight, judgment, and planning*: Note in history taking.
7. *Calculation*: Note performance on cerebral function test.

II. Speech, language, and voice
   A. *Dysphonia*: Neuromotor difficulty in producing voice (cranial nerve X).
   B. *Dysarthria*: Neuromotor disorder of articulation and voice.
      1. Labials (cranial nerve VII).
      2. Velars and velopharyngeal closure (IX and X).
      3. Linguals (XII).
   C. *Dysphasia*: Cerebral disorder of understanding and expressing language (give aphasia-screening test).
      1. Fluent. (Give screening aphasia test.)
      2. Nonfluent. (Give screening aphasia test.)
   D. *Dyspraxia*: Cerebral disorder of articulation and prosody and/or disorder of oral movement.
      1. Dyspraxia of speech.
      2. Oral dyspraxia.
   E. *Dementia*: Cerebral disorder of language or intellectual deficit.
      1. Presenile.
      2. Senile
   F. *Disorganized language*: Cerebral disorder of language or confusion.
   G. *Dysphagia*: Neuromotor disorder of swallowing (V, VII, IX, X, and XII).

III. Cranial nerves for speech and hearing
   A. *Speech* (V, VII, IX, X, XII, and XI).
      1. V: Inspect masseter and temporalis muscle bulk; palpate masseter when the patient bites.
      2. VII: Evaluate forehead wrinkling, eyelid closure, mouth retraction, whistling or puffed out cheeks, wrinkled skin over neck (platysma), and labial articulation.
      3. IX and X: Evaluate phonation, hypernasality, swallowing, gag reflex, and palatal elevation.
      4. XII: Evaluate lingual articulation and midline and lateral tongue protrusion; inspect for atrophy and fasciculations.
      5. XI: Inspect sternocleidomastoid and trapezius contours; test strength of head movements and shoulder shrugging.

6. Test for pathologic fatigability by requesting 100 repetitive movements (for instance, eye blinks) if the history suggests myopathic or myoneural disorder.

B. *Hearing* (VIII).

1. Evaluate for threshold and acuity, including adequacy of hearing for conversational speech.
2. If history or preceding observation suggests a deficit, do air-bone conduction audiometric screening.

IV. Motor system

A. *Inspection.*

1. Take history, including initial appraisal of the motor system; inspect the patient for postures, general activity level, tremors, and involuntary movements.
2. Observe the size and contour of the muscles, looking for atrophy, hypertrophy, body asymmetry, joint misalignments, fasciculations, tremors, and involuntary movements.
3. Evaluate gait, including free walking, tandem walking, and deep knee bend.

B. *Palpation*: Palpate muscles if they seem atrophic or hypertrophic, or if the history suggests that they may be tender or in spasm.

C. *Strength.*

1. *Upper extremities:* Test biceps.
2. *Lower extremities:* Test knee flexors and foot dorsiflexors if necessary and feasible.
3. *Pattern:* Discern whether any weakness follows a distributional pattern, such as proximal-distal, right-left, or upper extremity–lower extremity.

D. *Muscle tone*: Move the patient's joints to test for spasticity, clonus, or rigidity.

E. *Muscle stretch (deep) reflexes*: Test jaw jerk (cranial nerve V afferent and efferent) as well as other MSRs, if necessary and feasible.

F. *Cerebellar system* (gait tested previously).

1. Evaluate finger-to-nose, rebound, and alternating motion rates.
2. Carry out heel-to-knee testing.

V. Sensory examination

A. Test superficial sensation by light touch with cotton wisp and pin prick on face.

B. Ask if the face feels numb.

C. Test superficial sensation on the tongue surface with swab stick unilaterally and bilaterally, anteriorly and posteriorly.

VI. Cerebral function

A. When the history or antecedent examination suggests a cerebral lesion, test for finger agnosia and right-left disorientation.

B. Have the patient do the cognitive, constructional, and performance tasks from standard aphasia or neuropsychological tests.

Source: Adapted from W. DeMyer, *Technique of the Neurologic Examination* (New York: McGraw-Hill, 1980).

Glossary

abduction: movement of a body part away from the midline.
acalculia: inability to do simple arithmetical calculation due to brain injury.
action potential: buildup of electrical current in the neuron.
acuity: sharpness or acuteness.
adduction: movement of a body part toward midline.
afferent: traveling toward a center.
agnosia: lack of sensory recognition as the result of a lesion in the sensory association areas or association pathways of the brain.
alexia: acquired disturbance of reading due to brain injury.
alexia with agraphia: classic neurologic syndrome of reading disorder in which there is damage to the angular gyrus and the surrounding areas.
alexia without agraphia: classic neurologic syndrome of reading disorder, usually caused by a left posterior cerebral artery occlusion in a righthanded person; the resulting infarct produces lesions in the splenium of the corpus callosum and the left occipital lobe.
alpha motor neurons: neurons allowing contraction of extrafusal fibers and that have their final common path in cranial and spinal nerves.
Alzheimer's disease: the most common type of dementia; its most striking feature is progressive deterioration of cognitive functions; its language disturbance is a major symptom.
angular gyrus: convolution in the left parietal lobe that is critical for language processing.
anomia: loss of the power to name objects or recognize and recall their names.
anoxia: absence of oxygen in inspired gases, arterial blood, or tissue.
anterior horn cell: cell in the ventral portion in an *H*-shaped body of gray matter in the spinal cord associated with efferent pathways.
apex: the extremity of a conical or pyramidal structure.
apraxia: a disorder of learned movement distinct from paralysis, weakness, and incoordination; results in a disturbance of motor planning.
apraxia of speech: disorder of programming the muscles of articulation in the absence of paralysis, weakness, and incoordination.
arcuate fasciculus: long subcortical association tract connecting posterior and anterior speech-language areas in the cerebrum.
association area of association areas: the area of the inferior parietal lobe where the visual, auditory, and tactile association fibers converge.

asymmetry: disproportion or inequality between two corresponding parts around the center of an axis.

asynergy: lack of coordination of agonistic and antagnostic muscles, particularly associated with cerebellar disorders.

ataxia: defect of posture and gait associated with a disorder of the nervous system; **sensory ataxia,** associated with dorsal column dysfunction, is distinguished from **cerebellar** or **cerebellar pathway ataxia.**

autism: major developmental disability marked by disturbed stereotyped behavior and language patterns; echolalic verbal behavior is often present, as are neurologic signs.

axon: literally, "the axis"—a straight, relatively unbranched process of a nerve cell.

basal ganglia: subcortical structures, part of the extrapyramidal system, associated with motor control of tone and posture.

bilateral: related to or having two sides.

border zone: the limit of the cerebral area served by either the anterior, middle, or posterior cerebral arteries.

bouton: from the French, meaning "button"—a synaptic knob.

brain scan: a neurodiagnostic tool utilizing a radioisotope to detect damaged brain tissue.

Broca's aphasia: common adult language disorder characterized by nonfluent speech and language, usually accompanied by hemiplegia and an anterior lesion of the brain.

Broca's area: major speech-language center in the dominant frontal lobe; important for expression of language.

capsular: referring to the internal capsule.

cerebral arteriogram: X-ray picture of the arteries of the brain after injection of a contrast medium.

cerebrum: the major portion of the brain, consisting of two hemispheres; contains the cortex and its underlying white matter as well as the basal ganglia and other basal structures.

chorea: disorder characterized by irregular, spasmodic, involuntary movements of the limbs or facial muscles.

choreiform: resembling chorea.

circumlocution: wordy and circuitous description of unrecalled terms.

clonus: form of movement marked by contractions and relaxations of a muscle occurring in rapid succession.

colliculi: little hills or mounds within the brain; the superior and inferior colliculi are found in the midbrain.

competence/performance: **Competence** refers to the innate rules of language that are presumably stored in brain tissue; **performance** refers to the overt use of the ruies of language in speaking, writing, and gesturing.

computerized tomography (CT): X-ray imaging technique in which the brain is viewed at different depths; the various views are correlated by computer to show structural lesions of the brain.

conduction aphasia: an adult language disorder in which auditory comprehension is good, but exact repetition is poor; the site of the lesion producing the syndrome is in debate, but it may interrupt the arcuate fasciculus.

confabulation: the verbal or written expression of fictitious experiences.

confusional state: acute symptoms of mental disorganization and agitation that may accompany head trauma or other medical conditions; the language is often marked by irrelevancy and confabulation.

connectionism: theory of brain function that gives prominence to the interconnections of the association fibers between brain centers.

construction disturbance: the inability to form a construction in space because of a cerebral deficit.

contralateral: related to the opposite side.

corpus callosum: the largest transversal commissure between the hemispheres; it is about 4 inches long.

corpus quadragemina: the two pairs of colliculi (superior and inferior) of the midbrain.

decussation: crossing over or intersection of parts.

deglutition: the act of swallowing.

dendrite: literally, "treelike"—the short branching processes of a nerve cell.

denervation: a cutting of the nerve supply by excision, incision, or blocking.

dentate nucleus: the largest and most lateral of the deep nuclei of the cerebellum.

dichotic listening: test situation in simultaneous auditory stimuli are presented to both ears at the same time; **ear preference** (right or left) is judged by which ear first recognizes the auditory stimulus.

diplegia: paralysis of corresponding parts on both sides of the body, with legs more impaired.

diplopia: double vision.

distal: away from the center of the body.

dysdiadochokinesia: the inability to perform and sustain rapid alternating movements; speech-language pathologists in particular apply this term to a motor deficit in the oral muscles; also called **alternate motion rate**; associated with cerebellar disorder syndromes.

dyskinesia: disorder of movement usually associated with a lesion of the extrapyramidal system.

dysmetria: the inability to gauge the distance, speed, and power of a movement.

dysphagia: difficulty swallowing.

dysprosody: disturbance of stress, timing, and melody of speech.

efferent: conducting (fluid or nerve impulses) outward from a given organ or part.

electroencephalogram: graphic record of electrical activity of the brain as recorded by an electroencephalograph.

encephalitis: inflammation of the brain.

encephalopathy: pathology of the brain.

equilibrium: the state of being balanced.

etiology: the cause of disease or damage.

extensor: a muscle, the contraction of which tends to shorten a limb; antagonist to flexors.

extraocular: adjacent to but outside the eyeball.

facilitation: process of making the nerve impulses easier by repeated use of certain axons.

fasciculation: involuntary contractions or twitches in a group of muscle fibers.

fasciculus: a nerve fiber bundle forming a connection between groups of neurons in the CNS (also known as a tract).

fissure: a groove on the surface of the brain or spinal cord.

flaccid: flabby; without tone.

fluent/nonfluent: a dichotomous classification of aphasic language on the basis of the type of conversational speech.

foramen: an aperture or perforation through a bone or a membranous structure.

frontal alexia: reading disorder known as the "third alexia"; associated with a lesion in the left frontal lobe; often accompanies a Broca's aphasia.

funiculi: aggregates of fiber bundles (or tracts) in the nervous system, as seen in the spinal cord; also called **columns**.

gamma motor neuron: neurons innervating the muscle spindle; they allow contraction of intrafusal fibers and increased sensitivity of the fibers to the muscle stretch reflex.

ganglia: nerve cells with common form, function, and connections that are grouped outside the central nervous system.

genu: any structure of angular shape resembling a flexed knee.

Gerstmann syndrome: a cluster of left parietal lobe lesion signs including finger agnosia, left-right disorientation, acalculia, and agraphia; developmental form of the syndrome has been described.

glial cells: cellular elements, of which there are several types, that support and expedite the activity of the neurons. Glial cells outnumber the neurons 10 to 1.

gray matter: the grayish substance of brain and spinal cord composed of neuronal and glial cell bodies, unmyelinated nerve fibers, and synapses.

gyrus: an elevation or ridge on the surface of the cerebrum.

hemianopsia: a visual-field defect of one-half of the eye field.

hemiplegia: paralysis of one side of the body.

hemorrhage: bleeding; a very profuse flow of blood.

Henschen's axiom: axiom stating that restitution of speech is due to the opposite hemisphere.

homunculus: literally, "little man"; caricature mapping the connections between the area of the motor or sensory cortex and the innervated body part.

hyperreflexia: a condition in which the deep tendon reflexes are exaggerated.

hypertonia: extreme tension of the muscles.

hypotonia: muscle flaccidity; a decrease in normal muscle tone when passive movement is performed.

ideational apraxia: disorder of motor planning in which complex motor plans cannot be executed, although individual motor components of the plan can be performed.

ideomotor apraxia: a motor disturbance in which there is inability to carry out motor acts on command, but some evidence is present that these motor acts can be carried out imitatively or automatically.

innervate: to supply with efferent nerve impulses.

internuncial: being functionally imposed between two or more neurons.

intervertebral foramina: the openings between the vertebrae of the spinal cord through which the motor and sensory roots exit and unite to form the spinal nerves.

ipsilateral: on the same side.

island of Reil: part of the cerebral cortex forming the floor of the lateral fissure; also known as **insula.**

kernicterus: a form of infantile jaundice in which a yellow pigment and degenerative lesions are found in areas of the intracranial gray matter.

lacrimal: related to the tears, their secretion, and the organs concerned with them.

language dominant: refers to the hemisphere that is the site for the major language areas and connections.

lesion: an area of damage in the body.

magnum foramen: opening in the base of the skull through which the spinal cord is continuous with the brain.

mamillary bodies: two nipple-shaped protuberances on the ventral surface of the hypothalamus; the mamillary nuclei inside have connections that are important to hypothalamic function.

masking: the "drowning" of a weak sound by a louder one.

mastication: the chewing of food.

minimal cerebral dysfunction (MCD):   a syndrome of neurologic dysfunction in children usually marked by impairments of fine coordination, clumsiness, and choreiform or athetoid movements; often associated with learning disorders.

mixed dominance: inconsistency in laterality of speech and related motor functions such as handedness, footedness, and eyedness in some individuals; sometimes associated with language and learning disorders.

monoplegia: paralysis of one limb.

motor integration: complete and harmonious combining of muscular elements of the nervous system.

myelin: the fatty substance surrounding some axons that speeds neural transmission; the myelin-covered areas are the white matter of the brain.

myelogenesis: the cyclic process of laying down of myelin on certain fiber tracts.

neologistic jargon: utterances that include meaningless, newly coined words.

neologistic jargon aphasia: a temporal lobe syndrome marked by newly coined words and unintelligible utterances.

neuron: nerve cell.

neural integration: complete and harmonious combining of components of the nervous system.

nystagmus: rhythmical horizontal, rotary, or vertical oscillation of the eyeballs.

obligatory: without an alternative path.

olfaction: the sense of smell.

olivary nucleus: oval elevations in the medulla that are way stations in the auditory pathways.

operculum: a lid or covering structure; part of the cerebrum that lies over the insula and which forms the lateral fissure.

optic chiasm: the structure located on the floor of the third ventricle composed of crossing optic nerve fibers from the medial (nasall) that is half of each retina and fibers from the lateral (temporal) half of each retina that do not cross midline.

oral apraxia: buccofacial apraxia; inability to program nonspeech oral movements.

organic brain syndrome: a psychiatric term used to describe deterioration of intellect and related functions due to brain dysfunction; **dementia** is the neurologic equivalent for the same condition.

palpate: to examine by feeling and pressing with the palms of the hands and fingers.

paraplegia: paralysis of both lower extremities and, generally, the lower trunk.

paraphasia: the substitution of words or sounds in words in such a way as to decrease intelligibility or obscure meaning.

parasympathetic: pertaining to that division of the autonomic nervous system concerned with the maintenance of the body; its fibers arise from the brain and the sacral part of the spinal cord.

perisylvian zone: an area on the lateral wall of the dominant hemisphere for language that includes the major centers and pathways for language reception and production.

phrenic nerves: nerves arising from the cervical spinal cord that supply the diaphragm.

plantar: relating to the sole of the foot.

plasticity: the concept that in the immature brain some functional areas are not established and that unestablished areas may assume any one of a variety of functions.

positron emission tomography: imaging technique that visualizes the functioning brain by showing its activity through blood flow and glucose metabolism.

postganglionic: pertaining to those nerve fibers in the autonomic nervous system that are exiting the ganglion.

praxis: the normal performance of a motor act.

preganglionic: pertaining to those nerve fibers in the autonomic nervous system that are going toward a synapse at a ganglion but have not reached it.

prematurity: a state of being born after fewer than 37 weeks of gestation (birth weight is no longer considered a critical criterion).

prone: lying face down.

prosopagnosia: a visual agnosia characterized by inability to recognize the faces of other people or one's own face in a mirror; associated with agnosia also for color, objects, and place.

proximal: toward the midline or center of the body.

pseudohypertrophy: increase in the size of an organ or part not due to increase in size or number of the specific functional elements; rather, due to increase in some other fatty or fibrous tissue.

pulvinar: the posterior end of the thalamus.

putamen: a part of the lenticular nucleus; a structure of the basal ganglia.

quadriplegia: paralysis of all four limbs.

reflex arc: a pathway leading from receptor of a sensory stimulus to motor response; the response is known as an **automatic reflex action**.

refractory period: momentary state of reduced irritation after a neural response.

secretomotor: stimulating secretion.

servomechanism: a control device for maintaining the operation of another system.

soft signs: minor and inconsistent neurologic signs often said to be associated with a diagnosis of minimal cerebral dysfunction; may indicate neurologic lesion or immaturity.

somatic: having to do with the structure of the body wall (muscles, skin and mucous membranes).

somesthesia: the consciousness of having a body.

somesthetic: pertaining to the senses of pain, temperature, taction, vibration, and position.

spasticity: syndrome of hypertonus with exaggeration of stretch reflexes following certain neural lesions.

splenium: the thickened posterior part of the corpus callosum.

split brain: a condition in which the corpus callosum has been surgically divided so that there is no information flow between hemispheres.

sublingual: below the tongue.

substantia nigra: a mass of gray matter extending from the upper border of the pons into the subthalamic region.

sulcus: groove on the surface of the brain or spinal cord; also known as **fissures**.

summation: the product of the neural impulses acting on a given synapse.

supine: lying on the back.

supramarginal gyrus: convolution in the inferior parietal lobe, surrounding the posterior end of the sylvian fissure.

sympathetic nervous system: that division of the autonomic nervous system concerned with preparing the body for "fight or flight"; its neurons arise in the thoracic and upper lumbar segments of the spinal cord.

synapse: a juncture or connection; the functional contact of one neuron with another.

tectum: roof of the midbrain; composed of the superior and inferior colliculi.

transcortical aphasia: several types of language disturbances whose causes are lesions outside the perisylvian area.

transitory: related to or marked by a transition.

tremor: a purposeless involuntary movement that is oscillatory and rhythmic.

triplegia: paralysis of an upper and a lower extremity and of the face or of both extremities on one side and one on the other.

uncus: the hooked extremity of the hippocampal gyrus.

vermis: the medial portion of the cerebellum between the two hemispheres.

vesicle: a blister or bladder; the intracellular bladder is believed to be filled with neurotransmitter substances.

volitional: voluntary.

Wernicke's aphasia: a common adult language disorder characterized by fluent, paraphasic speech and language; the patient is free of hemiplegia, and the lesion is usually in the temporal lobe.

Wernicke's area: a major speech-language center in the dominant temporal lobe, important for comprehension of language.

white matter: substance of the brain and spinal cord consisting of myelinated fibers and containing no neuronal cell bodies or synapses; in a freshly sectioned brain it glistens white due to the high content of lipid-rich myelin.

Index

Abbs, J. H., 168
Abducens nerve (VI), 142
Abortive clonus, 117
Absolute refractory period, 70
Acalculia, 22, 220, 230
Accessory. *see* Spinal Accessory nerve (XI)
Acetylcholine (ACh), 71, 124
Acoustic nerve, 148–150
Acoustic nerve. *see* Vestibular-acoustic
    nerve (VIII)
Acquired childhood aphasia, 262–263
Action current, 69
Action potential, 69–70
Action tremor, 127, 180
Acute confusional states, 237
Adamovich, B. L. B., 238
Adiadochokinesia, 134–135
Affective aprosodia, 246
Afferent nerve fibers, 48
Afferent neuron, 42
Agnosia, 6, 31, 62, 216–220
    auditory, 31, 218–219
    auditory nonverbal, 218–219
    auditory verbal, 31, 218–219
    color, 218, 244
    finger, 22, 220
    Gerstmann syndrome, 220
    tactile, 31, 90, 219–220
    visual, 31, 218
Agrammatism, 205
Agraphagnosia, 244
Agraphia, 32, 197, 220, 229, 232–233
    alexia with, 22, 230–231
    alexia without, 229–230
Akathisia, 129
Akinesia, 124–125
Alar plate, 44
Albert, Martin L., 4
    Manual of Aphasia Therapy (with
        Nancy Helm-Estabrooks), 4
Albert, M. L., 247

Alberts, M. J., 169
Alexander, M. P., 199, 212
Alexia, 197, 205, 228–229
    with agraphia, 22, 230–231
    anterior, 231
    aphasic, 197, 229, 230, 231
    central, 230
    frontal, 197, 231
    literal, 228
    occipital, 229
    parietal, 230
    phonological, 231–232
    posterior, 229
    pure, 228–229
    verbal, 228
    without agraphia, 229–230
Alpha motor neurons, 118
Alternate motion rate (AMR), 135
Alzheimer's disease, 215, 234–235
Amacrine cells, 96
Amatruda, Catherine S., 272
    Developmental Diagnosis
        (with A. Gesell), 272
American Sign Language, 17
Amygdala, 32, 51
Amygdaloid nucleus, 26
Amyotrophic lateral sclerosis (ALS), 174–176
    neurologic characteristics, 174
    oral musculature, 174–175
    speech characteristics, 175
    swallowing, 175–176
Analgesia, 89
Anarthrias, developmental, 272
Anatomical direction, 12
Anatomical orientation, 13–14
Andrews, G., 184
Anesthesia, 89
Angular gyrus, 22, 32, 197
Annulospiral endings, 119
Anomia, 22, 209–210
    color, 218

Anomic aphasia, 209–210
Anosognosia, 244
Anosmia, 31
Ansa Cervicalis, 156
Anterior alexia, 231
Anterior aphasia, 205
Anterior cerebral artery, 57
Anterior communicating artery, 57
Anterior corticospinal tract, 86, 109
Anterior, defined, 12
Anterior horn cell, 47
Anterior lobe, 131
Anterior root, 47
Anterior spinothalamic tract, 86
Anterior subcortical aphasia syndrome, 211
Anterior temporal association area, 24
Aphasia, 5, 6
  acquired childhood, 262–263
  anomic, 209–210
  anterior vs posterior, 205
  bilateral tactile, 219–220
  border zone syndromes, 209
  Broca's, 6, 196, 202, 205–206, 207
  childhood, with abnormal EEG
    findings, 263
  classification, 204–216
  conduction, 196, 205, 206–208
  expressive, 205
  fluent, 205
  global, 205, 208
  language functions, 217
  localization in the central language
    mechanism, 214
  models, 204–205
  motor, 196, 205
  neologistic jargon, 206
  nonfluent, 205
  pharmacology, 246–248
  posterior, 205
  progressive, 210–211
  receptive, 205
  sensory, 31, 196, 205
  subcortical, 199, 211–213
  tactile, 219–220
  testing, 213–216
  total, 208
  transcortical, 205, 209, 210
  Wernicke's, 6, 196, 202, 206, 207–208
Aphasia Language Performance Scales, 216
Aphasia quotient (AQ), 215
Aphasic agraphia, 232–233
Aphasic alexia, 197, 229, 230, 231
Aphemia, 224
Aphonia, 128

Apraxia(s), 6, 220–227
  buccofacial, 223–224
  callosal, 223
  construction, 227
  ideational, 226–227
  ideomotor, 221–222
  limb, 222
  limb-kinetic, 223
  oral, 223–224
  speech, 224–225, 272
  sympathetic, 223
  trunk, 222
Aprosodia, 245
  affective, 246
  motor, 245
  sensory, 246
Arachnoid mater, 52
Arcuate fasciculus, 25, 196–197
Areflexia, 113
*Arizona Battery for Communication
  Disorders of Dementia*, 236
Arm ataxia, 136
Aronson, A. E., 9, 167, 175, 181, 183,
  184, 187, 188
Articulatory undershoot, 178
Ascending reticular activating system, 243
Aspiration, 169, 171, 173, 175, 179,
  182, 185
Association area(s), 27
  cortical motor speech, 29–31
  function, 28–29
  master, 258
  sensory, 31–32
Association cortex, 24
Association fibers, 25
Association pathways, 34–43
Association tracts, 25
Astereognosis, 90
Astrocytes, 80
Asymmetrical cerebral hemisphere
  function, 260
Asymmetrical tonic neck reflex (ATNR),
  116, 278–279
Asynergia, 131
Ataxia, 134, 273
Ataxic dysarthria, 135–136, 185–187
  etiology, 186
  neurologic characteristics, 186
  speech characteristics, 186–187
Athetosis, 128, 182–185, 273
  etiology, 182
  neurologic characteristics, 182–183
  speech characteristics, 183–184
  swallowing, 185

Atopognosis, 89
Atrophy, 113
Attention deficit-hyperactivity disorder, 265–266
 signs of, 266
Auditory agnosia, 31, 218–219
Auditory nonverbal agnosia, 218–219
Auditory physiology, 101–103
Auditory radiations and cortex, 100
Auditory receptor cortex, primary, 30
Auditory system. *see* Central auditory nervous system
Auditory verbal agnosia, 31, 218–219
Autism, childhood, developmental language disability and, 267
Autonomic nervous system, 50–52
Axon, 67

Babinski, Joseph, 243–244
Babinski sign, 116, 274
Basal ganglia, 20, 34–35, 122–125, 176
Basal plate, 44
Bashir, A. S., 289
Basilar artery, 58
Bassich, C. J., 184, 189
Bayles, K. A., 236
Beauvois, M. F., 219, 232
Bell, Charles, 139
Bell's palsy, 190
Bender-Gestalt tests, 228
Benson, D. F., 32–34, 197, 209, 220, 231, 233, 235
Benton, A. L., 215
Berry, K. E., 228
Bilateral speech motor control, 61
Bilateral symmetry, 110
Bilateral tactile aphasia, 219–220
Bipolar cells, 96
Bite reflex, 292
Blitzer, A., 183
Blonsky, E. R., 177
Bloomfield, L., 3
Blumback, R. A., 265
Body sway test, 90
Border zone aphasic syndromes, 209
Borkowski, J. G., 236
Boshes, B., 177
Bosma, J., 185
Boston Diagnostic Aphasia Examination (BDAE) 9, 215, 228
Botulinum-A injection, 184
Bouillaud, Jean, 262
Brachium conjunctivum, 133
Brachium pontis, 132

Bradykinesia, 176
Brain, 18, 19–20
 development, 45–46
 measurement of metabolic activity, 10–11
 neurodiagnostic imaging, 9–11
 protection and nourishment, 52–56
 weight, 18, 19
Brain growth, 256–257
 differential, 257–259
Brain injury, traumatic, 237–241
Brainstem, 20, 35, 36–39
 lower, 37
 upper, 37
Brain weight, 256–257
Branchial cranial nerves, 140
Brassell, E. G., 216
Brazer, S. R., 171
Brin, M. F., 184
Broca, Pierre Paul, 5, 27, 32, 195, 213, 224
Broca's aphasia, 6, 196, 202, 205–206, 207
Broca's area, 6, 18, 22, 30, 78
 and central language mechanism, 196, 197, 199
 development, 258–259
Brodmann, Korbinian, 27, 29
Brodmann's areas, 27, 29, 30, 99
Bromocriptine, 247
Brownell, H., 245
Brown, J., 9, 167, 175, 177, 181, 187, 188, 238
Bruhn, L., 265
Bruhn, P., 265
Buccofacial apraxia, 223–224
Buckingham, H. W., 195
Bulb, 38
Bulbar palsy, 169, 172 *See also* Flaccid dysarthria
Bundle, 13
Butenica, N., 228

Calcarine sulcus, 24
Callosal apraxia, 223
Capildeo, R., 176
Caplan, D., 77–78, 203
Carhart, Raymond, 83
Cauda equinas, 45
Caudate nucleus, 35, 122, 123
Celesia, G. G., 178
Cellular electrical potentials, 69–70
Central alexia, 230
Central auditory nervous system, 100
 auditory physiology, 101–103
 auditory radiations and cortex, 100
 brainstem level, 101

Central auditory nervous system—*cont.*
cranial nerve level, 100
lesions, 103
receptor level, 100
Central autonomic network, 51
Central language disorders, 216–244
acute confusional states, 237
agnosia, 6, 31, 62, 216–220
agraphia, 32, 197, 220, 229, 232–233
alexia, 197, 205, 228–232
apraxias, 6, 220–227
constructional disturbances, 227–228
dementia, 233–237
Gerstmann syndrome, 220
parietal alexia, 230
right-hemisphere lesions, 241–244
traumatic brain injury, 237–241
Central language mechanism, 195
model for language and its disorders,
195–204
See also Acute confusional states;
Agnosia; Agraphia; Alexia; Aphasia;
Apraxia(s); Constructional
disturbances; Dementia; Right-
hemisphere lesions
Central nervous system, 19–20
Central pattern generator (CPG), 161
Central sulcus, 21
Cephalic, defined, 12
Cerebellar dysfunction syndrome, 136
Cerebellar syndrome, 136
Cerebellar system, 35–36, 130
anatomy, 130
cerebellar syndrome and dysarthria, 136
clinical signs of dysfunction, 134–136
lesions, 185–187
lobes, 131
peduncles and pathways, 132–133
role in speech, 133–134
synergy and asynergy, 131
Cerebral blood supply, 56–60
Circle of Willis, 57, 59–60
internal carotid artery, 56–57
vertebral artery, 58–59
Cerebral connections, 25
Cerebral cortex, 34
association area, 24, 28–29
auditory radiations and, 100
cortical motor functions, 29
cortical motor speech association
areas, 29–31
development of, 45–46
heteromodal, 33
organization, 61–63

Cerebral cortex—*cont.*
other association areas, 32–33
paralimbic areas, 32–33
premotor area, 21, 29
primary auditory receptor, 30
primary visual, 98–99
sensory association areas, 31–32
septal area, 32
supplementary motor area (SMA), 29
visual association, 99
Cerebral dominance for language, 260–262
Cerebral lobes, 20–24
Cerebral palsy, 273–274
classification, 273–274
Cerebral plasticity, 259–260
Cerebrospinal fluid (CSF), 52, 56
Cerebrum, 20
Cerenko, D., 159, 161, 162
Charcot, Jean, 7, 9, 187
Chemical transmission disorders, 72–73
Cherney, L. R., 171
Cherniack, L., 161
Cherniack, R., 161
Chewing. *see* Mastication
Childhood aphasia, with abnormal EEG
findings, 263
Childhood autism, developmental
language disability and, 267
Childhood language disorders, 262–264
acquired childhood aphasia, 262–263
attention deficit-hyperactivity disorder,
265–266
childhood aphasia with abnormal EEG
findings, 263–264
developmental dyslexia, 228, 267–268
developmental language disability,
263, 264, 267
minimal cerebral disorders/attention
deficit-hyperactivity disorder,
265–266
Childhood suprabulbar palsy,
congenital, 275
Childhood suprabulbar paresis, 274–275
Childhood suprabulbar paresis
syndrome, dysarthria in, 275
Chomsky, Noam, 3–4, 8, 203, 204
Syntactic Structures, 3
Chorda tympani, 145
Chorea, 127, 180–182
Huntington's, 180–182
neurologic characteristics, 181
oral musculature, 181
speech characteristics, 181
Sydenham's, 180, 181

Choreoathetotic movements, 128
Choroid plexus, 54
Churchland, P. M., 203, 204
Circle of Willis, 57, 59–60
Circulus arteriosus, 59–60
Circumlocution, 210
Clark, R., 8
Clasp knife reaction, 115
Clasp knife spasticity, 115
Claustrum, 35
Clinicopathologic method, 9
Clonus, 117
  abortive, 117
Closed head injury (CHI). *see* Traumatic
  brain injury (TBI)
Closed-loop control system, 76
Cochlear branch, 100, 149
  See also Vestibular acoustic nerve (VIII)
Code, C., 203
Cognitive-communicative disorder, 238
Cognitive deficit, generalized, 267
Cognitive language model, 203
Cognitive neuropsychology, 202–203
Cogwheel rigidity, 176
Collateral circulation, 59–60
Collicular pathway, 98–99
Colliculus, 38
  inferior, 38
  superior, 38
Color agnosia, 218, 244
Color anomia, 218
Coltheart, M., 202, 203
Column, 13
Commissural fibers, 25
Commissurotomy, 26–27
Competence and performance, 202
Computerized axial tomography (CT)
  scanning, 9–10
Conduction aphasia, 25, 196, 205, 206–208
Cones, 96
Confabulation, 237
Confrontation naming, 206, 208
Congenital aphasia, 264
Congenital childhood suprabulbar palsy, 275
Congenital word blindness, 267–268
Connectionist language model, 203
Connective pathways, 12–13
Constructional disturbances, 227–228
Construction apraxia, 227
Contingent negative variation (CNV),
  78, 79
Contralateral innervation, 110–111
Contralateral motor control, 60
Contralateral red nucleus, 133

Conus medullaris, 44
Convergence, principle of, 75
Coronal section, 14
Corona radiata, 107
Corpus callosum, 20, 25–26
Corpus quadrigemia, 38
Corpus striatum, 35
Cortex. *see* Cerebral cortex
Cortical deafness, 219
Cortical motor functions, 29
Cortical motor speech association areas,
  29–31
Cortical organization, 61–63
Cortical quotient (CQ), 216
Corticobulbar tract, 107, 109–110, 141
  bilateral symmetry, 110
  contralateral and unilateral
    innervation, 110–111
  and cranial nerves, 141
Corticofugal pathways, 107
Corticopontine tract, 107
Corticopontocerebellar fibers, 133
Corticopontospinal tract, 107
Cough reflex, 161
Crago, M., 4, 265
Cranial, defined, 12
Cranial nerves, 18–19, 49–50
  corticobulbar tract and, 141
  descending tract, 91–92
  embryological origin, 140–141
  function for oral musculature, 163–165
  and modified feeding, 294–298
  names, 139–140
  for smell and vision, 141–142
  somatomotor cranial nerves, 140
  somatosensory cranial nerves, 140
  for speech and hearing, 142–150
  swallowing, 158–162
Cranium, 20
Cremasteric reflex, 117
Critchley, MacDonald
  Aphasiology, 256
  The Divine Banquet of the Brain, 1
Crosson, B., 199
Crus cerebri, 38
Cummings, J. L., 233, 235

Damasio, A. R., 10
Damasio, H., 10
Daniel, G., 178
Darley, F., 9, 167, 181, 187, 188, 236
Darwin, Charles, 3
Darwinian principle of natural selection, 3
Dawson, G., 267

Deafness
  cortical, 219
  pure word, 218–219
Decomposition of movement, 134
Decussation, 109
Dedo, H. H., 184
Deep dyslexia, 231–232
Deglutition, 158–161
  assessment, 161–162, 293–298
Dejerine, Joseph J., 6, 197, 229, 230, 231
Dementia, 177, 233–237
  assessment of communication
    disorders in, 235–237
  cortical, 233–234
  management of communication
    disorders, 236–237
  management of swallowing disorders,
    236–237
  mixed, 233
  of the Alzheimer's type (DAT), 233–235
  subcortical, 233–234
DeMyer, W., 215–216
Dendrites, 67
Denervation, 112
Denial, 243–244
Dentate nucleus, 133
Dentatothalamic pathway, 133
Dermatomes, 48, 88
Descending motor pathways, 107
Descending tract of cranial nerve V, 91–92
Deutsch, G., 201
Developmental anarthrias, 272
Developmental aphasia, 264
Developmental apraxia of speech,
    225–226, 272–273
Developmental dysarthrias, 272–274, 276
Developmental dyslexia, 228, 267–268
Developmental Gerstmann syndrome, 220
Developmental hearing loss and
    language disorders, 266–267
Developmental language disability, 263,
    264, 267
Developmental motor speech disorders,
    272–273
  cerebral palsy, 273–274
  childhood suprabulbar paresis, 274–275
  muscular dystrophy, 115, 275–277
*Developmental Visual Motor Integration
    Test,* 228
Diaphragma sella, 52
Diencephalon, 37, 39
Diffuse axonal injury (DAI), 238
Diffuse deficits, 230
Dilapidation, 234

Direct activation pathway, 112
Divergence, prinicple of, 74–75
Diversions of the nervous system, 18–19
Dominance
  cerebral, 260–262
  mixed, 262
Dopamine, 29
Dopamine deficiency
  in dyskinesias, 126
  in Parkinsonism, 126, 176
Dorsal column(s), 87
  lesions, 90
  modalities, 88
Dorsal, defined, 12
Dorsal nucleus, 152
Dorsal plate, 44
Dorsolateral fasciculus, 84
Double simultaneous stimulation, 243
Drager, G., 189
Dronkers, N., 225
Duchenne dystrophy, 275–276
Duffy, J. R., 112, 121–122, 168, 171, 178, 187
Dura mater, 52
Dysarthrias, 7, 9, 81, 246
  ataxic, 135–136, 185–197
  and cerebellar syndrome, 136
  in childhood suprabulbar paresis
    syndrome, 275
  defined, 167
  developmental, 272–274, 276
  dyskinetic, 176–185
  flaccid, 171–173
  hyperkinetic, 180
  hypokinetic, 176–179
  mixed, 187–191
  spastic, 168, 169–171
  spastic-ataxic, 188–189
Dysdiadochokinesia, 134–135, 186
Dyskinesias, 124–126, 273
  caused by dopamine deficiency, 126
  and dysarthria, 176–185
  nonspeech, 129
  orofacial, 129, 185
  tardive, 129, 185
  types, 126
Dyslexia, 228
  classification of, 231–232
  deep, 231–232
  developmental, 228, 267–268
  surface, 231–232
Dysmetria, 134
Dysphagia, 142, 173, 182, 185, 236
  and speech, 288–289
Dysphasia, 264

Dysphonia, spastic (SD), 128, 180, 183–184
Dystonia, 128, 182–185
  Botulinum-A injections, 184
  etiology, 182
  musculorum deformans, 128
  neurologic characteristics, 182–183
  speech characteristics, 183–184
  swallowing, 185
Dysynergia, 131

Ear advantage, 262
Early language models, 6–8
Echolalia, 209
Effector, 42
Efferent fibers, 47
efferent neuron, 42
Egggert, G., 195
Eisenson, J., 8, 215
Electrical potentials, cellular, 69–70
Electroencephalography (EEG), 77
  abnormal findings in childhood
      aphasia, 263
Ellman, J. L., 204
Empty speech, 206
Encephalon, 20
Eppiglottis, 152, 159, 160
Essential tremor, 180
Esthesiometer, 93
Evatt, M. L., 169
Event related potential (ERP), 77–78, 79
Evoked potentials, 77–79
Examining for Aphasia, 215
Excess and equal stress, 187, 189
Expectancy waveform, 78
Explosive speech, 187
Expressive aphasia, 205
Exteroceptors, 83
Extinction, 243
Extrafusal fibers, 118
Extrapyramidal system, 121
  anatomy, 121–122
  athetosis, 128
  basal ganglia, 122–125
  chorea, 127
  dyskinesias, 125–126
  dystonia, 128
  indirect activation pathway, 121–122
  myoclonus, 128–129
  orofacial dyskinesia, 129
  tardive dyskinesia, 129, 185
  tremors, 126–127

Facial nerve (VII), 145–148
  anatomy, 145–146

Facial nerve (VII)—*cont.*
  function, 146–147
  innervation, 146
  testing, 147–148
Facilitation, 74
Falx cerebri, 52
Fasciculations, 113, 172
Fasciculus, 13, 25
  arcuate, 25, 196–197
  dorsolateral, 84
  inferior longitudinal, 34
  occipital-frontal, 34
  superior longitudinal, 25, 34, 197
  uncinate, 34
Fasciculus cuneatus, 87
Fasciculus gracilis, 87
Feedback, 76
  negative, 76–77
  positive, 76
Feedforward, 76
Feeding, modified, 294–298
Feeding reflexes, 289
Festinating gait, 177
Fiberoptic Endoscopic Examination for
      Swallowing (FEES), 162
Fibrillations, 113
Fight-or-flight system, 50–51
Finger agnosia, 22, 220
Fisher, H. B., 177, 178
Fissure, 20
  Rolandic, 21
  Sylvian, 21
Fitzgerald, M., 226
Flaccid dysarthria, 171–173
  etiology, 171
  neurologic characteristics, 172
  oral musculature, 172
  speech characteristics, 172–173
  swallowing, 173
Flaccid paralysis, 113, 172
Flocculi, 131
Flocculonodular lobe, 131
Flower spray endings, 119
Fluent aphasia, 205
Focal deficits, 238
Folger, W. N., 168
Folstein, M. F., 236
Foramen magnum, 52
Form perception, 86
Fovea centralix, 96
Freud, Sigmund, 6
Friedman, S. G., 237
Frontal alexia, 197, 231
Frontal lobe, 18, 20–21, 62

Frontal operculum, 29
Functioning language models, 200–201
Funiculus, 13

Gag reflex, 292
Gait ataxia, 136
Galanthamine, 247
Galant reflex, 284–285
Gamma loop system, 120
Gamma motor neurons, 118, 120
Ganglion cells, 96
Gasserian ganglion, 91, 92
General senses, 84
Gerstmann, Joseph, 220
Gerstmann syndrome, 220
  developmental, 220
Geschwind language model, 202
Geschwind, Norman, 2–3, 4, 6, 8, 202,
  203, 217–221, 223, 258
  Cortex, 195
Gesell, Arnold, 278
  Developmental Diagnosis (with C. S.
  Amatruda), 272
Gilles de la Tourette's syndrome, 190–191
Glia, 40, 80
Global aphasia, 205, 208
Global attention, 243
Global Deterioration Scale, 236
Globus pallidus, 35, 122, 123
Glossopharyngeal nerve (IX), 150–152
  anatomy, 150–151
  function, 151
  innervation, 151–152
Glutamate, 124
Gnosis, 29
Golgi tendon organs, 121
Goodglass, H., 9, 215, 228
Gopnik, M., 4, 204, 265
Gowers, William R., *A Manual of Diseases
  of the Nervous System*, 7, 167
Greater petrosal nerve, 145
Grozinger, B., 78
Gyrus, 20
  angular, 22, 32, 197
  Heschl's, 24, 28, 30, 31
  inferior frontal, 197
  opercular, 29
  parahippocampal, 30
  postcentral, 22
  precentral, 21
  supramarginal, 22, 32, 197
  temporal, 122

Haberman, S., 176

Hagen, C., 241
Hagerman, E. L., 288
Halperin, H., 237
*Halstead-Wepman-Reitan Aphasia
  Screening Test*, 215–216
Hamm, A., 8
Hand preference, 262
Harman, D. E., 183
Harmtman, D. E., 168
Harper, C. R., 265
Harris, R. A., 3
Head, Henry, 7, 47, 213
Hearing loss, developmental, language
  disability and, 266–267
Hebb, D. O., 74
Heilman, K. M., 203
Heimer, L., 51
Helm-Estabrooks, Nancy, 4
  Manual of Aphasia Therapy
  (with Martin L. Albert), 4
Hemiballismus, 129, 190
Hemiparalysis, 109
Hemiparesis, 109
Hemiplegia, 109
Henderson, J. A., 238
Henderson, L., 265
Henschen, Salomon E., 242
Henschen's axiom, 242
Heredofamilial tremor, 180
Hersch, T., 162
Heschl's gyrus, 24, 28, 30, 101
Heteromodal cortex, 33
Hippocampus, 32, 74
Homeostasis, 51
Homunculus, 22
Horizontal cells, 96
Horizontal plane, 14
Hormones, 39, 51
Horner, J., 171
Hough, M. S., 245
Howie, P. M., 184
Hubel, D. H., 98
Huntington's chorea, 180–182
Hurford, J. R., 4
Hyperalgesia, 89
Hyperasthesia, 89
Hyperkinesia, 125
  slow, 182
Hyperkinetic dysarthria, 180
  chorea, 180–181
  dystonia and athetosis, 182–185
  tardive dyskinesia, 185
Hypernasality, 168, 170, 173, 175, 178,
  181, 184, 186, 188–189

Hyperprosody, 245
Hyperreflexia, 115
Hypertonia, 115
Hypoalgesia, 89
Hypoesthesia, 89
Hypoglossal nerve (XII), 155–158
  anatomy, 155
  function, 156
  innervation, 155–156
  testing, 156–157
Hypoglossal nucleus, 155
Hypokinesia, 125, 126
Hypokinesia dysarthria, 176
  Parkinsonism, 176–179
Hyporeflexia, 113
Hypothalamus, 39
Hypotonia, 113, 135, 136
Hypoxia, 128

Ideational apraxia, 226–227
Ideomotor apraxia, 221–222
Impaired emphasis, 189
Inattention, 245
Indirect activation pathway, 121–122
Inferior cerebellar peduncles, 38, 132
Inferior colliculus, 38
Inferior, defined, 12
Inferior frontal gyrus, 197
Inferior longitudinal fasciculus, 34
Inferior parietal lobule, 32, 62, 197
Information processing language model,
  202–203
Innervation, contralateral and unilateral,
  110–111
Insula, 24, 33
Intention tremor, 127
Internal capsule, 107
Internal carotid arteries, 56–57
Interneurons, 73
Interoceptors, 84
Intrafusal fibers, 118
Involuntary movement disorders, 125
Ipsilateral motor control, 60
Irregular articulatory breakdown, 181–182
Island of Reil, 24, 33
Isolation of speech area, 209

Jackson, John Hughlings, 221
Jackson, R. T., 159, 161
Jaw reflex, 92
Jones, L. V., 215

Kagel, M. C., 182
Kandel, E. R., 74

Kaplan, E., 8, 215, 228
Keenan, J. S., 216
Kent, R., 184
Kent, R. D., 274
Kertesz, A., 215
Kirshner, H. S., 29, 179, 211, 212
Kleist, Karl, 227
Koppitz, E. M., 228

Lacrimal nucleus, 145
Landau-Kleffner syndrome, 263
Lang, A. E., 124
Langmore, S., 162
Language
  dominance development, 260–262
  myelination for, 259
Language disability, developmental, 263,
  264, 267
Language disorders
  childhood, 262–264
  childhood, classification, 268
  differential diagnosis, 266–267
Language impairment in traumatic brain
  injury, testing and treating, 241
Language mechanisms, unilateral, 261
Language Modalities Test for Aphasia, 215
Language model. *see* Central language
  mechanism
Larson, C., 161
Laryngeal
  closure, 152–153, 159–160, 179
  elevation, 143, 146, 156, 160, 171
  sensation, 161
Lateral corticospinal tract, 86, 109
Lateral, defined, 12
Lateral geniculate body, 97
Lateral lemniscus, 101, 149
Lateral spinothalamic tract, 84–86
Lateral sulcus, 21
L-dopa, 247
Left-handedness, 241–242, 263
Lemniscus, 13, 84
  lateral, 101, 149
  medial, 87
Lenneberg, Eric, 4, 8, 106, 261–262
  Biological Foundation of Language, 4
Lenticular nucleus, 123
Lentiform nucleus, 35
Leopold, N. A., 182
Lesion(s), 48
  basal ganglia, 124, 176
  of central auditory system, 103
  cerebellar pathway, 185–187
  dorsal column, 90

Lesion(s)—*cont.*
lower motor neuron, 171–174
mixed dysarthrias, 187–191
mixed upper and lower motor neuron, 174–175
right hemisphere, 241–244
Levitsky , W., 8
Levitt, L. P., 188
Liepmann, Hugo, 6, 221, 223, 224, 226
Limb apraxia, 222
Limbic lobe, 32
Limb-kinetic apraxia, 223
Limb position, inability to recognize, 90
Lip
movement, 140, 143, 153
sensation, 143
Lissauer's tract, 84
Literal alexia, 228
Literal paraphasia, 206
Lobe(s), 131
anterior, 131
cerebellar, 131
cerebral, 20–24
flocculonodular, 131
limbic, 32
Localization of function, 5
Logemann, J., 173, 177, 178, 179
Logorrhea, 205
Long term potentiation (LTP), 74
Lou Gehrig's disease. *see* Amyotrophic lateral sclerosis (ALS)
Lou, H. C., 265
Love, R. J., 224, 226, 245, 277, 288, 289
Lower brainstem, 37
Lower motor neuron (LMN), 112
lesions, 171–174
lesions, mixed upper, 174–176
paralysis, 112–115
Ludlow, C., 189
Ludlow, C. L., 184
Lumbar puncture, 56
Luria, Alexander, 247

Macula, 96
Magnetic resonance imaging (MRI), 9, 10, 169
Magnum foramen, 40
Magnus, Rudolph, 277
Malkmus, D., 241
Mamillary bodies, 39
Mantle plate, 44
Marin, O. S. M., 203
Marsden, C. D., 124–125
Marshall, J. C., 203, 231

Masked facies, 177
Massey, E. W., 171
Mastication, 143–144, 160, 293–298
Mayo Clinic, 9, 167, 175, 181, 184, 187, 188
McAdam, D. W., 78
McBride, Katherine, 205
McConnel, F., 159, 161, 162
Medial, defined, 12
Medial lemniscus, 87
Median fissure, 38
Median plane, 14
Medulla oblongata, 37, 38
Meige syndrome, 129
Meninges, 52–54
Mental retardation, developmental language disability and, 267
Mesencephalon, 37, 38
reticular formation, 123
Mesulam, M. M., 32–34, 99–100
Metter, E. J., 199
Meyer, L. A., 274
Meyer's loop, 97–98
Meyers, P. S., 246
Meynert, Theodore, 6
Micrographia, 177
Middle cerebellar peduncle, 132
Middle cerebral artery, 57
Miller, A. J., 161
Milner, B., 241
Mimura, M., 247
Minimal cerebral dysfunction (MCD), 265–266
Mini-Mental Status Exam, 236
Minnesota Test for Differential Diagnosis of Aphasia (MTDDA), 9, 204, 215
Mixed dementia, 233
Mixed dominance for language, 262
Mixed laterality, 262
Mnemonic device, cranial nerves, 139
Mobius syndrome, 171
Model(s), language, 200–203
cognitive, 203
connectionist, 203
functioning, 200–201
Geschwind, 202
information processing, 202–203
usefulness, 202
Modified feeding, 294–298
Monoloudness, 169, 170
Monrad-Krohn, G. H., 245
Moro reflex, 116, 285–287
Moss, S. E., 203
Motor aphasia, 196, 205

Motor aprosodia, 245
Motor control
  bilateral speech, 61
  contralateral, 60, 109
  ipsilateral, 60
Motor endplate, 71
Motor equivalence, 120
Motor nucleus, 146
Motor speech disorders, developmental,
  272–273
Motor strip, 21
Motor unit, 113
Mueller, K., 184
Multiple sclerosis (MS), 80–81, 187–189
  etiology, 187
  neurologic characteristics, 187–188
  speech characteristics, 188
Multiple stretch reflex (MSR), 115, 135
Muscle spindles, 95, 118, 119
Muscular dystrophy, 115, 275–277
  psuedohypertrophic, 275–276
Myasthenia gravis, 72, 115, 171
  speech characteristics, 173–174
Myelin, 79–81
  development of, 80
  disorders, 80–81
Myelination, for language, 259
Myelogenesis, 259
Myoclonus, 128–129
  palatal, 129
  palato-pharyngo-laryngeal, 190
Myopathy, 115
Myotomes, 48

Naesar, N. A., 199, 212
Naimark, A., 161
Naming. see Anomia
Nasal fibers, 96–97
Natural selection, Darwinian principle
  of, 3
Naunton, R. F., 184
Negative feedback, 76–77
Neglect, 242–243
Neocerebellum, 131
Neologistic jargon aphasia, 206
Nerve block, 93–94
Nervous system, 17–18
  development, 43–46
  divisions, 18–43
  See also Autonomic nervous system;
    Brain; Central nervous system;
    Peripheral nervous system
Nervus intermedius, 145
Netsell, R., 178, 184

Neural tube, 44
  alar plate, 44
  dorsal plate, 44
  mantle plate, 44
Neuraxis, 19
Neuroimaging techniques, 9–11, 169
Neurolemma, 79
Neurological exam
  bedside, 308–309
  screening for speech-language
    pathology, 310–313
Neurologic disorders
  diagnosis with primitive reflex, 277–298
  diagnostic technique, 77–79
  prevalence, 300–302
Neuromuscular transmission, 73
Neuron, 67–69
Neuronal operation
  principles of, 74–75
  servomechanism theory, 76–79
Neuropathy, 115
*Neurosensory Center Comprehensive
  Examination for Aphasia*, 215
Neurotransmitter(s)
  acetylcholine, 71, 124
  dopamine, 29, 126, 176
  glutamate, 124
  types, 73
Newcombe, Freda, 231
Nociceptive receptors, 84
Nodes of Ranvier, 79
Nodulus, 131
Nonfluent aphasia, 205
Nonfocal brain disease, 210
Nuclear bag fibers, 118
Nuclear chain fibers, 118
Nuclei of origin, 141
Nuclei of termination, 141
Nucleus ambiguous, 151, 152
Nucleus solaritarius, 51, 151, 152
Nystagmus, 135, 136

Obligatory reflex response, 278–279
Occipital alexia, 229
Occipital-frontal fasciculus, 34
Occipital lobe, 20, 24, 62
Oculomotor nerve (III), 142
Ogle, William, 6
Oldring, D. J., 184
Olfactory nerve (I), 141–142
Olfactory receptor cortex, primary, 30–31
Oligodendroglia, 80
Olivary nucleus, 38
Olives, 38

Olivopontocerebellar atrophy, 191
Olsen, N., 162
Open-loop control system, 76–77
Opercular gyrus, 29
Ophthalmic artery, 57
Optic chiasma, 39, 96
Optic disk, 96
Optic nerve (II), 142
  pathway of, 96–98
Oral apraxia, 223–224
Oral and pharyngeal reflexes, 287–288,
  287–290
  bite reflex, 292
  feeding reflex, 266
  gag reflex, 292–293
  rooting reflexes, 290
  sucking reflex, 290–291
  swallowing reflex, 292
  tongue reflex, 292
Oral sensation, 90
  sensory pathway of cranial nerve IX, 92
  sensory pathway of cranial nerve V, 91–92
  See also Sensation, bodily
Oral sensory receptors, 93
  oral proprioceptors, 93
  oral sensation studies, 93–94
  sensory control modalities, 94
  speech proprioception, 95
Organic voice tremor, 180
Orofacial dyskinesia, 129
Orthostatic hypotension, 189
Orton, Samuel Terry, 7
Overshooting, 136

Palatal myoclonus, 129
Palato-pharyngo-laryngeal myoclonus, 190
Paleocerebellum, 131
Pallie, W., 8
Pallilalia, 179
Palumbo, C. L., 199
Papagno, C., 199
Parahippocampal gyrus, 30
Paralimbic areas, 32–33
Paralysis, 109
  flacid, 113, 172
  lower motor neuron, 112–1115
  uppper motor neuron, 115–117
Paraphasia, 206
  literal, 206
  verbal, 206
Parasympathetic nervous system, 50, 51
Parasympathetic nucleus, 146
Paresis, 109
Parietal alexia, 230

Parietal lobe, 18, 20, 22
Parietal temporal-occipital association
  area, 24
Parkinsonism, 176–179
  dopamine deficiency, 126, 176
  neurologic characteristics, 176–179
  oral musculature, 177
  speech characteristics, 177–179
  and swallowing, 179
Pascal, G., 228
Pathologic tremor, 126
Pendular reflexes, 135
Penfield, Wilder G., 8, 29, 39, 198–199, 262
  Speech and Brain Mechanisms, 8
  The Cerebral Cortex of Man, 8
  The Second Career, 17
Perception, 28, 86
  form, 86
  visual, 99, 100
Performance and competence, 202
Periaqueductal gray, 51
Perikaryon, 67
Peripheral nerves, 40
Peripheral nervous system, 41, 47–52
Perisylvian zone, 195, 201, 205
Peterson, S. I., 79
Pharyngeal clearing force, 159, 161
Pharyngeal gag, 151
Pharyngeal reflexes. *see* Oral and
  pharyngeal reflexes
Phenothiazines, 129
Phonological alexia, 231–232
Phrenic nerves, 48
Physiologic tremor, 126–127
Pia mater, 52
Pierce, R. S., 245
Pill rolling tremor, 176
Pinker, S., 3
Planum temporale, 261
Platt, L. J., 184
Polyneuritis, 190
Pons, 37, 38, 133
Porch, B., 9
*Porch Index of Communicative Ability
  (PICA)*, 9, 204, 215
Positive feedback, 76
Positive support reflex (PSR), 279–280
Positron emission tomography (PET),
  10–11
Postcentral gyrus, 22
Posterior alexia, 229
Posterior aphasia, 205
Posterior cerebral arteries, 58
Posterior communicating arteries, 57

Posterior, defined, 12
Posterior lobe, 62, 131
Posterior root, 47, 48
Posterior root ganglion, 48
Postganglionic fibers, 51
Postsynaptic potential, 73
  excitatory (EPSP), 73, 74
  inhibitory (IPSP), 73, 74
Precentral gyrus, 21
Prefrontal association area, 24
Preganglionic fibers, 51
Premotor area, 21, 29
Pretectal nuclei pathway, 98–99
Primary auditory receptor cortex, 30
Primary motor cortex, 21
Primary motor projection areas, 27–28
Primary olfactory receptor cortex, 30–31
Primary sensory receptor area, 27–28
Primary visual cortex, 98–99
Primary visual pathways, 98–99
Primitive reflex, 277–278
  asymmetrical tonic neck reflex
    (ATNR), 278–279
  diagnosis of neurologic disorder with,
    277–278
  galant reflex, 284–285
  Moro reflex, 284–285
  positive support reflex (PSR), 279–280
  segmental rolling (SR) reflex, 282–284
  symmetrical tonic neck reflexes
    (STNR), 279
  tonic labyrinthine reflex (TLR), 280–282
Progressive aphasia, 210–211
Progressive supranuclear palsy, 191
Proprioception
  oral, 95
  pathways, 86–87
  speech, 95
Proprioceptors, 83–84
Prosodic insufficiency, 178
Prosopagnosia, 244
Prostigmine, 73
Pseudobulbar palsy, 169, 170
Pseudohypertrophic muscular dystrophy,
  275–276
Ptosis, 142, 173
Pulvinar, 39
Pure alexia, 228–229
Pure word deafness, 218–219
Putamen, 35, 122, 123
Pyramidal system, 21, 106–107
  corticospinal tract, 107
  decussation, 109
  descending motor pathways, 107–109

Pyramidal system—*cont.*
  paralysis, 109
Pyramids, 38, 109

Rancho Los Amigos Levels of Cognitive
  Recovery, 241
Rate disorder, 178
Readiness potential, 78
Reading disability, specific, 267
Rebound, 135
Receptive aphasia, 205
Receptive fields in vision, 98
Receptor, 42
Red nucleus, 123, 133
Reflexes, 42–43
Reflexes. *see* Oral and pharyngeal
  reflexes; Primitive reflexes
Reisberg, B., 236
Relative refractory period, 70
Restiform body, 132
Resting potential, 69
Rest tremor, 127
Reticular formation of mesencephalon, 123
Retina, 95–96
Retinal fibers, 96–97
Rhinencephalon, 20, 35
Right-hemisphere lesions, 241–244
Right-left disorientation, 220
Rigidity, 125, 176
  cogwheel, 176
Rivers, D. L., 245
Robbins, J., 169, 173, 179
Roberts, Lamar, 198–199, 262
Rodriguez, M., 187
Rods, 96
Roeltgen, D. P., 203
Rolandic fissure, 21
Roland, P. E., 68, 74
Romberg test, 90
Rooting reflexes, 290
Rose, F. C., 176
Rosenfield, D. B., 183, 184
Rostral, defined, 12
Rothi, L. G., 203
Rubrospinal pathway, 133

Sagittal plane, 14
St. Vitus Dance. *see* Sydenham's chorea
Salivation, 145, 151, 292
Saltatory transmission, 79
Scanning speech, 7, 187
Schatz, K., 162
Schuell, H. M., 9, 216
Schwann cells, 79

Secondary motor area (SMA), 29
Secondary trigeminothalamic tract, 92
Segmental rolling (SR) reflex, 282–284
Seizures, epileptic, surgery, 26–27
Senile tremor, 180
Sensation
  anatomy, 84
  and anterior spinothalamic tract, 86
  classification, 83
  and lateral spinothalamic tract, 84–86
  proprioception pathways, 86–87
Sensation
  Sherrington's scheme, 84–86
  See also Oral sensation; Oral sensory
    receptors
Sensation, bodily, 83–87
Sensory aphasia, 31, 196, 205
Sensory aprosodia, 246
Sensory association areas, 31–32
Sensory control modalities, 94
Sensory examination, 87–90
  light touch, 89
  pain and temperature, 89
  two-point discrimination, 89
Sensory nucleus, 146
Sensory strip, 22
Septal area, 32
Servomechanism theory, neuronal
    function, 76–79
Shane, H. C., 289
Sherrington, Charles, 48, 74, 75, 83–84,
    95, 112
Sherrington's scheme, 83–84, 84–86
Shy-Drager syndrome, 189–190
  etiology, 189
  neurologic characteristics, 189
  speech characteristics, 189–190
Shy, G., 189
Simple reflex arc, 42
Single photon emission tomography
    (SPECT), 11
Smell and vision, cranial nerves, 140
Solely special sensory cranial nerves, 140
Soma, 67
Somatomotor cranial nerves, 140
Somatosensory cortex, primary, 30
Somites, 140
Somitic cranial nerves, 140
Spasmodic dysphonia (SD), 128, 180, 183–184
Spastic-ataxic dysarthria, mixed, 188–189
Spastic dysarthria, 168, 169–171
  etiology, 109
  neurologic characteristics, 170
  oral musculature, 170

Spastic dysarthria—*cont.*
  speech characteristics, 170–171
  swallowing, 171
Spastic dysphonia (SD), 128, 180, 183–184
Spasticity, 170, 273
Spastic paralysis, 115
Spatial organizational deficits, 244
Special senses, 84
Specific-event related electrical
    potential, 77
Specific language impairment (SLI),
    264–265
Specific reading disability, 267
Speech
  apraxia, 224–225
  cerebellar role, 133–134
  and dysphagia, 288–289
  explosive, 187
  neurologic control, 106
  proprioception, 95
  scanning, 7, 187
Speech area, 205
Speech-language, and evoked potentials,
    77–79
Speech-language, and brain science
    development, 5–11
Speech-language pathology, 8, 11
Speech mechanism, sensory innervation, 91
Speech motor control, bilateral, 61
Speech zone, 62
  See also Perisylvian zone
Sperry, Roger, 8
Spinal accessory nerve (XI), 154–155
  anatomy, 154
  function, 154–155
  innervation, 154
  testing, 155
Spinal cord, 18–19, 39–42
  development of, 44–45
Spinal nerves, 18–19, 40–41
Spinal tap, 56
Spinocerebellar tract, 86
Spinothalamic tract
  lateral, 84–86
  ventral, 86
Spiral ganglion, 84, 100, 149
Split-brain research, 26–27
Spreen, O., 215
Springer, S. P., 201
Striate area, 30
Stroke, 168
Stuttering, 7
Stylopharyngeus muscle, 151
Subarachnoid space, 54

Subcallosal gyrus, 32
Subcortical aphasia, 199, 211–213
Subcortical dementia, 233, 234
Subcortical mechanisms, and language, 197–201
Subcortical structures, 34–35
Subdural space, 53
Substantia innominata, 32
Substantia nigra, 35, 38, 123
Subthalamic nuclei, 35
Subthalamus, 123
Suckling reflex, 290
Sulcus, 20
  calcarine, 24
  central, 21
  lateral, 21
Sulcus limitans, 44
Superficial abdominal reflex, 117
Superior cerebellar peduncle, 133
Superior colliculus, 38
Superior, defined, 12
Superior longitudinal fasciculus, 25, 34, 197
Superior salivatory nucleus, 145, 146
Supplementary motor area (SMA), 29
Suprabulbar palsy, childhood, 275
Suprabulbar paresis, childhood, 274–275
Suprabulbar paresis syndrome, childhood, 275
Supramarginal gyrus, 22, 32, 297
Surface dyslexia, 231–232
Suttel, B., 228
Swallowing, 158–161
  and amyotropic lateral sclerosis, 174–176
  assessment, 161–162
  and cerebrovascular accident, 169, 173
  and chorea, 182
  and dystonia, 185
  and flaccid dysarthria, 173
  and Parkinsonism, 179
  and spastic dysarthria, 171
  unilateral reflex, 169
Swallowing center, 161
Swallowing reflex in infants, 292
Sydneham's chorea, 180, 181
Sylvian fissure, 21
Symmetrical tonic neck reflexes (STNR), 279
Sympathetic apraxia, 223
Sympathetic nervous system, 50–51
Sympathetic trunk, 51
Synapse, 70–73
Synaptic cleft, 71
Synaptic excitation and inhibition, 73–74
Synaptic knob, 71

Synaptic plasticity, 74
Synaptic transmission, 73
Synaptic vesicles, 71
Synergy, 131
Szekeres, S. F., 238
Szinles, J., 78

Tactile agnosia, 31, 90, 219–220
Tactile aphasia, 219–220
  bilateral, 219–220
  unilateral, 219
Tardive dyskinesia, 129, 185
Taste, 145–146, 148, 162
Tauc, L. L., 74
Tectal pathway, 98–99
Tectospinal tracts, 98
Tectum, 38
Temporal fibers, 96
Temporal lobe, 18, 20, 22, 62
Temporal loop, 97–98
Tensilon, 73
Tentorium cerebelli, 52
Thalamic aphasia, 199
Thalamic radiations, 28
Thalamus, 39
Tiami, E. G., 288
Tomoeda, C. K., 236
Tongue
  movement, 156–180, 295–296
  sensation, 145, 151, 160, 162
  thrusting, 292, 295
Tongue, atonic, 172
Tongue driving force, 159, 161
Tongue reflex, 292, 295
Tonic labyrinthine reflex (TLR), 280–282
Tonic neck reflex, asymmetrical (ATNR), 116, 278–279
Tonus, 115
Topognosis, 89
Total aphasia, 208
Tract, 40
  defined, 13
Tractus solitarius, 145
Transcortical aphasia, 205, 209, 210
Transcortical motor aphasia, 201, 209
Transcortical sensory aphasia, 201, 209
  mixed, 209
Transverse cut, 14
Traumatic brain injury (TBI), 237–241
  cognitive impairment, 239–240
  neurobehavioral sequelae, 238
  testing and treating language impairment, 241
Travis, Lee Edward, 7

Trigeminal nerve (V), 142–145
  anatomy, 142
  function, 143
  innervation, 143
  testing, 143–144
Tremor(s), 126–127, 135
  action, 126–127
  essential, 180
  heredofamilial, 180
  intention, 127
  organic voice, 180
  pathologic, 126
  physiologic, 126–127
  pill rolling, 176
  rest, 127
Trochlear nerve (IV), 142
Trunk apraxia, 222
Tupper, D., 266
Two-point discrimination, 86, 89
  disorder, 90
Two-point sensitivity, 86

Uncinate fasciculus, 34
Uncinate fits, 31
Uncus, 30, 32
Unilateral inattention, 243
Unilateral innervation, 110–111
Unilateral tactile aphasia, 219
Upper motor neuron (UMN)
  lesions, 168–171
  lesions, mixed lower, 174–176
  paralysis, 115–117
  stroke, 168

Vagus nerve (X), 152–154
  anatomy, 152
  function, 152
  innervation, 152
  testing, 153–154
Van den Burg, W., 188
Vaughan, H. G., 78–79
Velopharyngeal closure, 140, 159, 184
Ventral, defined, 12
Ventral spinothalamic tract, 86
Ventricles
  fourth, 55
  lateral, 54
  third, 39, 55
Ventricular system, 54, 55
Ventrolateral nucleus, 133
Verbal agnosia, auditory, 1, 218–219
Verbal alexia, 228
Verbal paraphasia, 206
Vermis, 130

Vertebral arteries, 56, 58–59
Vestibular-acoustic nerve (VIII), 148–150
  anatomy, 149
  function, 150
  innervation, 149–150
  testing, 150
Vestibular branch, 100, 148–150
  See also Vestibular-acoustic nerve (VIII)
Vibration, 86
Vibratory sensibility disorder, 90
Viscera, 23
Vision, cranial nerves for smell, 141–142
Visual agnosia, 31, 218
Visual association cortex, 99
Visual integration, 99–101
Visual-perceptual and reading deficits, 244
Visual system, 95–100
  optic nerve path, 96–98
  primary visual cortex, 98–99
  retina, 95–96
  visual association cortex, 99
  visual integration, 99–101
Vocabulary development, 258
Voice tremor, organic, 180
Von Cramon, D., 170

Wada, J. A., 8
Wada test, 241
Wallesch, C. W., 199
Wallman, J., 18
Webb, W. G., 179, 224
Wechsler Adult Intelligence Scale, 236
Wechsler, D., 236
Weil, L., 159, 161, 162
Weinberg, W. A., 265
Weiner, H. L., 188
Weiner, W. J., 124
Weisenburg, Theodore, 205
Wepman, Joseph, 8, 215
  Recovery from Aphasia, 8
Wernicke, Carl, 6, 195, 207, 209
Wernicke's aphasia, 6, 196, 202, 206, 207–208
Wernicke's area, 6, 24, 31, 196, 199
  development, 258
  function, 196
Western Aphasia Battery (WAB), 215
Westlake, Harold, 8
West, Robert, 8
Whitaker, H. A., 78, 200, 202
Wiesel, T. N., 98
Wilde, Oscar, 67
Wilson, F. B., 184
Witelson, S. F., 8
Wood, B. I., 263

Word-blindness, 228
Word-blindness, congenital, 267–268
Workinger, M. S., 274
Worster-Drought, C., 275

Ylvisaker, M., 238, 241

Zeigler, W., 170